SPORT MINDSET FOR EXCELLENCE

THE ULTIMATE MANUAL OF SPORT MENTAL COACHING FOR SPORT CHAMPIONS AND ELITE PROFESSIONALS

JOE SANTANGELO

This Book is a work of fiction. Names, characters, businesses and organizations, places, and events if they may happen. It is the author's imagination that has been created. Has no bearings on the living or the dead? Any clashes would be entirely incidental.

Ordering Information:

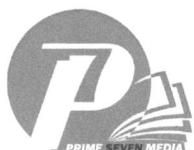

Prime Seven Media
518 Landmann St.
Tomah City, WI 54660

Printed in the United States of America

Table of Contents

Author's Dedication

This volume is dedicated to those who are unsatisfied and those who push hard as they can to achieve the highest results. This is dedicated to those athletes who know and feel inside that they can turn themselves into champions, but do not know what to do or how to achieve, and so they are bogged down in the ocean of mediocrity and ordinariness. This volume is dedicated to you, who are reading right now. If you want to work hard to overcome yourself, if you feel the fire of aspiration and ambition burning continuously inside, if you can see yourself on the highest podium, then don't hesitate. This book is for you, I know you can get great benefits from it.

The Author

Thankfulness

My first thanks and gratitude are for my *sports discipline*.

I guess I owe almost everything to my commitment and my devotion, but I also know that I had fallen in love with my sports practice since I was a teenager and then I didn't ever quit dreaming to become a champion and I have never diverted from my pathway. Such kind of love was reciprocal, as always happens between lovers. My sport taught me everything I could learn and even more. Taught me how to live honestly and never give up. I was imprisoned and became a means through which my sports discipline would have affirmed itself: I realized such an emotional kidnapping and I accepted the challenge and now I am here and I feel honored for talking about the secrets I have learned. I can assure you all that the process of training, learning, and improving my skills was much better and satisfactory than becoming the World Champion. No way: sport is bigger than success.

My immense gratitude also goes to those people who have allowed me to excel in sports. I am not necessarily referring to great coaches and national team leaders, but rather to those athletes and all those humble and generous people who offered me their great wealth without asking for anything in return.

Thanks to my lovely students, readers, and coaches.
This book was just written for you.

www.joe-santangelo.com
mail@: joes.ps.mail@gmail.com

Volume Introduction

When I started my sports career, I was only 13 and I just didn't know yet I was starting, nor that I would have fallen in love with a sports discipline, a passion that moves me and motivates most of my actions and decisions still now, forty years later. I entered the gym alone and stared looking at the athletes. They were so beautiful to my eyes, I felt a kind of embarrassment and excitement at the same time. A strange struggle started inside: I wanted to do something, but I felt I was inadequate. I was the kind of boy who is destined to be bullied and that was what happened to me, that far. I was blond-haired, blue eyes, and very thin: I would probably seem a girl as much as a boy and my closed and introspective character, in addition to my natural inclination to non-conformity, made things much more difficult. What should I do? I wanted to do something to become stronger and respected by other people and thought I found my chance, but I was not sure I would have deserved it, for I felt inadequate. The struggle was torturing me, but after a few weeks I realized that my mind could become stronger than my body and made my decision: I accepted the challenge and I bet on my achievement. Later on, in an unknown future, I would have become a champion: that was my commitment, my dream. After such a decision I was only in need of time, the bigger size of time my routine could offer me to train, to dedicate the whole of myself to my sports discipline, to my physical empowerment, and, finally, to my strategic mindset. That's what I realized at the age of thirteen: I guess I was lucky, but also a kind of precocious: I understood very quickly that my mind could have strived, moved, and motivated my body and granted appropriate growth, and that's what happened.

Soon I got addicted to my discipline: the training sessions became holy: the gym was my church and I used to go there as I was a religionist who had to commit himself to his religion. I became familiar with the whole of the technical gestures and used to strive hard and consume all my energy to comprehend the movements, and the techniques, integrate them into my body, and mix them in a set of ordinary and routine moves. I got addicted to my sport and there was nothing more important, for me than completing my school homework, which allowed me to reach the gym and work hard for two sessions, at least: amateurs (boys) and professionals (adults). I took an old bike and made my 5 kilometers every day, with a big heavy bag held on my shoulders. I clearly remember that I felt happy, even though my training commitments were really hard to drive because no one believed in me yet, but I didn't have any idea of quitting. I held a dream, a big dream in my heart and I always found the strength and energy to overcome the humiliations and the absence of any real attainment.

When I was 17 a few important things happened. I significantly increased the time for my training. I used to train 10 times per week, Saturday and Sunday included: I was given the key to the Gym by my coach and used to go there alone to improve some gestures and empower my body during the night and on the weekend. I used to do that secretly: I didn't want any other people to catch my real intentions. I had never declared officially my inner aim and ambitions, for I thought they were too big and I didn't want any confrontation with anyone on this subject. I knew from the start there were four factors, which I had to handle: there was my mind, my body and there was another strange force within, which wanted to prevent me from taking charge of my dream. Finally, there was me: the main actor of this movie, the person destined to find a compromise with that strange individual – my internal enemy – and to drive body and mind towards success. I knew it was very hard and I used to feel a sense of responsibility for such a challenge and this dramatically changed my personality.

Some significant successes arrived and, at the age of 21, I entered the national team to represent my country in the European Championship to be held in England. I was so happy, astonished. I guessed the whole of my efforts were coming back in terms of chances. I could have had a real chance, that time, to prove myself I was right. My inner dream began to push: he wanted to get out and declare itself to the outside world, but I managed to keep it silent.

At that time, I didn't have a coach. I left my first sports school for my former coach didn't want me to follow my natural propensity to experience adjacent styles: this would have meant attending other schools, following other recommendations, and learning different styles and gestures. I was alone, but I was not scared. I was sure that I could have overcome such an event. I quit my former school and, as a consequence, I was suspended for one year from any national and international tournaments. I thought I was ready, I had been the many times national champion, and I deserved such a chance, but I could not take part in the European Championship. At the age of 21, I only had one certainty: an official suspension of 1 year, because I decided to switch from the old team to the new team. That was the punishment from my former coach. And this became my primary, strongest motivation to strive harder and harder. I had a deal with a new team: I would have become one of their athletes the upcoming year, meantime I could have entered their facilities any time, any day of the year. Suspension: I couldn't perform officially, but I had one entire year to empower my physical capabilities, enrich my tactical and strategic competencies, to fill all the technical gaps. And that's what I did, that year.

Things were changing inside, something radical. I learned how to deal with my internal enemy: all of a sudden, I took the power away from him and reduced him to silence. My dream broke through and began to yell: *I want to become World Champion in my sport, I want to be number one.* I was so embarrassed. Nobody could hear such a scream but me. Whenever I repeated such a commitment in my head, I felt a physical vibration and my inner soul started to shake. It was right: I wanted to be a World Champion, but I also knew *I had to become* a World Champion before winning. So I switched to an upper level and the whole of the training and the preparation switched with me.

I was seeking improvement, I pushed my training session to my possible best, and I became much more constant and perseverant, I simulated tournaments, performances, and scores, I used to train myself with any athlete who wanted me as a partner or a companion: older, smarter, stronger than me, without being envious, embarrassed, without feeling humiliated, ever. I was seeking improvement, I just wanted to push forward my technicalities and my mindset.

One year passed by, and I come back to tournaments. I won all the national championships in different disciplines and officially re-entered the National Team. I didn't have a coach. I used to teach as a coach in three different gyms and I trained myself some kind of 4 hours per day, while I was still studying at the University. I knew I was in need of a coach, but it was very difficult to coach me because I was already a certified coach, a national team athlete and I had my own ideas on training, methodologies, and models of action during a match. So, what really could I do? I got an additional switch and became my personal coach of myself. I started studying anything I could on the subject, utilizing any kind of chances and tools to do that: interviews with sports champions whom I personally knew, books, articles from specialized magazines, VHS, and emulation. Coaches, master classes, additional certifications. I wanted to fill the gaps which I knew I had. I wanted to be complete, quiet and lucid, and elegant while performing, strong, powerful, creative. I wanted to become a model for myself, as an athlete, and as a man, and I spent all the money and all the energy to achieve this target.

At the age of 24, I had my chances. I become a European silver medalist: I remember that I cried when I was in the Hotel, that night. I knew I was stronger than my opponent, but something happened to my mind, from the very moment I saw the microphone coming down from above, into the ring. I was not ready enough and that affected my resources and jeopardized the whole performance. I thought that I had to show up my entire arsenal, that I was a superstar, in a sense, and I was punished by my ego. The year after I was appointed as the Captain of the National Team. I was really honored by such an appraisal and tried to do my best with my companions. I was a bronze medalist and clearly realized that I was in lack of something which I could not even define, so how could I achieve more? I got in my mind that if you want to become the Champion you need to accomplish the appropriate mindset of the Champion. No way, no excuses: the tournament is won on execution, not on emotions. I made my decision and opened a new wave. On one side I started training according to the usual standard protocols, on the other hand, I began studying myself, my reactions, my delusion, my motivations, my will to survive, to succeed, to overcome issues, my will to improve myself, my attitude not to feel satisfied, neither when I failed nor when I succeeded. The whole of such a hard study was performed in comparison to the attitudes, habits, and skills of the champions: I had to understand the gaps and I had to fill those gaps, at any cost. I resolved that *Mindset* was the real element I still lack, to succeed. I continued my study while performing officially in tournaments. I won several championships and many elements came, naturally, and instinctively: discipline, perseverance, calmness, lucidity, internal LOC, resilience, fair play, humility, self-confidence, performance flow, courage, the propensity to risk, will to face problems and issues, technical bilateralism, will to train harder and harder, will to compare my performance to champions', imagery, creativity, uniqueness, patience, learning from failures, goal setting. The Champion which was inside me was there to come out and reveal his real talent to the other competitors, to coaches and referees, and to the media. It was not a matter of being provided with a strong will: everyone has it, at a professional level. I realized I had to free the champion who was imprisoned in myself.

I was confirmed as Captain of the National Team. I won the European Championship. Then I became World Champion for the first time. Then I won again the tournament and was confirmed Elite World Champion. I took an additional day in the Hotel to celebrate myself. I was alone, in the hotel room. I had my gold medal in one hand and the World Champion Belt on the table. I felt satisfied for the first time in my sports career. I questioned myself while drinking a glass of red wine. *How long... How hard, stressful, and humiliating was my trip?* I would have been so grateful to anyone if he had told me and taught me kind of so important recommendations before. I would have been so grateful if someone had approached me long before to tell me *"Good Joe, you're on the right way, you're doing good. Be patient, do not give up, do not quit, everything will happen whenever you're ready".* I was forced to learn my lesson by myself, on the basis of failures, humiliations, hard work, and huge sacrifices. That day, when I was in the hotel room, I had all the answers to my questions. My life gave me back something great: the dream of that wand-scared boy had been accomplished.

That's the reason why I have decided to talk about these recommendations I myself wanted to be given in the past. The *8 Pillars Model* which I present in this book includes the whole of the elements which a Sports Champion must have to accomplish and maintain his position. It is based on an academic model mixed with my personal experience as a Coach and as a Sports Professional. No magic, no mysteries, no genius or talent, or superhuman skills are required to become a Peak-Performer: only hard work. You ought to work for a strong physical shape, to enrich and empower a tactical and strategic mentality, and, finally, a robust Sports Mindset, which, in my personal opinion, means the most of it all.

Joe Santangelo
April 3th, 2023

Preface

Nobody is a champion *before becoming* a champion.

Sport is highly democratic, much more than any other kind of activity or business in this world. Just think it over a bit: no other person but you can give you the honor, the respect, and the glory of being the World Champion. It's only up to you. This has always been for centuries – back to the Greek Olympiads and Roman Coliseum games – and this will always be.

This only means one true thing: nobody is born a champion, but anyone can become a champion if he/she truly deserves that.

Any champion has started to practice a sports discipline, then something happened in his/her psyche and a big switch occurred: the decision to devote anything, any kind of energy, to become a champion, one day. So any champion has learned the lesson, has trained hard for decades, has failed, and has had the nerve to get up and keep fighting to make a dream come true, the big dream.

So what I want you to keep clearly in your mind is that becoming a champion is up to you. You ought to understand what makes an athlete a champion so that you can decide to switch your psychology and strive hard to make your dream come true. Or maybe you'll decide to take your time and apply the whole of the methodology step by step, slowly, and see what happens. Or you can decide that you're not that kind of person, so you quit and continue to practice for your own personal relaxation. The choice is yours, that switch is up to you. No one can empower your aim and motivation, no one can transform your brain: is a personal business.

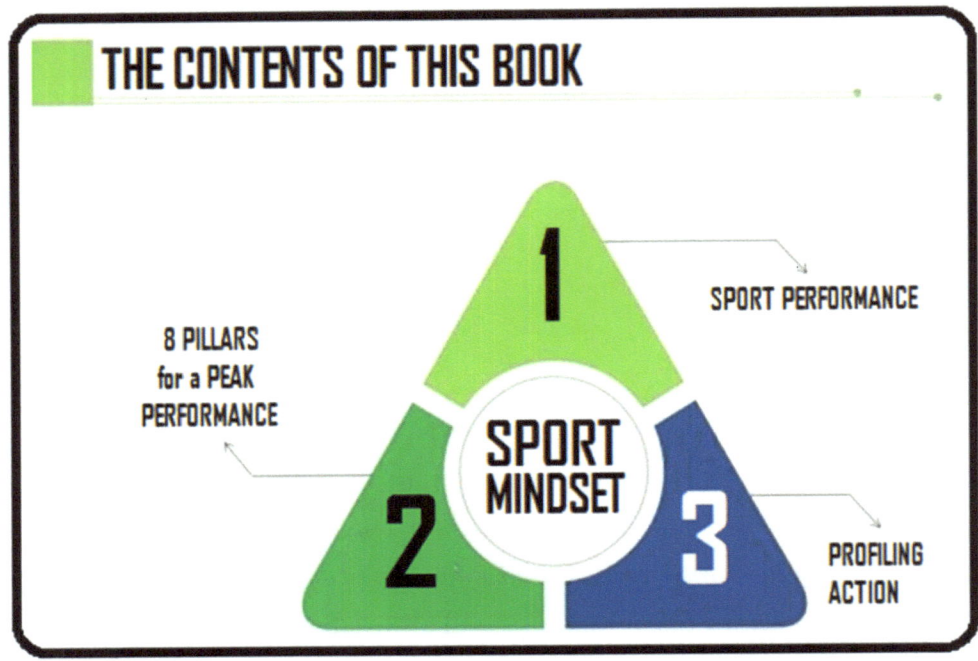

This book is divided into three parts:

In the first one, we will examine the model for finalizing the Sports Peak Performance, which can be defined as that special state in which the athlete performs to the maximum of his/her ability, characterized by subjective feelings of confidence, effortlessness, and total concentration on the task. The first chapter deals with this topic and is basically funded on Sports Training Theory studies which are universally accepted by both medical science and sports coaches' associations.

In the second one, we will explore the Sport Mindset of a Peak Performer. After a deep detection of the peculiar sub-elements which compose the mindset's area, we will go through the whole of these elements according to a special pattern which will include 9 declinations of the topic: *1 – Definition; 2 – Contextualization; 3 – Factors; 4 – Threats; 5 – Opportunities; 6 – Methodologies; 7 – Practical Techniques; 8 – Powerful Questions; 9 – Instructions & Recommendations.* Every paragraph will be tagged with a specific icon, to facilitate your learning process. This second is the core part of this book and consists of 8 chapters (*Chapter 2 → Chapter 9*). Each of these chapters is focused on one of the 8 Mindset Pillars: *1 – Physical Training; 2 – Tactical/Strategic Training; 3 – Sports Code of Ethics; 4 – Goal Setting; 5 – Clarity; 6 – Self Consciousness; 7 – Adaptation; 8 – Courage.*

ICON	PARAGRAPH	MEANING
	DEFINITION	A modern definition of the topic, according to the current trend of Psychology and Psychodynamics
	CONTEXTUALIZATION	Contextualization of the topic into the general framework of Psychic Skills of the Athlete
	FACTORS	The Sub-Elements which are included into the topic. Each Pillar is a Multifactor element
	THREATS	The negative events which might impact the Performance if the factors are neglected or absent
	OPPORTUNITIES	The positive advantages which are determined by a strong control of the factors
	METHODOLOGIES	The methodologies used to strengthen or to develop the factor, if absent
	PRACTICAL TECHNIQUES	The practical and empirical techniques which are used to strengthen the factor
	POWERFUL QUESTIONS	A short list of *Effective Questions* to the Athlete, used to unlock and enable different perspectives
	INSTRUCTIONS & RECOMMENDATIONS	A short list of technical and psychic methodologies to strengthen and improve the factor

The third and last part consists of a *call to action*: that includes practical and methodological recommendations and instructions to utilize all the contents which have been developed in the 8 previous chapters. It only consists of two chapters (Chapters 10 and 11). Chapter 10 includes a presentation of the profiles of the Peak-Performer and relevant recommendations per each of them, while chapter 11 completes the analysis and presents a *Call-2-Action* for both Athletes, Coaches, and Sports Educators. I wish you a good reading and a good workout.

Good luck.

Joe Santangelo

Elective Addressees

*S*ports *Mindset* for Peak Performers is a special mix of several elements which need to be present at a specific percentage. Is a magic potion which-with any top performer belonging to any kind of discipline drives the performance, at any time. Mindset is everything for any kind of athlete. For this reason, this book has been conceived and written for **Athletes**, primarily. For all those athletes who have decided not to settle for being second, in the tournament. For all those athletes who have realized they have a special talent, but yet really do not know how to unlock their potential, completely. For those athletes who want to express their creativity and want to offer their opponents the best shape of themselves, and for those who cannot manage to understand which additional ingredient is still missing. For those athletes who have a strong desire to excel.

Competition sports reality does not make any difference between routine endurance disciplines and situational, between individual and collective sports, between Olympics and non-Olympics. Mental toughness is the only unique guide that drives any athlete to victory. Any World and Olympics Champion is provided with a strong and tough mindset, no matter sex, age, specialty, or discipline: he/she is simply driven to perform at his best thanks to his/her competitive, strong, and strategic mindset.

This book has also been written for **Mental, Life, and Sports Coaches**, all professionals who can take huge advantage from studying how a sports champion mindset works and can be empowered, if weak, to determine a better performance. Apart from Sports Science literature, this book provides easy examples of both patterns of applications and real experiences taken from the sports arena, from sports events, and from facts. Practicality is one of the pluses which I offer to them.

Sport Managers can also be advantaged because they can catch a general overview of this significant topic so that they can better assess the skills and the profiles of their technology partners and of the coaches whom they are selecting and who will be recruited and engaged in the sports association/corporation they lead.

As a matter of fact, also **Business Man** can take profit from this book because the rules for success are absolutely the same: it has been proven that Managers who are used to practicing a competitive sports discipline perform better than others and that's enough, in my view, to offer the contents of this book to such kind of readers' segment.

Any individual who wants to learn how to manage his personal resources and push them to an extreme level of performance cannot ignore his/her mindset, so this book is for him/her.

Labor omnia vincit improbus

The phrase is adapted from Virgil's Georgics, Book I lines 145–6

(*Anything can be achieved if proper work is applied*)

SPORT MINDSET FOR EXCELLENCE

## CHAPTER ONE

The Sport Performance

1 – Definition

The ultimate goal of this book is the exploration and description of the peculiar factors and elements which enable a strong athlete to become a champion. My goal is that you catch and understand what you have to do and how you have to train yourself, from now on, to perfect your gestures and to perform at your possible best, in the next crucial tournaments, so that you can periodize your training, plan your training sessions and achieve. Before exploring such peculiar factors, we need to get a general overview of the topic. We need to know what a generic performance is and which are the primary factors that actually influence a performance.

Sports Performance: Sports Performance is a complex mixture of biomechanical functions, emotional factors, and training techniques.

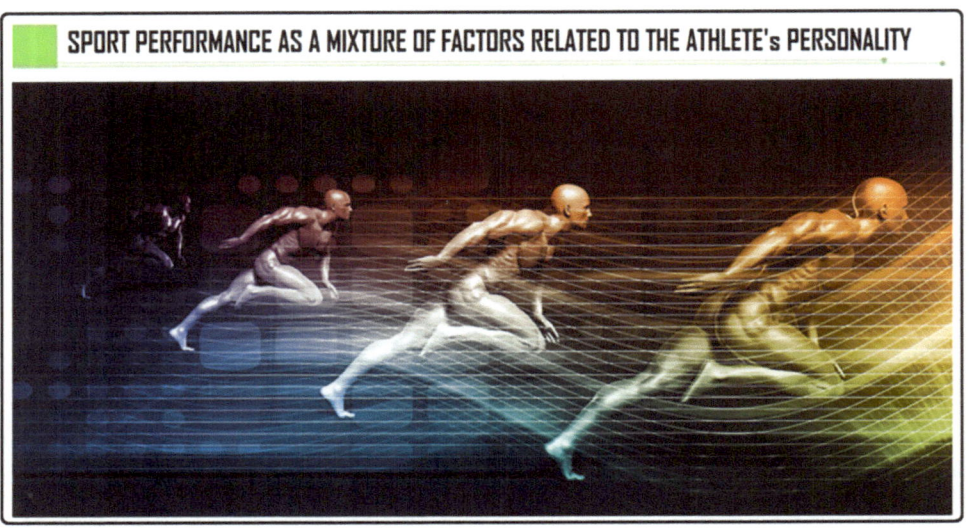

SPORT PERFORMANCE AS A MIXTURE OF FACTORS RELATED TO THE ATHLETE's PERSONALITY

In fact, any kind of athlete offers a performance, when attending any kind of tournament, both as an amateur and as a professional. Neither matters the discipline he/she is practicing nor matters the level of the competition: the behavior of any athlete, during a regulated competition, is outputting a performance.

What you first have to understand is that the quality of this performance is quite often connected with the result achieved, but there is no identity between the two. An average performance can drive the athlete to victory and an excellent performance might be returned by failure. The level of competition is the real discriminant. The best scenario would always be to express yourself at your possible best (which means: utilizing and expressing the whole of your internal and external resources at their maximum level and potential), but even if you perform at your best this does not mean that you deserve to win the competition. It's a matter of the level of competition and of synch between this level and the competitive quality of the athlete. From another hand, you can even offer a lower performance, if compared to your personal best (potentials), and win an important tournament. The sports performance is plainly connected to the final result, but, at the same time, does not ensure the achievement of this result. On the other hand, the performance of a professional and high-level quality athlete always determines the final result. This is the reason why we need to catch, understand and master the factors which determine this performance.

QUALITY	PERFORMANCE	RESULT
Low quality athletes *Amateurs*	Low/High	NOT GUARANTEED *Disconnected*
Average quality athletes *Semi-Professionals*	Low/High	NOT GUARANTEED *Disconnected*
High quality athletes *Peak-Performers*	High	GUARANTEED *Highly correlated*

All of that said, you must accept that there is no hidden secret that will enable you to quicken any learning process and there is no magic potion that will ensure you will become the champion you want to be. Anything depends on you and on your technical and physical states: technicalities and body training are the two areas that Sport theory names *"controllable"*. This means that you can manage the twos and that you can control both: these two areas will define the base upon which you will build your UPP: *Unique Performance Proposition*, what you offer to contrast your opponent to win the competition.

So training is nothing but learning how to control the *controllable*, the two basic areas to which you must apply systematically: physical and technical.

2 – Factors Affecting the Sports Performance

Sports Theory, Sport Psychology, and Psychology of Sports Performance strongly agree in defining the areas which affect and determine the Sports Performance of a generic athlete:

1) *Technical and Tactical skills.* The sports technique can be defined as the effective and rational execution of an exercise that leads to good results in sports competitions. The most important technical qualities are the ease, lightness, and economy of the movement without superfluous muscle tensions. Technical perfection directly affects the success of a sports performance and, in order to have an effective technique, one of the most important elements to be developed is the balance of the body in the position required for that peculiar exercise. In this regard, when the analysis of the technical elements is started that a discipline entails, one must first examine the possible positions in which the center of gravity is located at the lowest point, managing to provide solid base support in executing the gesture. We can define tactics as the set of methods applied to reach the ultimate purpose. Starting from here we can fix the tasks for a certain competition in a concrete way, fixing the general plan of the athlete and the team for the competition and the development of a specific action plan to achieve a victory, exploiting the weaknesses of the opponent and our best qualities. The quality of tactical actions depends on multiple factors, including the level of preparation (psycho-physical and technical) of the athlete, the number of known tactical variants, and the improvements of resources and structures that can directly influence the outcome of a competition.

2) *Coordinative capabilities and motor skills.* Motor skills are those factors that affect performance and can be improved, educated, processed, and maintained through various forms of movement. These skills are multiple and it should be remembered that they do not intervene separately, but they are part of a unitary process that has continuous dynamic interchanges. These interconnections must be carefully considered and evaluated in the programming and determining the workload. Coordinative capabilities are the set of capabilities used to learn, control and organize (adapt and transform) a movement. They represent the basis for learning and improving technical skills and work in close interaction with conditional capacities. The development of coordinative skills is strictly dependent on the nervous system, in particular: (1) the perceptive apparatus (view, hearing, tact) – (2) the sense-motor apparatus (balance, perception of space and time) – (3) the communication and face expression capabilities (body language). There are 2 kinds of Coordinative Capabilities: (1) Basic: learning, organization, and motor control – (2) Specials: belonging to each particular sports discipline.

3) *Conditional capabilities.* Conditional capacities allow you to improve physical performance through training. They are divided into *conditional capabilities* and *coordinative capabilities.* The conditional abilities are based on energy processes and are dependent on the anatomical and physiological characteristics of some peculiar human sub-systems. The main motor forms are represented by *resistance, strength, rapidity, arms mobility, flexibility,* and *speed.* They compose the fundamental assumptions for learning and performing physical motor sports actions. The conditional capabilities are mainly based on energy processes: they are physical abilities that depend on energy availability, physical status, and the metabolism of the athlete. The *force* is the energy of the muscles that allow the muscles to contrast external resistances, which is often considered the ability to win. It depends not only on muscle mass but also on the capacity of the nervous system to stimulate a lot of tension into the muscle itself. In order to use higher degrees of strength, in fact, the nervous system increases the frequency of pulses by activating as many as possible muscle fibers. The conditional abilities are linked to the coordinative ones, three basic strength types can be identified: *speed* is the capacity of the athlete to perform motor actions in a minimum time. Speed includes the motor reaction time, the speed of a single movement, and the frequency of the movements. Resistance is the body›s ability to program and endure prolonged work over time by contrasting and overcoming the arrival of fatigue, keeping unchanged the quality of muscle action. *Arms/articular mobility* is that quality that allows movements to be carried out with the greater possible amplitude. The body speed is the ability to carry out motor actions in a given time.

4) *Psychic skills and competencies.* The three bundles of skills that have been described above are not enough and ought to be supported and driven by a fourth set of competencies: psychic skills and competencies. This volume exactly explores these invisible and intangible features. The correct mix of the appropriate 4 bundles of skills generates the IPS, e.g. the *Ideal Performance State* of the athlete: it consists of the mix of physical and psychic shapes which grants the player to perform at his/her optimum with ultimate calm, confidence, and health. By definition "*IPS is reached when an individual achieves*". In the next chapters, we will go through the whole of the psychic skills needed to achieve such a state, preliminary to becoming a champion.

THE 4 MAIN-FACTORS AFFECTING THE SPORT PERFORMANCE

1	TECHNICAL AND TACTICAL SKILLS AND COMPETENCES	SPECIFIC DISCIPLINE (INDIVIDUAL/COLLECTIVE)
2	COORDINATIVE CAPABILITIES AND MOBILITY SKILLS	AGILITY - FLEXIBILITY MOTOR-FANTASY
3	CONDITIONAL CAPABILITIES AND SKILLS	STRENGH - RESISTENCE SPEED - POWER
4	PSYCHIC SKILLS AND COMPETENCES	8 PILLARS OF THE PEAK PERFORMANCE

3 – Sports Performance Model

A few models have been developed to instruct Sports Coaches, Gym Teachers, and Sports Pedagogues to facilitate the Athlete's process of learning, both related to Motor Capabilities (e.g.: *Coordinative + Conditional Capabilities*) and Technical and Tactical competencies. The Psychic Factor is usually neglected for a couple of reasons: (1) the sport mindset is a peculiar mix that is very difficult to manage from the outside (Coach); (2) the sport mindset requires specific exercises and efforts to be properly developed, which are directly connected to the peculiarity of the sports discipline.

Any Model of Performance Development presents a common basic structure. The basis of the Athlete's arsenal consists of Motor Capabilities; Technical competencies are built upon this first layer of skills. Tactical is built upon technicalities because the technical skills actually influence the number of tactical possibilities. As a final achievement, the Psychic and Strategic competencies complete this vertical structure:

1) *Coordinative capabilities* — } FIRST STEP
2) *Conditional capabilities* —

3) *Technical competences* — } SECOND STEP
4) *Tactical competences* —

5) *Strategic competences* — } THIRD STEP
6) *Psychic competences* —

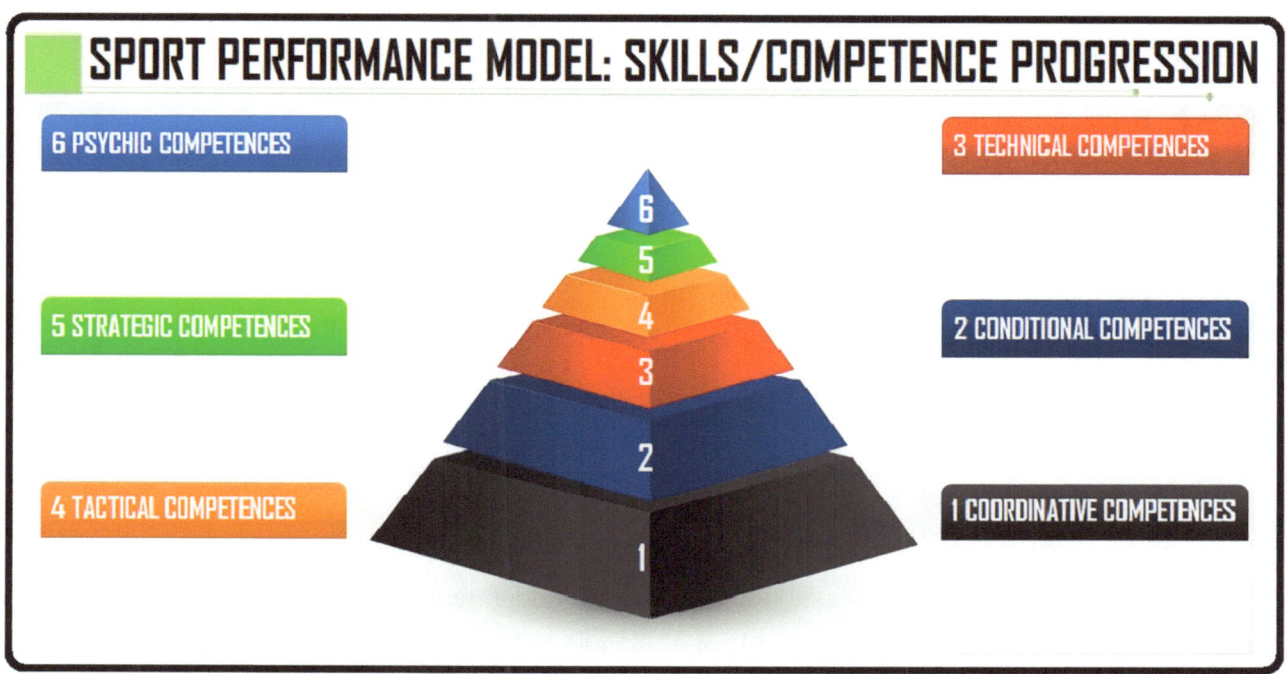

The Athlete sports personality (*resources + arsenal*) is expected to grow up according to this special scale. The process of physical empowerment is preliminary to the conditional process and both are preliminary to the acquisition of psychic skills, which are the real focus of our exploration. You have to accept that you cannot achieve a strong psychic attitude if there are still a lot of technicalities that you have to learn and automatize: physical, technical, and tactical completeness define the limitation of your ascent to success.

Except for the *Peak-Performance*, any other behavioral set of actions must be considered a performance; in most cases, these performances are based on the mix of the first 4 areas: *Coordinative + Conditional + Technical + Tactical*. A low/medium performance does not need any additional skill to take place: many competitors win or lose the tournaments without caring about mindset.

Unlike what just said, the Peak-Performance model defines the Mindset as the only crucial discriminant between the average performance and the performance of a high-level performer (the Champion): as you can see in the graph below, tactical, strategic and psychic training push a normal performance to excellence.

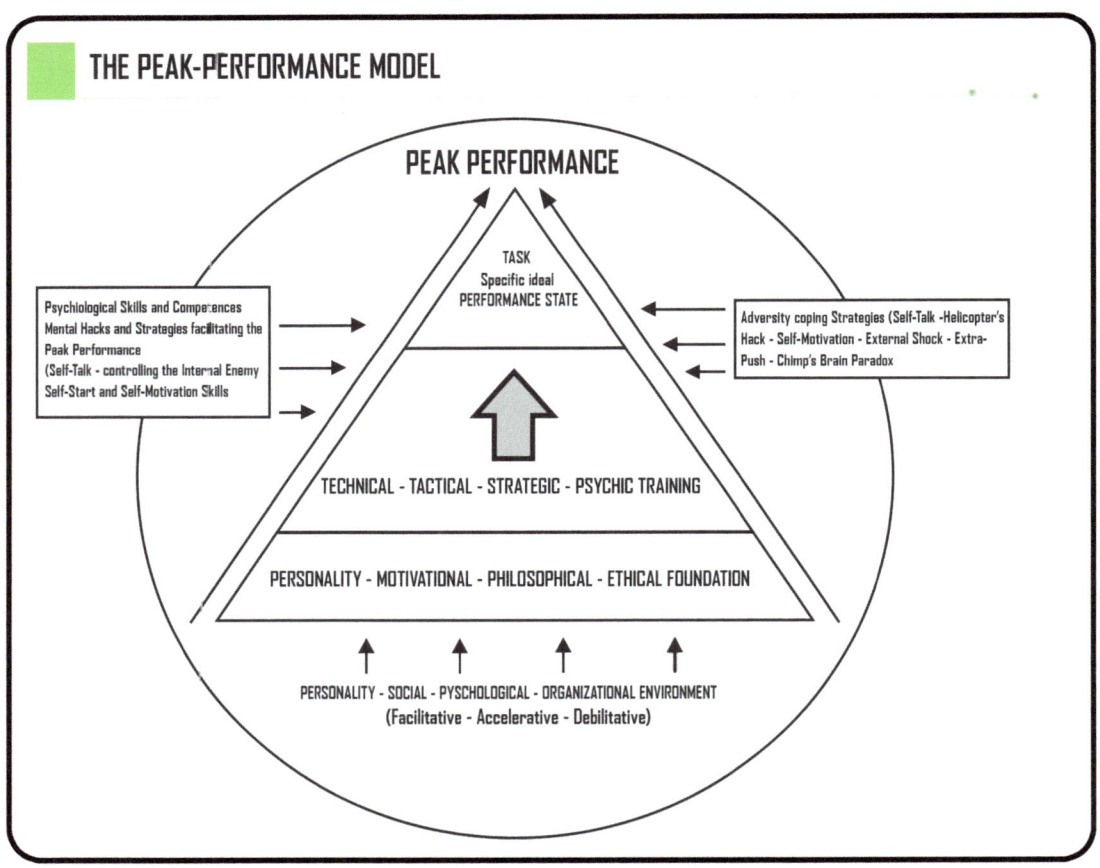

From a practical perspective, you need to know that even in a low/medium performance some kind of sport mindset is exploited. I developed a short study to understand the impact of the three areas on the performance of the three ordinary levels of performance, connected to the same number of quality levels of the athlete and something very interesting emerged as a result.

1) *Amateur Athlete*: The Sport Mindset is almost irrelevant, but when present doesn't score much more than 5%:

    a. Sport Mindset incidence: (max) 05%

    b. Other areas incidence: (max) 95%

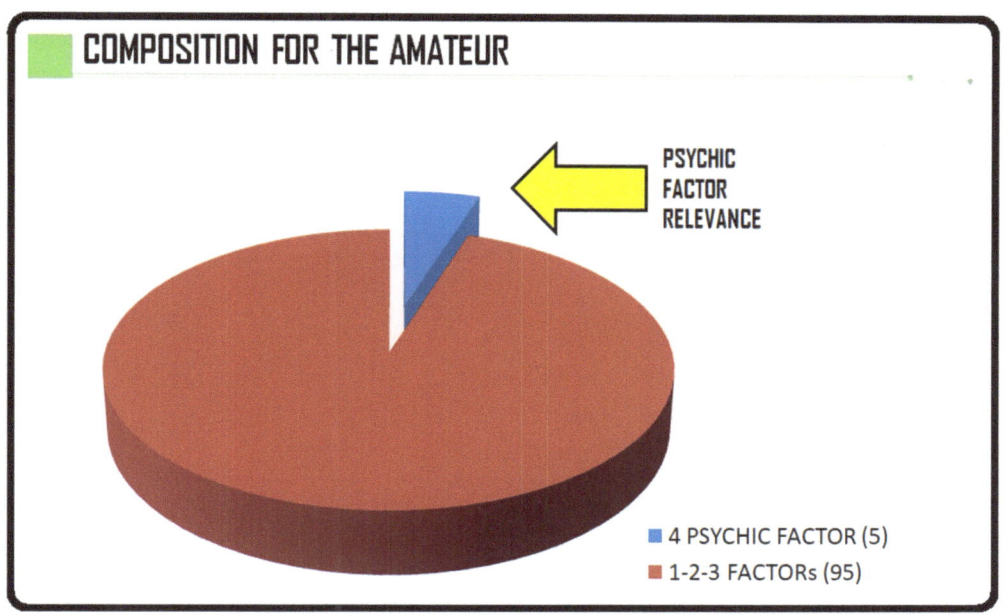

2) *Average Professional Athlete*: The Sport Mindset starts to be remarkable and scores 6 to 15% of the whole performance:

    a. Sport Mindset incidence: (max) 15%

    b. Conditional competencies incidence: (max) 35%

    c. Coordinative competencies incidence: (max) 25%

    d. Techno/Tactical competencies incidence: (max) 25%

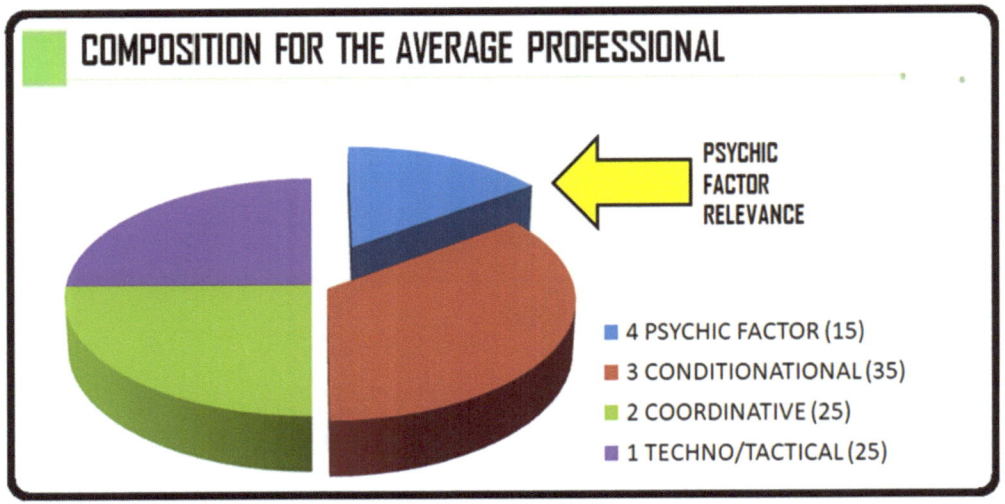

COMPOSITION FOR THE AVERAGE PROFESSIONAL

PSYCHIC FACTOR RELEVANCE

- 4 PSYCHIC FACTOR (15)
- 3 CONDITIONATIONAL (35)
- 2 COORDINATIVE (25)
- 1 TECHNO/TACTICAL (25)

3) *Peak-Performer*: The Sport Mindset scores a very significant impact on the whole performance:

    a. Sport Mindset incidence: (max) 30%

    b. Conditional competencies incidence: (max) 35%

    c. Coordinative competencies incidence: (max) 10%

    d. Techno/Tactical competencies incidence: (max) 25%

What we have to understand is that technical, tactical, and physical competencies and abilities must be considered already developed and consolidated to the athlete's arsenal, according to his/her quality (level) and to the level of competition they currently belong to. This means that for a Peak-Performer the techno/tactical competencies must be considered "*integrated*" into their arsenal at the highest levels; at the same time, they mark only 25% of incidence out of the total, while Sport Mindset marks 30%.

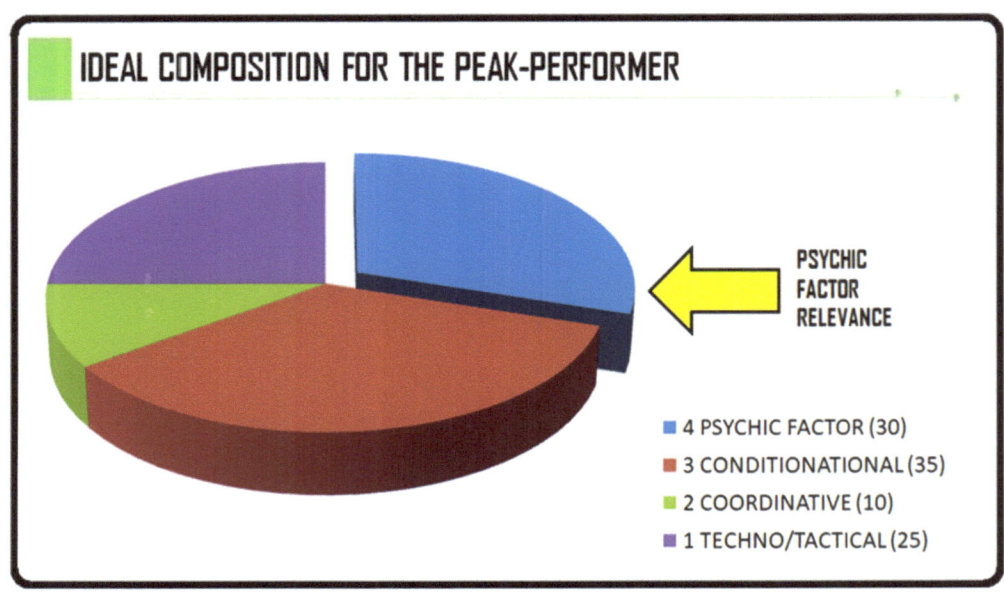

IDEAL COMPOSITION FOR THE PEAK-PERFORMER

PSYCHIC FACTOR RELEVANCE

- 4 PSYCHIC FACTOR (30)
- 3 CONDITIONATIONAL (35)
- 2 COORDINATIVE (10)
- 1 TECHNO/TACTICAL (25)

The IPS (*Ideal Performance State*) of a Peak-Performer is a mental condition which may be achieved after many years of training, practice, passion, and devotion to your discipline. In the chart below it is possible to get an overview of the average time needed to switch from the original state (*Amateur*) to the ultimate (*Champion*).

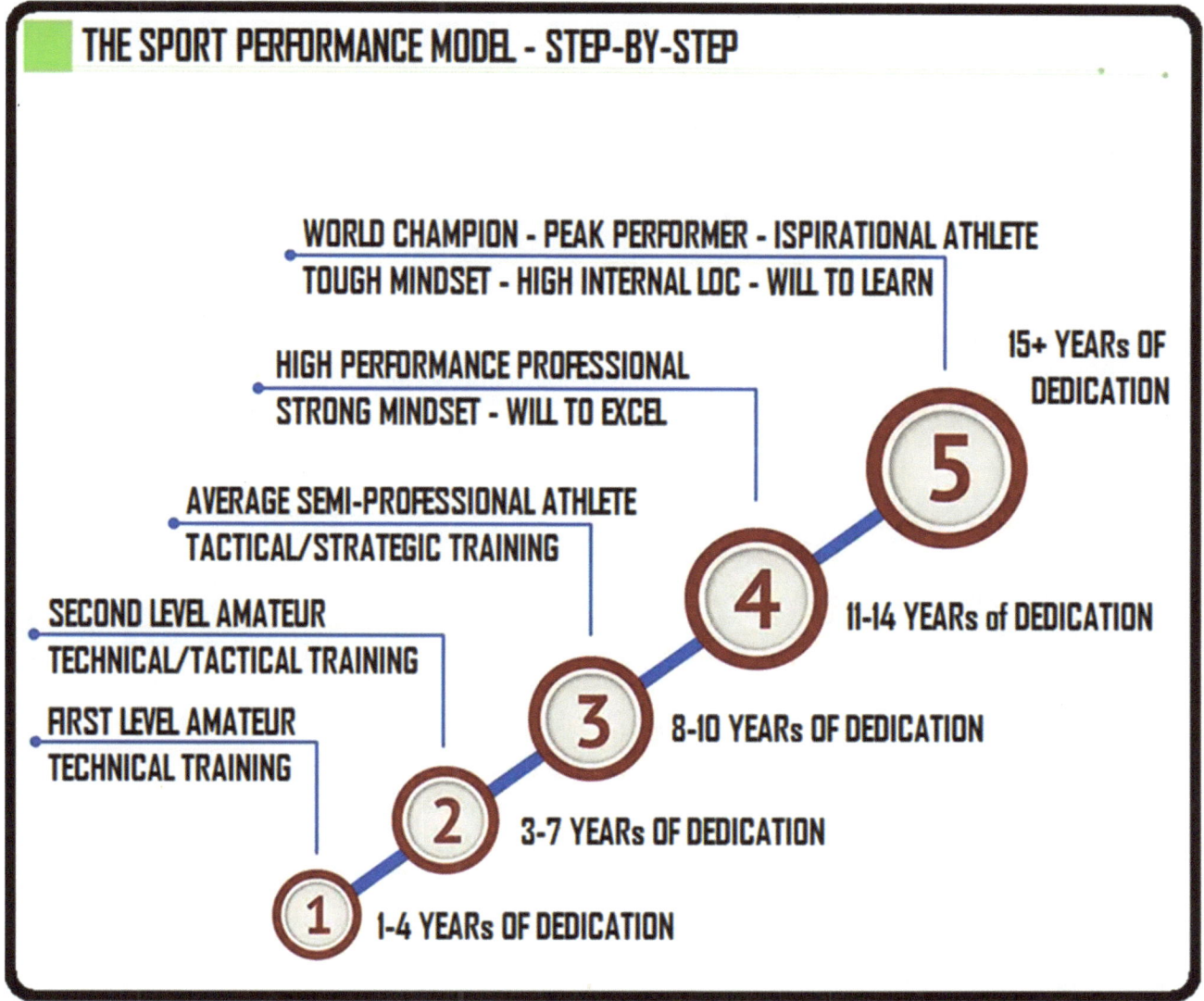

THE SPORT PERFORMANCE MODEL - STEP-BY-STEP

WORLD CHAMPION - PEAK PERFORMER - ISPIRATIONAL ATHLETE
TOUGH MINDSET - HIGH INTERNAL LOC - WILL TO LEARN

15+ YEARs OF DEDICATION

HIGH PERFORMANCE PROFESSIONAL
STRONG MINDSET - WILL TO EXCEL

AVERAGE SEMI-PROFESSIONAL ATHLETE
TACTICAL/STRATEGIC TRAINING

SECOND LEVEL AMATEUR
TECHNICAL/TACTICAL TRAINING

FIRST LEVEL AMATEUR
TECHNICAL TRAINING

5

4 — 11-14 YEARs of DEDICATION

3 — 8-10 YEARs OF DEDICATION

2 — 3-7 YEARs OF DEDICATION

1 — 1-4 YEARs OF DEDICATION

4 – Mindset and Peak-Performance

From a generic perspective we have to consider 3 levels of competition:

1st level: *Technical* – Low level of competition, low profile, and amateur athletes → *You win only after you compete.*

2nd level: *Tactical* – Intermediate level of competition, average and semi-professional athletes → *You compete after winning* (you win before, according to a strong tactical approach).

3rd level: *Strategic/Spiritual* – Top performer athletes, Champions, professionals → *You compete after winning – You win without competing.*

The discriminant amongst these three scenarios is the level of engagement of psychic skills (the mindset). At 1st level, the psychic skills have very little impact on performance (0-5/7%). At the 2nd level, the percentage is a bit higher (7-15%). At 3rd level, which is the one we have to consider if we really want to achieve peak performances, is definitely superior: 16-30%.

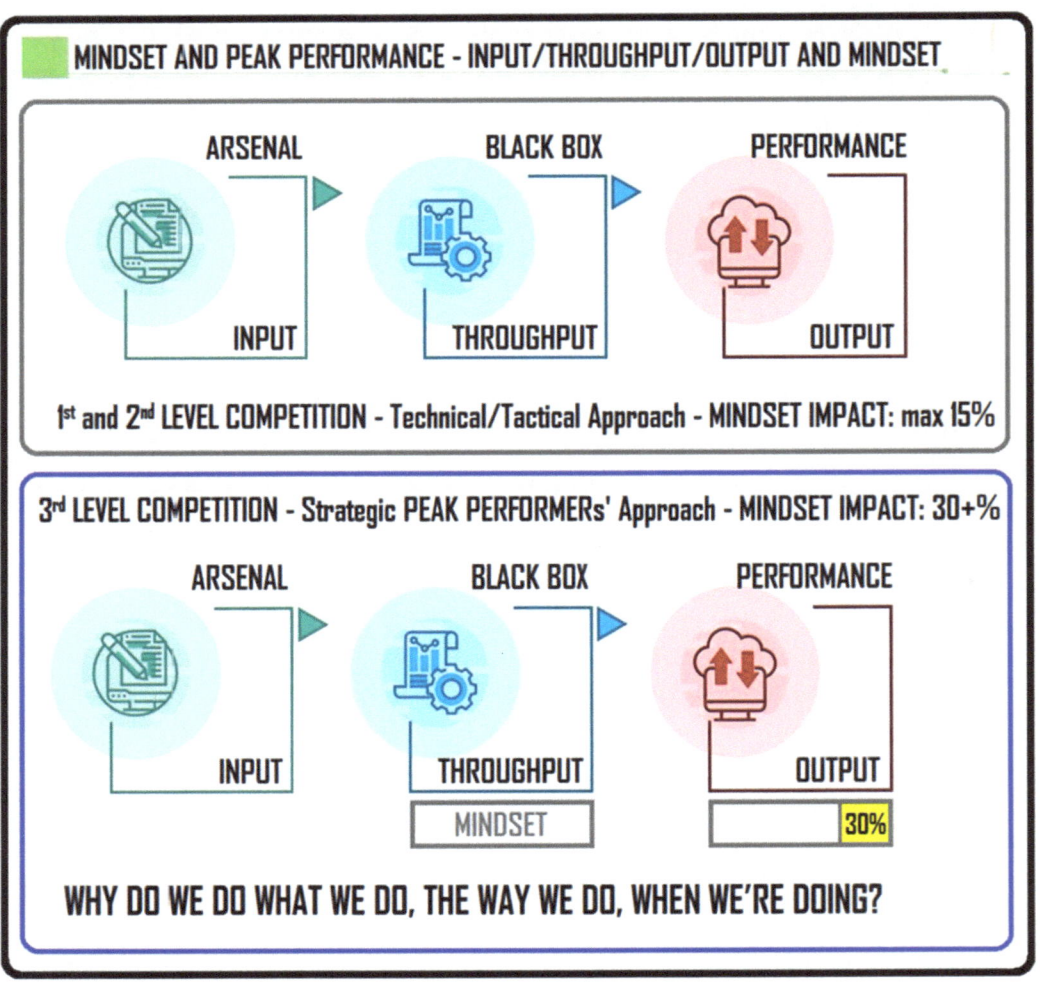

The level of engagement of Sport Mindset, finally, makes the real difference amongst the athletes and their performances.

The PROs attitude, which includes the Champions and Peak-Performers', always embodies the empowerment of mindset. Such an approach is omnipresent. They instinctively and naturally involve psychic skills and engage several of their mindset elements even while only footing, training, eating, relaxing, and competing. The mindset becomes *second nature* for the champions because their experiences have proved their actual effectiveness, then the personality of an athlete integrates these into other primary elements, a mix that is built to last.

The Peak-Performers' mindset is based on the *Principle of Consciousness*. They want and always need to know the reason why they are doing something. Such awareness enables their training in a different way, for their psyche is always working and every technical gesture they learn or perfect is coherently incorporated into the arsenal. This is a kind of application of the known proverb *"Knowledge is the power"*, to whom I would add *"Action based on knowledge is the power"*. All of that said, let's have a look at the three sentences, which easily describe the three levels of competition to whom the level of mindset engagement is connected:

1st level (Technical) → *WHAT*
"What do we do when we do what we're doing?"
2nd level (Tactical) → *HOW*
"How do we do what we do, when we're doing?"
3rd level (Strategic) → *WHY*
"Why do we do what we do, the way we do, when we're doing?"

You need to know everything about your training session so that you can consolidate any lesson you learn into a coherent framework of actions and instructions and exploit it whenever needed.

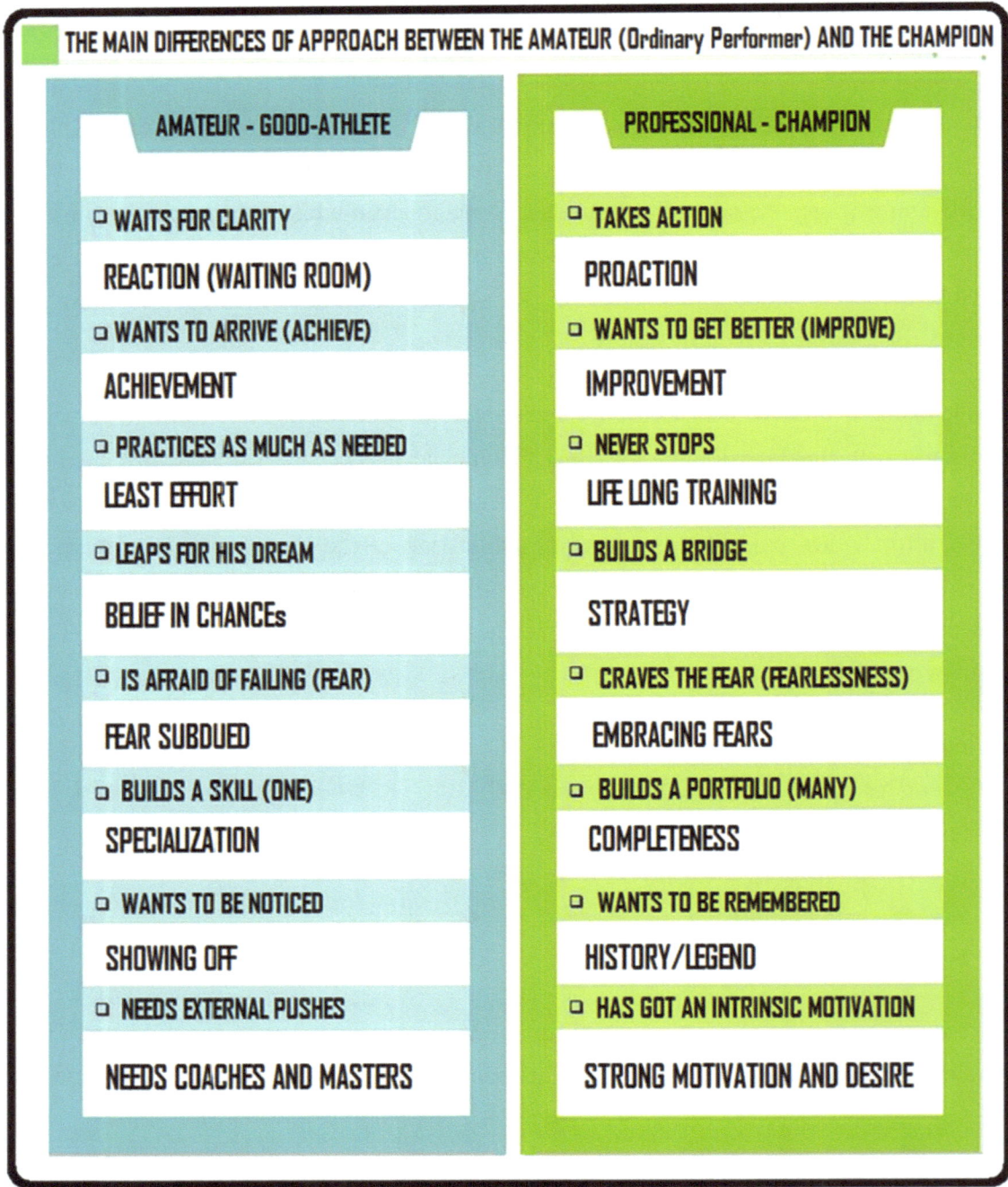

THE MAIN DIFFERENCES OF APPROACH BETWEEN THE AMATEUR (Ordinary Performer) AND THE CHAMPION

AMATEUR - GOOD-ATHLETE	PROFESSIONAL - CHAMPION
□ WAITS FOR CLARITY	□ TAKES ACTION
REACTION (WAITING ROOM)	PROACTION
□ WANTS TO ARRIVE (ACHIEVE)	□ WANTS TO GET BETTER (IMPROVE)
ACHIEVEMENT	IMPROVEMENT
□ PRACTICES AS MUCH AS NEEDED	□ NEVER STOPS
LEAST EFFORT	LIFE LONG TRAINING
□ LEAPS FOR HIS DREAM	□ BUILDS A BRIDGE
BELIEF IN CHANCEs	STRATEGY
□ IS AFRAID OF FAILING (FEAR)	□ CRAVES THE FEAR (FEARLESSNESS)
FEAR SUBDUED	EMBRACING FEARS
□ BUILDS A SKILL (ONE)	□ BUILDS A PORTFOLIO (MANY)
SPECIALIZATION	COMPLETENESS
□ WANTS TO BE NOTICED	□ WANTS TO BE REMEMBERED
SHOWING OFF	HISTORY/LEGEND
□ NEEDS EXTERNAL PUSHES	□ HAS GOT AN INTRINSIC MOTIVATION
NEEDS COACHES AND MASTERS	STRONG MOTIVATION AND DESIRE

Amateur, low-quality athletes, and even semi-PRO athletes have a low commitment: they often approach their sports discipline like a hobby and really think that it would be nice (and acceptable) to achieve their goals as long as it does not get too uncomfortable, risky, or painful. Professional athletes, champions, and peak/top performers have a completely opposite approach: the "*do-or-die commitment*". They behave at a different level of awareness: they approach their task and pathway towards victory as a war. Whilst amateur and semi-PRO always question the price they have to pay for success, champions, and peak performers pay whatever price it takes to win and they also prefer to pay in advance. They do not have any debit with both their sport and fortune: their focus and commitment cannot afford such a negative balance. They prefer paying in advance and keep waiting for their chance to come, calmly, hopefully.

5 – Mindset Factorization

This book analyses the whole of the factors and sub-elements which determine a strong and winning sport mindset (the so-called PPSM: *Peak-Performance Sports Mindset*). Each of these factors affects the performance according to special connections which have to be clearly explored; that's why I have segmented each of the Pillars into several factors (from 5 to 10 per each). These factors (or sub-elements) need to be caught, known, explored, and canceled or overturned if we realize they are set in the wrong direction. In fact, these elements are strictly connected to psychic and emotional factors which are very peculiar and require a specific set of exercises to be assessed, controlled, and empowered/overturned. In this book, we will go through all of that, as a piece of evidence. But there is still something missing that I want you to know and deeply understand in advance. Sport Psychodynamics specialists, Sport Psychologists, and Mental and Sports Coaches declare they possess the secrets to overcome any issue and illness which affect emotions, brain, and mind and they offer hacks, methodologies, exercises, and any other way to heal this malady. This book is nothing but a structured model based on the results coming from such studies so far, which also includes recommendations and instructions based on practical experiences (*athlete*) and effective methodologies, which have been tested on myself and on dozens of high-profile students (*coach/athlete*). All of that enabled a normal and average athlete to become a world champion. And still, there is something missing that I cannot neglect to affirm, here.

Hard training is the answer. Whenever you, as a coach or as an athlete, are questioning motivation, tactics, ambition, resilience, and perseverance, then remember that *hard training is the answer.*

Hard training is the cure. When you're looking for a specific medicine to heal depression, the consequences of failure and the idea of quitting, then remember that *hard training is the cure.*

And when you're trying to understand how a specific situation might be overturned, you have to fix in your mind that hard training is the magic drug, the secret to overcoming, the golden rule, the ultimate medicine to everything.

Training, practice, and direct experience: everything is connected to this. The Sports Mindset segmentation we offer in this book is just a scientific way to explore and better understand how several issues, hurdles, and problems which affect performance are connected to training. We do not look for and find something astounding, which we want to reveal. We only explain the way hard training empowers the greatest athletes' arsenal, mindset included.

All of that said: you will find factorizations, segmentations, and breakdowns. You will find relationships, connections, instructions, exercises, and recommendations. You will find some powerful questions finalized to push yourself opening your mind to different perspectives. All of that is finalized to unlock your potential and enable you clearly see your hidden talent to work on it. But finally, you have to come back to training. You will be most powerful, more motivated, more conscious, more ambitious, and more prepared to achieve your goals. You'll become much more self-confident and you will start feeling that *you can do that*, that one day you will become the champion. But nothing happens if you do not apply yourself to pain and fatigue, nothing will ever happen if you do not train yourself like hell, every single day of the week of every month of the year. Because hard training is the answer, anytime, anywhere for any sports discipline.

Let's start, now, by exploring the 8 specific areas which make up your sports mindset and trying to understand together how you can assess and manage each of them, to develop and reinforce your brain and your mindset driving your body to victory.

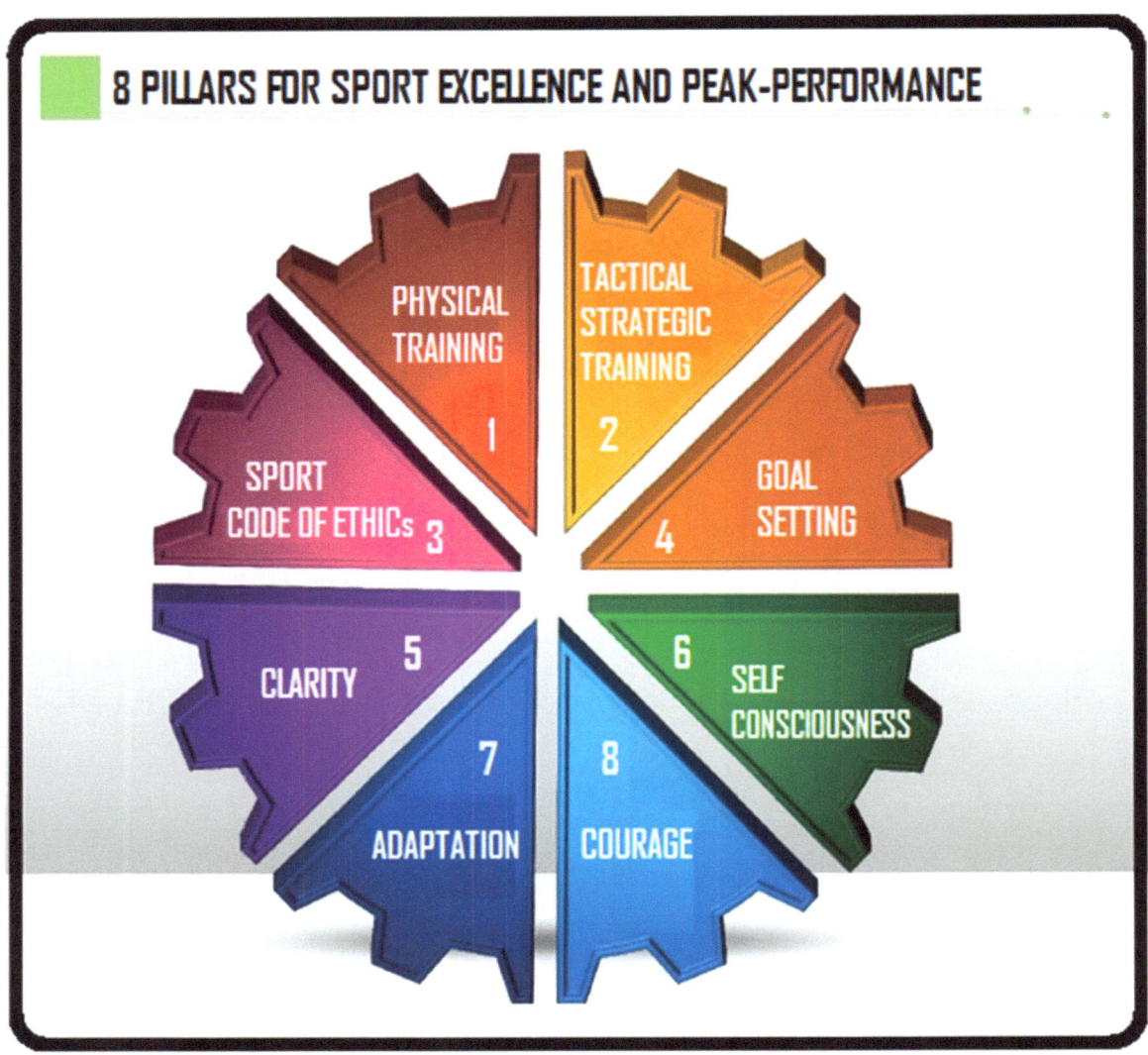

We will start from the first and we will apply the same pattern of analysis for each Pillar. Each sub-element declined will be unveiled and made susceptible to be managed.

8 PILLARS FOR A PEAK PERFORMANCE - SUB-ELEMENTS FACTORIZATION

1 PHYSICAL TRAINING	2 TACTICAL/STRATEGIC	3 CODE OF ETHICS
PASSION	TACTICS	HONESTY
STEADYNESS – PERSEVERANCE	STRATEGY	FAIRPLAY
CONTENTMENT	EMULATION	INTEGRITY
ENDURANCE	VISION	COHERENCE
SACRIFICE	RESPONSIBILITY	PROGRAMMING
	SELF-TALKING	DIVERSION

4 GOAL SETTING ATTITUDE	5 CLARITY OF DESTINATION	6 SELF CONSCIOUSNESS
SPORTS GOAL	SITUATION DEFINITION	SELF CONFIDENCE
MONITORING	EXPECTATIONS MANAGEMENT	CRITICISM MANAGEMENT
MOTIVATION	HERE AND NOW FOCUS	STRONG WILL
SELF-IMPROVEMENT	SENSATIONS MONITORING	RESISTENCE TO FLATTERY
EXCELLENCE	CONCENTRATION	UNIQUENESS
PROGRAMMING	SW-ANALYSIS	FRAMING THE FAILURE
PERIODIZATION	EMOTIONS CONTROL	AMBITION
PERFORMANCE DEVIATION		FRAMING THE VICTORY
METHODOLOGY	B-PLAN ATTITUDE	INNER SELF VULNERABILITY
		MANAGING THE INTERNAL ENEMY

7 ADAPTATION	8 COURAGE	
LEARN FROM FAILURES	PROPENSITY TO RISK	
SUSPENSION	RISK MANAGEMENT	
INJURY	NON-CONFORMITY	
HURDLES	INTERNAL LOC	
RESILIENCE	FEARLESSNESS	
	RESPONSIBILITY	

As preliminary information, you have to know that the whole of these Pillars, and the relevant skills and competencies which they include, present a specific degree of importance for the performance: some of them are actually more important than others. At the same time, they also present a different level of difficulty both related to the natural availability of the skills in the athlete's mindset, and to the development of the same ones. For such a reason I have developed a matrix that includes all the Pillars and easily highlights those which include the skills which can be considered as a *"Must-have"* for the top performer: difficult to develop and very crucial for the performance. I am talking about the Pillars which are present in quadrant #2: *Crucial Items.*

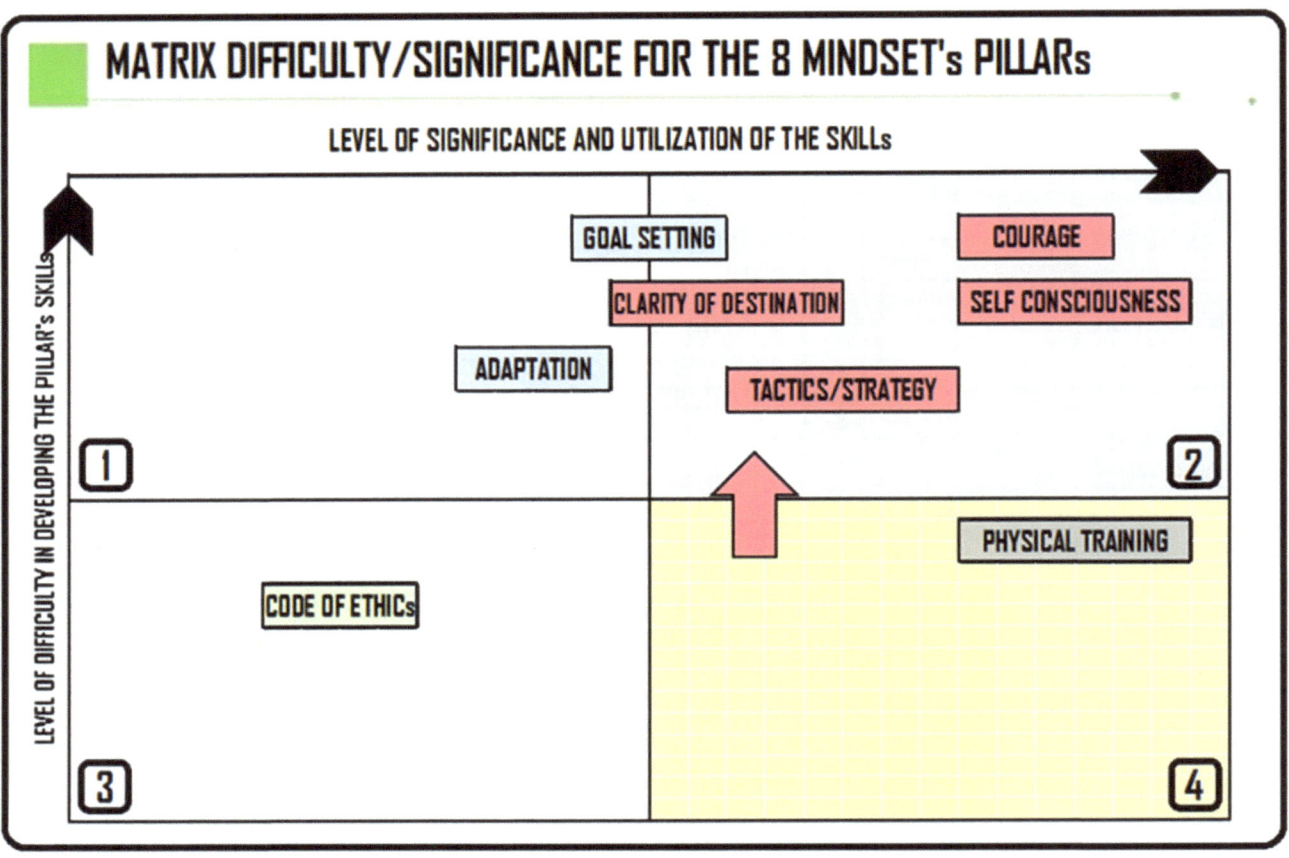

## CHAPTER TWO

Physical Training

6 – Definition

What we have to clearly understand is that hard training is nothing but building a foundation to last as long as possible. Is carving your body in rock. It means building your castle on the rock of the mountain.
Physical Training: The systematic use of exercises to promote bodily fitness and strength, cardiovascular and strength training and its related minimum standards and scores, used to determine standing for positions.

Training is a special activity that distinguishes athletes from ordinary people. The amount of training, finally, is the discriminant: what actually distinguishes the athletes based on quality and on level of professionalism:

	WHO	NO TRAINING	TRAINING	HARD TRAINING	HARD TRAINING + TACTICS	WORK LIKE HELL
INDIVIDUAL	Ordinary	X				
	Amateur		X			
	Semi Professional		X	X		
	Professional			X	X	
	Peak Performer				X	X

Table title spanning the columns: **AMOUNT OF TRAINING – DIFFICULTY OF TRAINING SESSIONs**

> Success isn't always about greatness. It's about consistency.
> Consistent hard work gains success. Greatness will come.
>
> [Dwayne "The Rock" Johnson – World Class Bodybuilder and Actor]

7 – Contextualization

Considered from the perspective of the *Training Theory, Physical Training* is a peculiar *"Process of Adaptation"*. The principle of adaptation refers to the process of the body getting accustomed to a particular exercise or training program through repeated exposure. As the body adapts to the stress of the new exercise or training program, the program becomes easier to perform and explains why beginning exercisers are often sore after starting a new routine, but, after doing the same exercise for weeks and months at the same intensity, the athlete experiences little, if any, muscle soreness. This reinforces the need to constantly vary the exercise and training routine if you want to maximize your results. This is the reason why the *Principle of Adaptation* is always coped and related to the *Principle of Progression.*

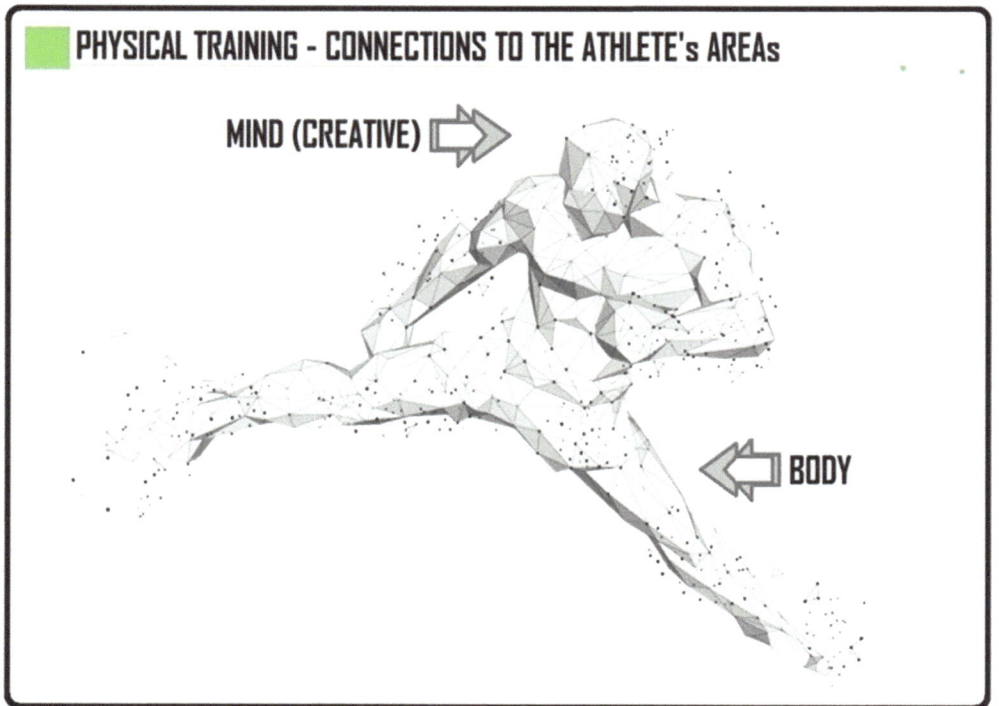

The human organism progressively adapts itself to the exercises. As a response, the body skills – coordinative and conditional capabilities – are enhanced and reinforced. This kind of physiological event is part of the bigger picture: the process of adaptation of humans to the external environment, which is determined by the *Principle of Survival* (the so-called: *"Instinct of survival and self-preservation"*). So Physical Training basically influences two areas:

a) The Body of the athlete
b) The Mind of the athlete

The mind is empowered due to the process of adaptation. The awareness of the connection between the progressive transformation of the body (strength, speed, power, resistance) and the adaptation itself is enough to hit the target: the athlete knows that the efforts are the real causes of this transformation and improvement (healthy state). On the other side, the evidence of this transformation facilitates the continuity of the efforts themselves, because it proves the ability to follow a training routine that comes from an arbitrary choice. The training activity, in fact, is nothing natural: the athlete makes the decision to create a problem (the exercise) and to solve this problem (application of the body to the exercise), in any single training session. This consciousness of such a choice empowers the athlete's mindset, day after day (*Principle Of Consciousness/Awareness*).

8 – Factors

Physical Training features, which are significant for the development of the Champion's Mindset, are 5: (1) Passion – (2) Steadiness/Perseverance – (3) Contentment – (4) Endurance – (5) Sacrifice.

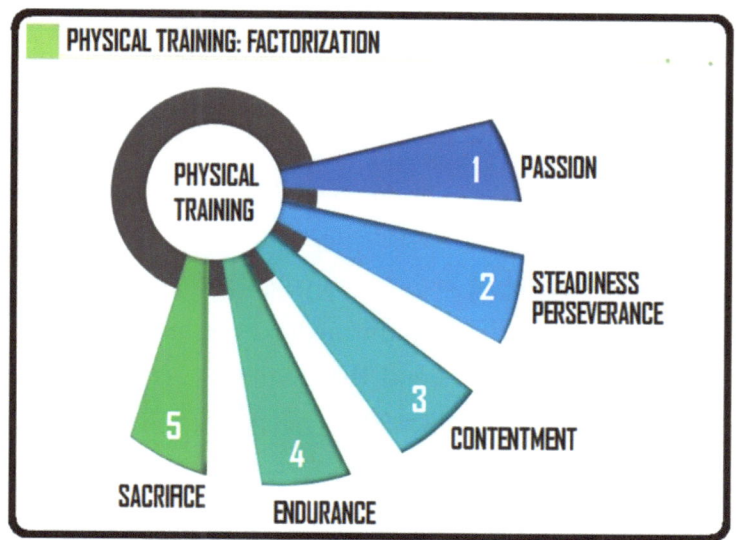

1. **Passion**: *This is a strong desire that can get you to do amazing things. Passion is an emotion to be acted upon. Without action, passion yields no worthwhile results. Passion is the fuel in the fire of action. When you have passion for something, you love it even when you hate it.*
   Passion is a fire constantly burning from the inside, something you cannot control, lock or ignore. Is stronger than pain, than fatigue, than rationality: that special something which deserves your complete commitment and sacrifice without you being aware. You have to recognize the passion, to learn how to master it (you don't have to be overwhelmed by your passion) and you need to drive it in the right direction; this means that, once you have become aware of your passion, you need to be able to switch your business from play to work. At the same time, you don't have to be overwhelmed: just keep doing what you love (and enjoy) and learn how to love what you do.

> I HAVE NO SPECIAL TALENTS. I AM ONLY PASSIONATELY CURIOUS.
>
> [ALBERT EINSTEIN – NOBEL AWARDED PHYSICIAN]

2. **Perseverance**: *A continued effort to do or achieve something despite difficulties, failure, or opposition.*
What you have to keep in your mind is that you can achieve your goals as long as you do not quit. Nobody can ensure you will succeed, neither your fans and coach nor your talent. You can be a *natural* (e.g.: naturally talented athlete), but this is not enough to succeed: you have to be there, to be trained, to be motivated, to be ready. There is plenty of *naturals* who held high hopes for their qualities, but never won anything of significance. They have been NCN: *Non-Champion Natural.* Passion ought to be managed and energy has to be distributed so that you can continue despite issues, injuries, threats, and any kind of external criticism. You have to introduce your constant training sessions into a sustainable routine which is coherent with all your residual goals and compliant with your personal ethics. Perseverance is strictly related to Resilience: is the first step to becoming a resilient individual. So you'd better develop a workout routine that can be introduced in a sustainable and coherent way with the rest: this will facilitate perseverance.

Persistence and perseverance are two primary skills of the great ones. You cannot achieve unless you train like hell, and you cannot train unless you are not persistent. You got to be there, anytime, any day, struggling, training, learning, and proving to yourself you can reach the target. As an amateur, you don't even know the meaning of being persistent, because you have never committed yourself for such a long time to a sport so much so you can catch what persistence really is. There is a threshold that requires your specific commitment. If you start empowering your commitment, you will intensify your training sessions and the frequency of your program, as a consequence. Physical stress, physical pain, and psychological pressure will come, and you will be surrounded by lots of doubts: *Should I continue or quit? Should I indulge such additional energy requirements or rather lighten my efforts?* This is the moment that requires you to become persistent. When mentally tough athletes determine their goals, they start burning their vision into their minds on a daily basis: they become obsessed with attaining the goal at almost any cost. From this stage on both persistence and perseverance become the very two factors to keep on the right track. You need to make your commitment and take action accordingly. You need to learn how to finish what you have started: a *do-or-die commitment*, in a sense. You will become unstoppable as far as you are convinced that you are destined for victory, that you cannot fail, only learn and grow. Persistence and perseverance are supported and fuelled by such an inner belief: *being destined to succeed*, in the long term.

> SUCCESS IS NOT FINAL, FAILURE IS NOT FATAL: IT IS THE COURAGE TO CONTINUE THAT COUNTS.
>
> [WINSTON CHURCHILL – ENGLISH POLITICIAN AND STATIST]

3. **Contentment**: *This is the state of being happy and satisfied.*
The presence of Contentment, which includes happiness and enjoyment, is the best proof that you started the right discipline and that you're on the right track. The practice of your sport discipline

SPORTMINDSETFOREXCELLENCE

is not an obligation: no one told you to do that; if someone did, then it is very likely that you're not enjoying your training sessions. So only the good emotions and positive perceptions of happiness may facilitate you entering the flow.

Contentment is an index that testifies whether you will be able to continue your discipline in the future (perseverance) or if you will not, in spite of problems. Is one of the inner motives which spurs you up and protects you from the outside chaos.

> I AM CONTENT, THAT IS A BLESSING GREATER THAN RICHES; AND HE TO WHOM THAT IS GIVEN, NEEDS ASK NO MORE.
>
> [HENRY FIELDING – ENGLISH NOVELIST, DRAMATIST AND MAGISTRATE]

4. **Endurance**: *The act, quality, or power of withstanding hardship or stress.*

From a strategic perspective Endurance is a crucial feature because enables the athlete to develop a long-term plan and apply this plan during the tournament. If an athlete is not provided with strong endurance, the organism will prevent him from performing according to a plan. The organism's needs will prevent the athlete from expressing the whole of both physical and techno/tactical resources (arsenal). Only a short-term plan would be applicable. In addition to that, a lack of endurance would prevent the athlete from completing the performance. Low-endurance athletes always rely on experience and fast completion of the competition, otherwise, the match is lost.

> ENDURANCE IS ONE OF THE MOST DIFFICULT DISCIPLINES, BUT IT IS TO THE ONE WHO ENDURES THAT THE FINAL VICTORY COMES.
>
> [GAUTAMA SIDDHARTHA BUDDHA – PHILOSOPHER, BUDDHISM FOUNDER]

5. **Sacrifice**: *A sacrifice is a loss or something you give up, usually for the sake of a better cause.*

Any time you select something, you are also sacrificing something else, which is not the favorite or the best choice: not according to your decision. Life's a matter of sacrifices because is a matter of choices. Your commitment requires you to neglect something (*present*) for something bigger to achieve (*future*). Your devotion requires you all (*now*) for a process of transformation: you will become something better (*future*). Your missionary attitude will require you to forget this world (*sacrifice*) and focus your attention and efforts only on useful activities and habits.

You have to understand if you are interested in pleasure, rather than gratification. Such a difference is really significant because defines the real distinction between an average athlete and the champion. Champions are only focused on *gratification-based activities* which normally take a huge amount of effort and time to be accomplished. Lots of champions and peak performers had to face external criticism due to such kind of long-term commitment: were ridiculed and criticized for investing so much time in the development of their core competencies and skills, whilst nothing good had happened so far meantime. Truth is that average people long for *immediate gratifications,* while champions neither require immediate compensation nor long for that: they only want to work hard to improve their arsenal, for they know that success will come, later on.

> THE GOOD AND THE GREAT ARE ONLY SEPARATED BY THEIR WILLINGNESS TO SACRIFICE.
>
> [KAREEM ABDUL JABBAR – WORLD CLASS BASKETBALL PLAYER]

9 – Threats

If you fail to focus on the features related to physical training, you're actually avoiding the basics of both your sports discipline and any generic sports activity. If you fail to apply yourself (*your time, your energy, your devotion*) to training sessions, you'd better prepare to fail as an athlete: no contest for you, no chance, and no good reputation. You are condemned to be a convolute, amateur, and average athlete. All your dreams of glory are nothing but lies you keep on telling yourself every day. You love *"the idea"* of being an athlete and you enjoy *"the idea"* of becoming a champion. You're on the ground level of the external exhibition of skills, competencies, and worthiness you are in lack of and that you do not deserve. The denial or neglect of these features determines the following threats:

#	FACTOR	POSSIBLE THREAT
1	PASSION	• Motivation decrease • Energy saving • Unwillingness to pain/sacrifice
2	STEADINESS – PERSEVERANCE	• Diversion • Quitting • Discontinuity
3	CONTENTMENT	• State of depression • Forcing
4	ENDURANCE	• Low performance • Demotivation • Quitting
5	SACRIFICE	• Amateur • Incoherence • Low profile and performance

1 Without a real passion you keep stuck in the illusion and delusion of your false desire. The desire is your propeller, makes you passionate. If you do not have any passion, then you will be a convolute athlete, stuck with your feet on the ground. Neither willing to sacrifice, nor to approach painful experiences.

2 Perseverance is the practical key to ensuring the appropriate training and conditioning. Perseverance comes from the mix of passion and desire, which is the discipline that obligates you from within. Without perseverance, you are condemned to be a low-level athlete. Perseverance keeps you far from diversion and discontinuity.

3 If you are not passionate, you're maybe equally not happy to join the gym, you are being forced by external mentors (parents/friends/coach/companions) or by yourself (your false self-image). No matter why: you have a serious problem which will lead you to depression, in the medium/long term.

4 Endurance enables you to express yourself and affirm your strategy and potential in the medium/long term. Without endurance, which is easily achievable through training and physical conditioning, you're condemned to be a low/average-quality athlete.

5 Physical conditioning, mental empowerment, and strategic approach may only be attained through hard work which requires you all. If you're not willing to do sacrifices, you are condemned to the level of amateur and low-profile athlete.

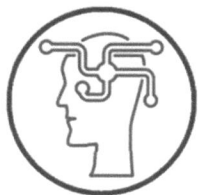

10 – Opportunities

Training will give you continuity, perseverance, and the chance to enhance your physical skills and competencies. Training means *building on rocks*: nobody can ever steal what you have done through sports training. Passion and enjoyment will enrich your inner being and will start the process of structuring your athlete personality, based on motivation and resilience. You will not feel the pain of sacrifice anymore, because sacrifice will become *second nature*. You will only feel satisfaction and gratitude for your discipline.

#	FACTOR	STRATEGIC ADVANTAGE
1	PASSION	• Motivation to train until excellence • Source of strength and motivation
2	STEADINESS – PERSEVERANCE	• Continuity • Several chances • Consistency
3	CONTENTMENT	• Energy and will to suffer • Training motivation
4	ENDURANCE	• High performances
5	SACRIFICE	• Learning any methodology to succeed • Hard training • Self-improvement • Overcoming problems and issues

1 Passion will give you the strength of continued motivation and will protect you from flattery, diversion, and big mistakes, in the long run.

2 Perseverance, together with passion, will keep you far from bad times and big mistakes. On the other hand, perseverance will offer many chances for the only easy reason that *"you are still there"*, working

hard. You are present and you will be in the right place at the right time. Perseverance will award you, in the future.

3 The contentment that you feel while practicing will fuel your dream, and will give you the energy to continue striving. Is your personal *"Training Motivator"*, in a sense. So do not lose such a desire to enjoy and to feel happy: is crucial.

4 Both the single competition and the training season are very long and hard to tolerate. If you want to achieve, you must enable your body to last as long as possible. Conditional skills ensure such an accomplishment and allow your brain to keep lucid and focused because resistance and power free your brain from the risk and the issue of fatigue. So, endurance is necessary for any discipline, not only for cyclic and non-situational (typically named *"Endurance Sports"*).

5 Only sacrifice ensures a real enhancement. Sacrifice means *"additional time"* which you can commit to your sport: training, additional sports activities, mental empowerment, trials and competitions, rest and sleeping, diet, Self-Autogenic Training, relaxation, massages, and mental coaching. When you are consciously sacrificing something, you are simultaneously gratifying another part of yourself and celebrating your sport.

11 – Methodology

The primary psychic factors related to Physical Training are the following:

- Perseverance —
- Endurance —
- Sacrifice —

The methodologies for empowering these factors are based on planning, programming, and tracking the progression of KPIs.

Perseverance is usually empowered through *"being perseverant"*, a kind of self-referential competence that ought to be applied like an obligation: you have to be present (during the training sessions), you have to train (more than expected), you have to keep in your mind that this is one of your main limitations.

Endurance works in the same way and recalls physical competencies, rather than psychic ones, but you need to reinforce your motivation to keep working on endurance. You need to constantly recall in your mind the original motivation that pushed you to start your sports: *"Why am I here for?"*.

Sacrifice attitudes need to be increased through a kind of planned self-indulgence: you must be perseverant, thus sacrificing lots of big times doing other things, but you can (and you have to) give yourself planned breaks and celebrate your freedom.

PILLAR # 01 - PHYSICAL TRAINING

	TOPIC	GOAL	ACTION	EXERCISE	REPETITION
1	PERSEVERANCE	Becoming incredibly constant in training and being focused on sports discipline	Train – Being present – Overwhelm any limitation	Planning – Programming – Tracking - Recovery	All life long
2	ENDURANCE	Becoming lucid and powerful during training sessions and performances	Challenging yourself when tired and demotivated	Train hard – Perform in spite of fatigue	1-2 times per week
3	SACRIFICE	Doing what planned – erasing other stuff and activities – love and passion for sport	Some activities as an award. when task completed	A complementary party/ vacation as a gift	1 time per month 1 time per 3 months

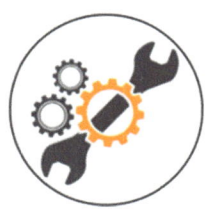

12 – Practical Techniques

Passion should be an innate skill for any serious athlete. Nevertheless, can be supported and endorsed effectively by keeping on the right track, which means strengthening the practice. You have to challenge yourself during the first stages of resistance due to (1) lack of technical knowledge – (2) lack of experience, in both gestures, environment, habits, and language – (3) false self-image – (4) shyness. So, take action and continue taking action in spite of hurdles, difficulties, and incompetence. Neither judge yourself nor listen to others' judgments and criticism.

To enhance Perseverance, you need to include in your training routine some specific additional exercises finalized to remind you of your will and ambition to be perseverant. Extend such activity for 4 weeks, at least, and consolidate your habits (at least 21/days or 21 times per month). So become perseverant acting *"as if"* you were already perseverant.

You need to enjoy your practice, every time you go to the gym or go on footing, fartlek, or whatsoever. This is a *"must"* for any athlete. Go into action to be happy and have fun, include friends and partners in your sports discipline and hide your dream, realize your healthy state, whilst practicing your favorite activity and focusing on that. Try to understand the inner sense of your sports discipline and become a missionary. Go and take your Contentment from your sports hobby.

To enhance your Endurance, you need to practice additional efforts and introduce new disciplines into your weekly routine. Once per week is enough: swimming, footing, biking. Enrich your training programs accordingly.

You need to discover the inner meaning of your commitment, its size, and its quality. You need to understand that for a Champion the sport is not only a kind of activity but even a mission. Take your time to explore the alibis which prevent you from doing with passion. The sense of your Sacrifice lies behind these alibis: you must catch and destroy these internal biases and barriers and you'll find all the energy you need.

13 – Powerful Questions

Use these questions to force yourself (as an athlete) or your coachees to switch to a higher mental perspective and unlock additional energy to keep being in the right direction. All the questions require specific and honest answers which may also take a few minutes or more, to be developed.

- ➢ 1.1 What are the real causes of your satisfaction and feelings you actually experience, while practicing your discipline?
- ✓ *You need to learn where your passion really originates from.*

❒

- ➢ 1.2 Explain the sense of completeness and internal fulfillment you feel. Where is it coming from? What kind of physical emotions and feelings does this generate?
- ✓ *Start detecting your inner emotions. Learn these emotions and start naming these emotions and imputing specific actions related to these emotions.*

❒

- ➢ 1.3 What are you willing to sacrifice in order to empower your training through additional time and training sessions?
- ✓ *You need to understand the size of your commitment, which is normally related to your willingness to sacrifice.*

❒

- ➢ 1.4 How hard do you feel hot and excited before you're going to join your training session?
- ✓ *Detect your burning heart, if present. Detect the real motivation which is testified by your excitement.*

❒

- ➢ 1.5 How do you figure out yourself when you're almost sleeping? What do you really feel? What are you imagining in your head?
- ✓ *The dreams and last pictures you figure out before sleeping testifies the size of your connection with your discipline and with your final purpose.*

❒

➤ 2.1 How much do you train weekly and why? Who is the person who recommended you this? Is it possible to increase such a figure? Do you think you could do better than this?

✓ *Get back to basics: there is no limit to training, but your body sensations and your commitment. Start developing a critical approach to ordinary training and conventional rhythms and pace and sync them to your skills and attitude to the effort.*

❐

➤ 2.2 What kind of commitment have you got with your discipline? What kind of commitment did you take to yourself?

✓ *A strong commitment enables you succeeding, in the long term, but also requires you quit deciding and start obeying your boss, which is your final Goal.*

❐

➤ 2.3 What might prevent you from training with perseverance? Why this factor may really break your training routine?

✓ *You need to detect which are the real threats that may lead you quitting, one day. You must predict such events in very advance and learn how to live with them.*

❐

➤ 3.1 Which are the sensations you feel inside, whenever you make and execute a physical gesture in the most appropriate way? Explain it and detail as much as you can and fasten it all in your mind.

✓ *Catch the real and tangible satisfaction of execution. Remember this perception and secure your body and mind.*

❐

➤ 3.2 Is there anything that gives you the same contentment and happiness that you feel during the practice of your discipline? Make a comparison and explain the possible causes for such an alignment.

✓ *Any alternative option is a threat and may become a current risk, in the future. You'd better understand honestly your preferences.*

❐

➤ 4.1 Which is the real cause that gives you the clear message that your fuel is finished? What really happens inside your body and your mind that causes you to quit, to give up the challenge if you're in a disadvantageous situation? Explore with details.

✓ *Start detecting the symptoms of a bad situation occurring and affecting your brain and your performance. Fatigue or fear of unpredictable events.*

❏

➤ 4.2 What really prevents you from insisting on *"5 seconds more"*? What really happened during those additional seconds? What may possibly happen?

✓ *The rule of "5 seconds more" can really help you raise back; in case you feel close to giving up. Use your brain, first, and then experience what may really happen if you apply such a hack. Then you can repeat a few times and you can overturn fatigue or bad occurrence.*

❏

➤ 4.3 List down the whole of self-talk which takes place in the 10 seconds which precede that moment you're almost quitting. Who is speaking?

✓ *You have to hunt down and flush out your alter ego. You need to know his language and the tone of his voice.*

❏

➤ 4.4 Why are you so sure that the person who is talking to you is right? Whom do you believe this person to be?

✓ *If you want to beat your enemy, you must be familiar with him. But before such a task, you must realize you have an adversary which cohabits with your same body and psyche.*

❏

➤ 5.1 What are your current priorities for the next 5 years in your personal life? What are your goals, in the next 5 years?

✓ *Start setting your goals and understand which are your goals, before planning a strategy to achieve them.*

❏

➤ 5.2 What do you believe you have been sacrificing in the last years of your life, to achieve your sports goals? Which kind of activities?

✓ *Shortlist the activities that you believe you have neglected. The sum of such activities is the size of your commitment to your goal.*

❏

➤ 5.3 Are you feeling okay with that? Why? Do you think you're postponing something? Is there any disappointment coming from any side? (*Family – Business – Study*).

✓ *According to an "Ecologic Vision" of goals, the whole of the targets must be coherent and susceptible to coexistence. Check if they really are, otherwise, your sports goal is not sustainable and will require more time than expected.*

❏

➤ 5.4 What are you currently not sacrificing, which you could, finalizing this additional time and energy to accomplish your sports career? Could you possibly plan your time accordingly?

✓ *The process of achieving a huge goal requires you to become radically essential: you only take care of activities that may get you closer to your objective and you neglect any other residual activity.*

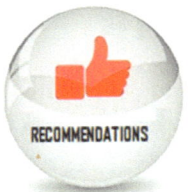

14 – Instructions & Recommendations

Take your passion and put it on top of your emotional priorities. Neither success nor fame can be compared to passion and its gifts. Let passion go through you and freely express as much as possible. Be always willing to let any piece of curiosity and any experience and any wish from your passion enter yourself and your inner spirit and feed the flow of your actions through your happiness and enjoyment. Progressively learn how to abandon yourself to training, efforts, sweat, and fatigue, how to take psychic advantage of the sense of being physically stressed, almost exhausted, and empty. Progressively learn how to challenge yourself while training and after you have trained: number of repetitions, number of series, number of training sessions, intensity and time spent, number of ordinary mistakes and fails. Passion leads to becoming familiar with challenges: welcome such a habit, rather than avoiding it. Small challenges prepare your body and your mind to apply for hard and crucial ones, when ready for that.

Challenge:

1) *your will* to train yourself (contrast your laziness);
2) *your body* limits;
3) *your technicalities*;
4) *tactical circumstances*;
5) *your mindset.*

Challenge yourself harder, as long as time goes by.

Passion can really support your perseverance, but your willpower will seriously be tested when a severe injury or a crucial problem which may divert you from training, would occur. In such a case you have to *re-engage yourself.* You need to apply visualization. You need to figure out the person that you want to become: that person needs you to be persistent *now*, there is no other way you can become that person but your efforts' revenge, in the present time. So, visualize this better version of yourself and re-engage your resources to keep on track. Do not be doubtful to apply the *helicopter hack*. Imagine you are slowly and progressively separating from yourself right now, you're moving up and you can observe yourself like you are on a helicopter. After a while you can get a clear vision of what is really happening, calmly, suspended. On the left side, there is your past, your place is the present and the right side represents the future. Your current problem is nothing but a moment of weakness in your life and career. Can you manage to figure out the future: how have you designed it in your mind? That future includes you, your survival, or your success: how important is what is currently happening to you now, for the future? Which is the evident size in the big picture? It's up to you. Then come down and land back to your current self and make your decision. You choose your reaction and your reaction will define your future.

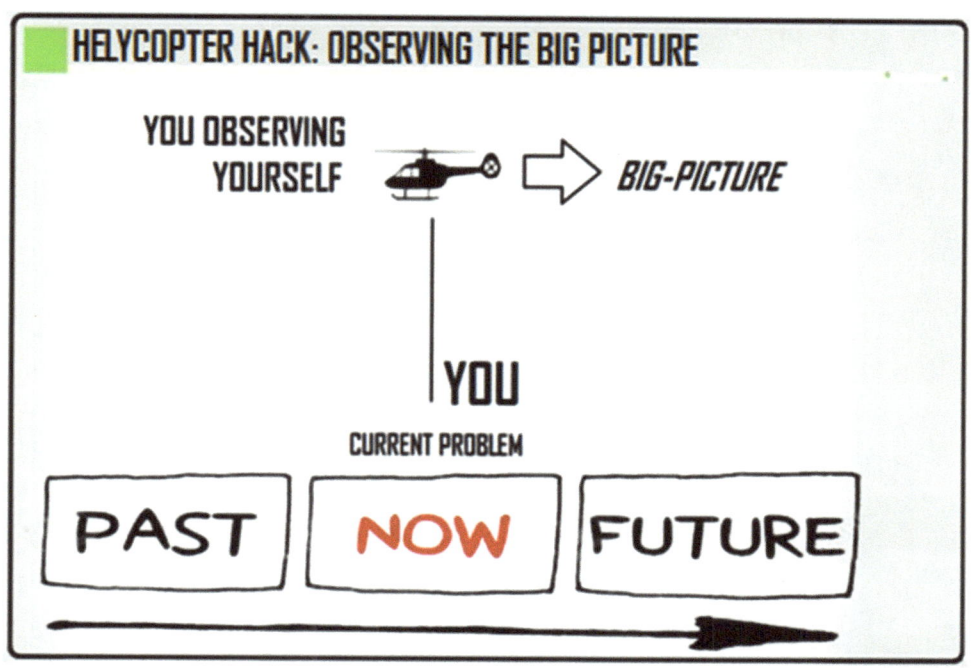

## CHAPTER THREE

Tactical/Strategic Training

15 – Definition

You can be a *"natural"*, you can be a strong and physically talented athlete, you can also be even rational, intelligent, and provided with spectacular skills and competencies, but without solid tactics and strategy, you cannot achieve in any sports discipline. Tactics and strategy are the primary resources for professional and semi-professional athletes: technical and physical skills should be considered consolidated and already integrated into the arsenal. As we already know, the presence and relevant exploitation of tactics and strategies define the level of the competition: 1st level: *strategic/spiritual level* – 2nd level: *tactical* – 3rd level: *technical*. The Peak Performers are provided with a strong strategic approach, which is directly related to a huge awareness of their own skills, what may happen, and what is actually happening during the tournament.

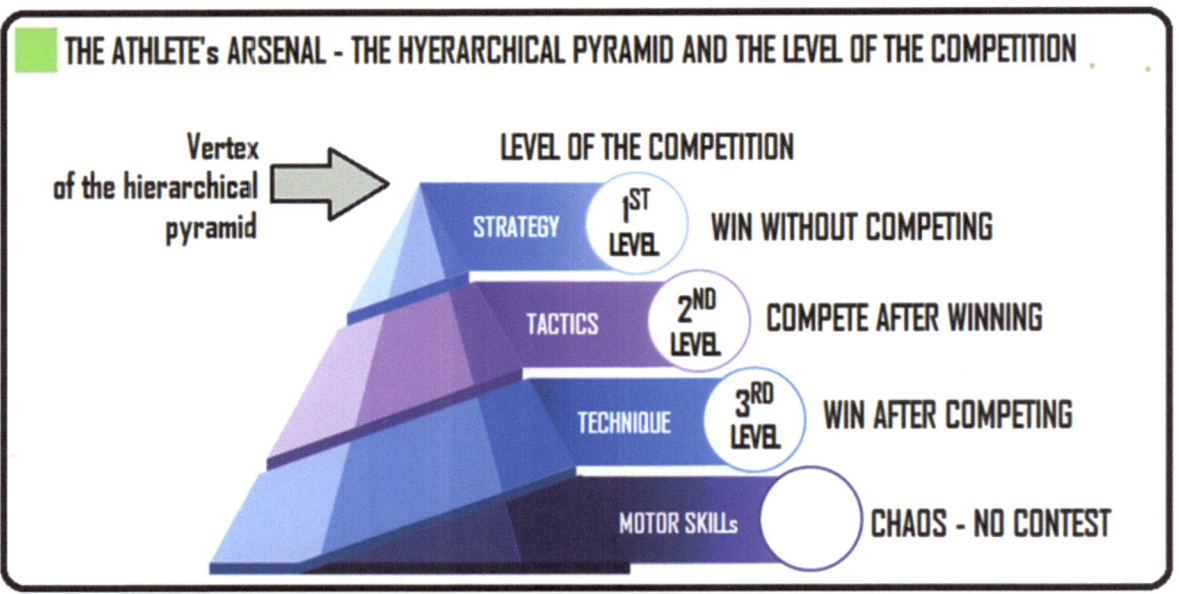

Tactical/Strategic Training: *Tactical and Strategic training and conditioning are applications of strength and conditioning principles in a tactical (e.g., military, law enforcement, sport) training environment.*

> TACTICS WITHOUT STRATEGY IS THE NOISE BEFORE THE DEFEAT.
>
> [SUN TZU – CHINESE MILITARY GENERAL, AUTHOR, PHILOSOPHER]

16 – Contextualization

The dimension of tactics and strategy is one of the most crucial for any sports professional who wants to get to the highest level. Strategy defines the highest level of competition. There is no high-level athlete who has achieved huge results without a strong and solid strategic approach. No matter the sports discipline: strategy is the vertex of any peak performance. On the other hand, a strong strategic plan for the competition actually requires that the athlete has developed strong skills related to self-awareness, mental presence, technical strengths/weaknesses, environmental threats, internal threats, opponent's potential, and other peculiar circumstances and features. For these two bundles of reasons, we can affirm that technical/tactical training directly affects:

a) The Mind of the Athlete (logic and strategic competencies)
b) The Spirit of the athlete (internal competencies and skills)

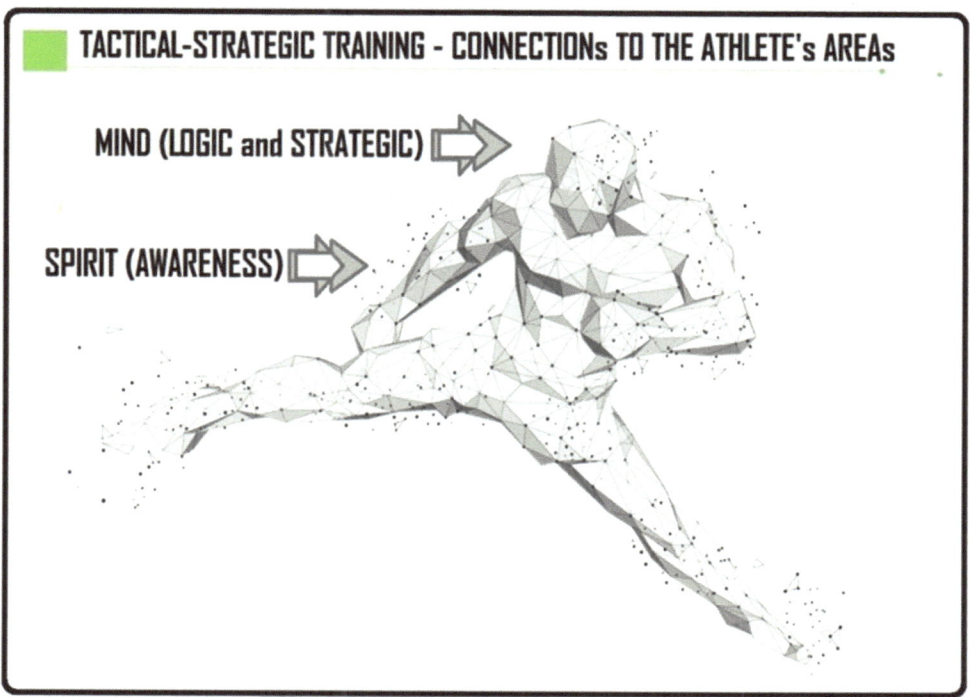

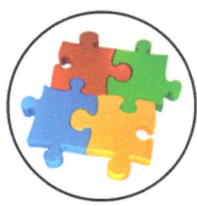

17 – Factors

Tactical/Strategic Training features, which are significant for the development of the Champion's Mindset, are 6: (1) Tactics – (2) Strategy – (3) Emulation – (4) Vision – (5) Responsibility – (6) Self-Talk.

TACTICAL/STRATEGIC TRAINING FACTORIZATION

1 TACTICS

2 STRATEGY

3 EMULATION

TACTIC/STRATEGIC TRAINING

4 VISION

5 RESPONSIBILITY

6 SELF TALKING

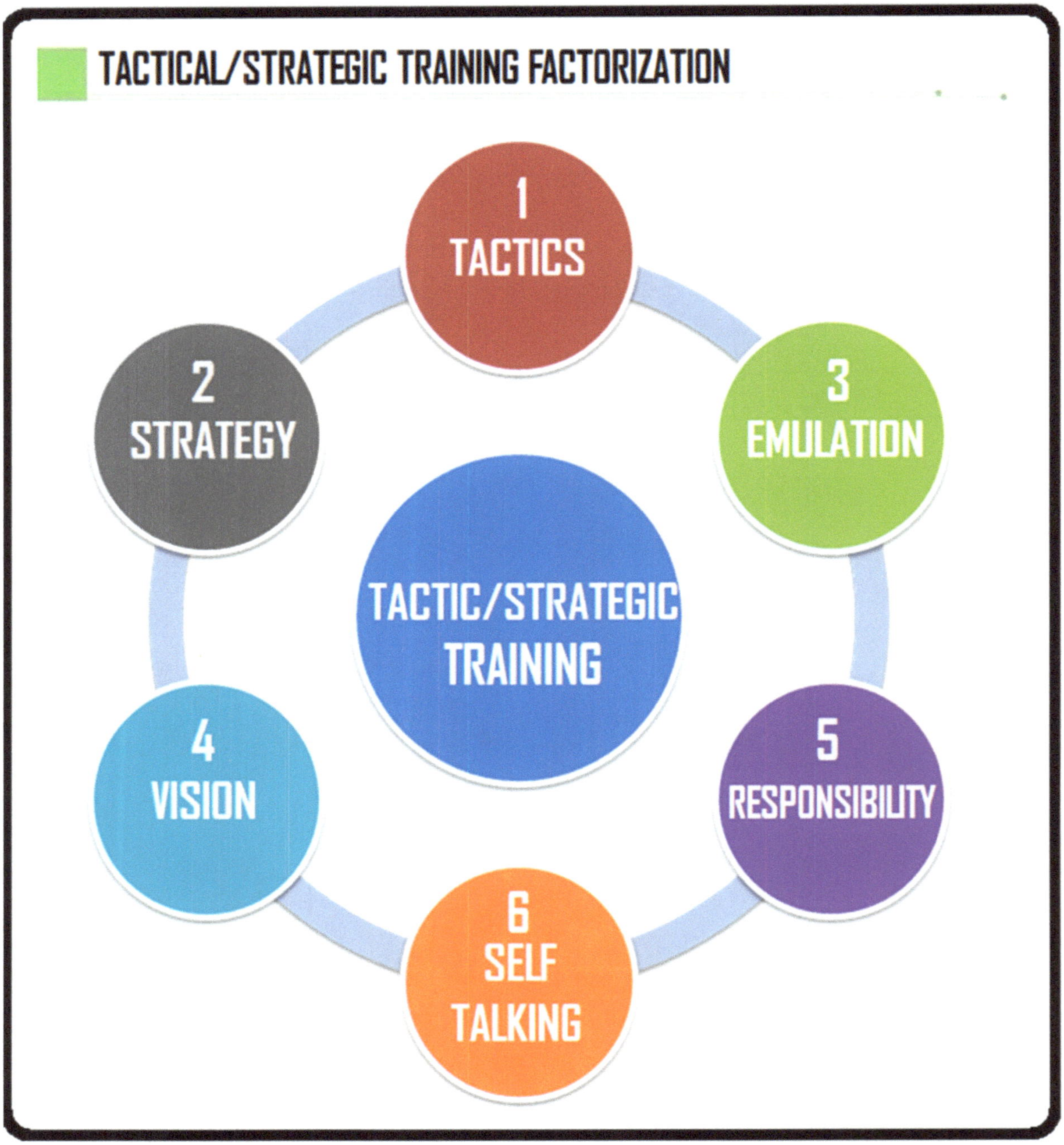

1) **Tactics**: *This is the science of planning the arrangement and use of military forces and equipment in war. The art or skill of employing available means to accomplish a specific purpose.*

If we frame the concept according to a competition perspective, the tactic should be considered as a set of recommendations that basically explain what to do and how doing. Tactics vary depending on the peculiarity of the discipline you practice: each sport presents special principles of tactical application. You can consider a tactic as a special way to apply a specific gesture or technical move. Champions and Peak-Performers are used to select a few tactics which are synched to their strong features and transform these tactics into *"special"*, which is a peculiar gesture/action finalized to overturn a bad situation. Tactics are directly connected to the Champion's mindset and to the chance to win the competition. Tactics are the dowels that determine the victory when placed in the correct sequence.

> TACTICS IS KNOWING WHAT TO DO WHEN THERE IS SOMETHING TO DO.
>
> [SAVIELLY TARTAKOWER – WORLDCLASS POLISH AND FRENCH CHESS PLAYER]

2) **Strategy**: *A detailed plan for achieving success in situations such as war, politics, business, industry, or sport, or the skill of planning for such situations.*

Similarly, if we adopt the same perspective of the competition, the strategy explains when and why doing what you have to do. There is no success without a strategy, but being provided with a strong strategy does not lead to success, necessarily. Lots of additional features are needed, but the whole of these is driven by a strong and accurate strategy, both contextual and preventive. What you have to know is that the perfect strategy actually does not exist, because no strategy can predict what contact with your opponent will lead to. This is the reason why a solid strategic plan ought to be 85% complete and let you improvise the residual 15%. No strategy can survive enemy contact, but your task consists of developing a strategy and learning how to apply it and when to switch to your B-Plan.

> STRATEGY IS KNOWING WHAT TO DO WHEN THERE IS NOTHING TO DO.
>
> [SAVIELLY TARTAKOWER – WORLDCLASS POLISH AND FRENCH CHESS PLAYER]

3) **Emulation**: *This is the process of copying something achieved by someone else and trying to do it as well as they have.*

A Champion is much more than a model, is an inspiring individual (and might become a mentor, in some cases). Very frequently occurs when a young athlete is influenced by a local champion (gym/ town) and this fatally becomes an idol and an idol becomes a limit. You need to select a strong model to whom you inspire your behavior, your training, and your vision. You need a great performer provided with talent and fair play. You have to investigate his/her mentality, to detect his/her training hacks, style, and resistance. Each champion has his/her story made of difficulties and hurdles which have been overcome. Select your favorite inspirer and get information regarding his/her attitudes, mental approach, methodology to react to problems, and even strategies, if available. Observe him/her in the movies. Find the gaps, study the gaps, and understand and fill the gaps.

> EMULATION IS A HANDSOME PASSION; IT IS ENTERPRISING, BUT JUST WITHAL. IT KEEPS A MAN WITHIN THE TERMS OF HONOUR, AND MAKES THE CONTEST FOR GLORY JUST AND GENEROUS. HE STRIVES TO EXCEL, BUT IT IS BY RAISING HIMSELF, NOT BY DEPRESSING OTHERS.
>
> [JEREMY COLLIER – ENGLISH THEATRE CRITIC AND THEOLOGIAN]

4) **Vision**: *This is the ability to imagine how your career will develop in the future and to plan it in a suitable way.*

A strategic attitude facilitates a high-level career. Push your mind to its stronger potential and figure out your sports career at its possible best. Try to visualize all the steps starting from your current state till your ultimate goal, the completion you long for. Design your pathway in your mind with lots of details, reasonable, sustainable, and crazy at the same time. Then switch it to action and follow it till the end. Every Peak-Performer is provided with a strong ambition and a vision when he/she started training. Any Peak-Performer has had the strength and the nerve to accept the intensive pathway which separated him/her from success and that way was run.

> A STRONG VISION WITH ACTION MAKES A POWERFUL REALITY.
>
> [RON KAUFMAN – AMERICAN BESTSELLING AUTHOR AND MOTIVATOR]

5) **Responsibility**: *This is the quality or state of being responsible: such as moral, legal, or mental accountability.* Nothing happens by chance, without a reason. All the issues, the problems, the victories, and the failures, are nothing but a sequence of events that resonates with your emotional and psychic state and with your level of responsibility. You need to know that being a champion is a matter of responsibility: you have to take responsibility for all the consequences of being a champion, a model, an inspiration, for the upcoming expectations, and for the respect of opponents and experts. Once you become the sole owner of your business, then you will only rely on your arsenal, neither on fate nor on your opponent's mistakes. The responsibility is a kind of peculiar resonance between your quality and your performance: the higher your quality, the highest your performance.

> EXCEEDING EXPECTATIONS IS WHERE SATISFACTION ENDS AND RESPONSIBILITY AND LOYALTY BEGINS.
>
> [RON KAUFMAN – AMERICAN BESTSELLING AUTHOR AND MOTIVATOR]

6) **Self-Talk**: *The act or practice of talking to oneself, either aloud or silently and mentally.*

We use to develop about 66 thousand thoughts every day and over 65% of these are negative thoughts because drive our self-talk to depression, demotivation, false predictions of difficulty, and hurdles that lead to failures. These negative thoughts are determined by fears, worries, lack of self-confidence, insufficient physical shape, pain, and other limiting beliefs. These thoughts are *"self-talk"* in a sense. Self-talk has a huge impact in initiating or quitting an action, but also in activating or deactivating the necessary resources for the relevant behavior (action). In short: thoughts start self-talk which enables you to make a decision and it also activates the resources needed to transform this decision into action. The self-talk drives the action, definitely. You have to select your thoughts, overturn the limited beliefs and switch them into self-talk which motivates you to follow the right vision and apply your workout routine. The attitude of overturning a negative situation is not natural: you have to develop it slowly and consolidate such skill into your arsenal. The self-talk actually starts here.

> LISTEN TO THE WORDS YOU SAY. THE VERY WORDS YOU SAY TO THEM ARE THE VERY WORDS YOU NEED TO HEAR. HUMANS TEND TO GIVE EACH OTHER WHAT THEY THEMSELVES NEED. SO TELL THEM THESE IMPORTANT THINGS AND THEN TURN AROUND AND TELL THEM TO YOUR VERY OWN HEART.
>
> [KATE McGAHAN – AMERICAN BESTSELLING WRITER AND PSYCHOLOGIST]

18 – Threats

The unwillingness and inability to explore and master tactical and strategic features of your sports discipline will move you away from success and will keep you to an average level: *winning after competing*. No certainty of results, no real enhancement at all. The incapacity of interpreting the match or the competition according to tactical/strategic patterns will lead you to find excuses, invent quick and childish alibis, and empower an external LOC which will become your boss. Your self-talk will follow accordingly and will include negative thoughts and negative sentences: *"I cannot"* – *"I'm inadequate"* – *"It's others' fault"* – *"The referees are unfair"*. The preliminary stage of the failure. Negation leads to the following:

#	FACTOR	POSSIBLE THREAT
1	TACTICS	• Improvisation • Confusion • Win after competing
2	STRATEGY	• Being a pawn • Improvisation • Failure
3	EMULATION	• Too few solicitations • Mental closure
4	VISION	• Goals postponement • Goals prevention
5	RESPONSIBILITY	• Believing in fate • Suffering others' decisions
6	SELF-TALKING	• Depression • Being stuck • Impostors' Syndrome

1 The lack of tactical competence leads to uncertainty. You are forced to use improvisation more than expected and quite often you find yourself in a state of confusion. You are condemned to the technical level of the competition: you must compete to win, but victory is never certain.

2 The lack of a strong, strategic approach, which depends on tactical weakness, leads to failure. You are condemned to play the role your strategic opponent has defined for you and you are forced to extemporize. You cannot create or build anything, for you are not provided with the tools for planning and programming.

3 You can get your job done simply by executing the instructions: this might be enough. Lots of mentally tough athletes do have not any mentor or idol to emulate, but they have a strong sense of action and huge self-confidence. Selecting a model can quicken the process of learning technical and tactical lessons.

4 If you do not have a strong vision, you cannot dream and you are condemned to procrastinate your goals. In fact, dreaming is a form of art: the dream of a pragmatic athlete is the most tangible thing the world has ever seen. The dreamer is able to visualize scenarios in detail before they actually happen if inspired by a strong vision and supported by a huge sense of responsibility. If you fail to dream you cannot develop a sustainable vision so you cannot define (and see) your goals. Without any vision, you are even prevented from succeeding, because things first happen in the invisible dimension (mind, imagination) and then in tangible reality.

5 Without a strong sense of responsibility you're condemned to be subdued to others' plans and decisions. You'll be strengthening your External LOC: complaints, alibis, childish excuses, mental barriers, and resignation.

6 When you tolerate or even undergo negative self-talk, you will be stopped and stuck by your Internal Enemy. In the long term, you may be affected by depression and may even quit training. You will be affected by the impostor's syndrome: even though you are ready and enough prepared for the higher level, you will feel (and confess to yourself) you are inadequate and do not deserve any kind of success.

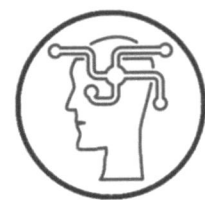

19 – Opportunities

Tactics and Strategy are *"Must Have"* for any sports professional. A strong strategic approach ensures huge chances of succeeding. The sense of responsibility, if correctly applied to training and competitions, will grant you a strong Internal LOC. Excellent performance will follow when you are ready for that.

#	FACTOR	STRATEGIC ADVANTAGE
1	TACTICS	• Compete after winning • Always knowing what to do
2	STRATEGY	• Planning and Programming • Strong approach to tournaments
3	EMULATION	• Mind Openness and inspiration • Learn as much as you can • Filling the gaps
4	VISION	• Direction • Ultimate clear goal
5	RESPONSIBILITY	• Internal LOC • Fearlessness • Self enhancement
6	SELF-TALKING	• Motivation • Relying on a loyal partner • Switching to a higher level

1 The professional is actually provided with tactical and strategic skills. The provision of a huge technical arsenal enables the athlete to select the best option for the specific circumstance. The level of competition is higher. *Compete after winning*: you enter the arena for competing, but thanks to your tactical approach you have already won.

2 Strategy enables the athlete to program, plan, developing the most effective and suitable solution to overwhelm the opponent(s). That's what is called the *"winning approach"* to the competition. A strong strategy may even enable you to *Win without competing* (3rd level of the competition).

3 A practice of emulation which is enough balanced, may quicken the pathway to excellence. You can learn by observing and studying and you can also fill your gaps before the opponent (competition) or the coach (gym) recommends such attainment.

4 A strong vision gives you a sense of direction which will drive your efforts towards the goal achievement. You cannot escape such a skill. This is a *"must-have"* quality of your being. Your ambition, your aim, and your desire: all these mixed up build your sports vision.

5 If you take full responsibility, you become the owner of your business. As the owner you cannot be scared by anything, for you already know all depends on you, even in collective and team sports disciplines. You start empowering your Internal LOC.

6 When you haunt down your Internal Enemy and force him to surrender, you're strengthening your self-confidence. You can rely on a very loyal partner, from that day on.

20 – Methodologies

The primary psychic factors related to Tactical/Strategic Training are the following:

- Tactics —
- Strategy —
- Emulation —
- Self-Talking —

The methodologies for empowering these factors are based on increasing the aware consciousness and the subconscious mind. You need to develop a kind of *"subconscious automated actionability"* in a sense, but to achieve such kind of competence you must be aware, in the preliminary stage.

Tactics and Strategies need awareness, understanding, planning/programming, and lots of scenarios planning, and of simulations that present the specific circumstances which you have to go through to improve your actions and reactions. It's a matter of defining the right conditions, including tactical boundaries and constraints, and exercising, repeating hundreds of times to secure this competence in your personal arsenal. *Create a scenario (full of constraints)* → *Plan an effective solution (which fits your arsenal)* → *Implement and apply (lots of times)* → *Achieve and succeed* → *Consolidate your arsenal.*

Emulation of inspirational models requires investigation, detection, understanding of attitudes and habits, surrounding with champions and peak performers, implementing a new and positive language, and visualizing your skills at their possible max.

Self-Talk, finally, requires your preliminary focus and attention: you ought to understand when/what/how this talk starts and why then you need to draft a script (sentences and statements) and you need to implement all of this stuff into your self-talk.

PILLAR # 02 - TACTICAL/STRATEGIC TRAINING

	TOPIC	GOAL	ACTION	EXERCISE	REPETITION
1	TACTICS	What to do When doing How to apply	Self-driven activation	Select – Isolate – Perform – Repeat Develop lots of Circumstances	Always, during training All life long
2	STRATEGY	Why doing Vision and Direction - Lucidity and clearness	Study schemes Study Adversary Strategy Plan and apply	Plan how to achieve Perform accordingly B-Planning	2 times per week Simulation Reinforcement Scenarios Simulation
3	EMULATION	Align to similar models Steal habits/secrets Steal Champions Mindset	Studying the Champion Ask, see and observe Following Champions	Isolate a specific skill and try to perform it	Consolidate 3 skills per year
4	SELF-TALKING	Controlling the Inner Enemy Motivational Talks Inspirational Talks	Ability to anchor memories Scripts – Compromise Win against	Use powerful self-talk and powerful sentences as proclaim and as motivational mantras	Every training session

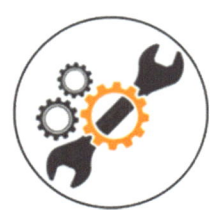

21 – Practical Techniques

To enhance Tactics, you need to practice tactical operations and become more familiar with a strategic perspective of the match. You need to: (1) create problematic situations, define the most appropriate solutions, and apply them until you're familiar – (2) observe your opponent's tactics and try emulating these tactics, securing to your arsenal, when fitting – (3) differentiate your training and start regularly applying tactics together with techniques (your gestures need to be joint to a tactical design).

To enhance Strategy, you must switch to a higher level of perception and understanding of the match. You need to: (1) dissect others' strategies and emulate what you understand – (2) find the inner sense of the victory – (3) plan a strategy and execute it both during official and unofficial competition – (4) study, explore and master the three basic methodologies of a strategic plan: a) *Attack* – b) *Defense* – c) *Counterattack*.

After you have accepted you are not a champion and that there are lots of lessons you can learn from others, you must select your Mentor and start your investigation of him/her. You need to study: (1) habits – (2) attitudes – (3) strategies – (4) approach to competition – (5) diet – (6) relationship with media. Try surrounding yourself with both Champions and others Peak-Performers to enrich your temper and personal attitudes. Emulation also goes through the study of any TOP-Performer you can explore through the internet (WEB).

From local to national to continental to world and Olympics: you need to become capable of figuring out your success escalation according to its natural progression. A strong and true Vision requires you to focus on your first target and then switch to the next. Details, precision, feelings: visualize your pathway to glory.

Responsibility is directly connected to your Internal-LOC, which ought to be pushed to its maximum potential, to achieve in sports. You need to enhance your sense of responsibility in just 9 steps: (1) take responsibility for your thoughts, feelings, words, and actions – (2) stop blaming – (3) stop complaining – (4) refuse to take anything personally – (5) make yourself happy – (6) live in the present moment – (7) use the power of intention – (8) feel calm and confident – (9) look for the good in people.

Self-Talk can be declined as follows: *Personalizing*: you blame yourself for everything. *Magnifying*: you focus on the negative aspects of a situation, ignoring any and all of the positive. *Catastrophizing*:

you expect the worst, and you rarely let logic or reason persuade you otherwise. *Polarizing*: you see the world in black and white, or good and bad. There's nothing in between and no middle ground for processing and categorizing life events. You need to manage or even master your self-talk so that you can exploit it before and during your performance. Take action against your hostile ego: (1) *Identify negative self-talk traps.* Certain scenarios may increase your self-doubt and lead to more negative self-talk. Work events, for example, may be particularly hard. Pinpointing when you experience the most negative self-talk can help you anticipate and prepare. (2) *Check in with your feelings.* Stop during events or bad days and evaluate your self-talk. Is it becoming negative? How can you turn it around? (3) *Find the humor.* Laughter can help relieve stress and tension. When you need a boost for positive self-talk, find ways to laugh. (4) *Surround yourself with positive people.* Whether or not you notice it, you can absorb the outlook and emotions of people around you. This includes negative and positive, so choose positive people when you can. (5) *Give yourself positive affirmations.* Sometimes, seeing positive words or inspiring images can be enough to redirect your thoughts. Post small reminders in your office, in your home and anywhere you spend a significant amount of time.

22 – Powerful Questions

Use these questions to force yourself (as an athlete) or your coachees to switch to a higher mental perspective and unlock additional energy to keep being in the right direction. All the questions require specific and honest answers which may also take a few minutes or more, to be developed.

> ➢ 1.1 Have you a clear perception that you know what you are doing, while you are performing during an official tournament? Is there any moment in which you feel confused? Explain and detail the reasons why.

> ✓ *As a professional you are strongly required to know exactly what you're currently doing, why are you acting that special way, and why you neglected alternative suitable solutions. If you do not start thinking and acting like a professional does, you cannot become a champion.*

❐

> ➢ 1.2 Explain and detail your tactics: attack – defense – counterattack – feinting, and enrich your explanations with reasons, goals, and tasks required for each of the four items.

> ✓ *You need to be provided with a mental pattern that includes objectives and methodology for each goal. You must break down your performance into a small set of instructions to ask for support when needed.*

❐

> ➢ 1.3 Don't you think there might be additional tactics that may enrich your personal arsenal?

> ✓ *Just start observing your idols and/or other high-level competitors. Try understanding which are the reasons which lay behind a gesture, an action, or a specific solution: the whole of their decisions is never made by chance. Each of them hides a tactical approach you may learn and emulate if fitting your arsenal.*

❐

> ➢ 1.4 Develop a plan so that you always know what you have to do, according to your tactical approach, when you are performing, something that includes your "specials" and your *Unique Performance Proposition* (UPP).

> ✓ *Such a plan prevents you from falling into the chaos trap of improvising. Improvisation leads to uncertainty, and tactics and strategy lead to victory.*

❑

➢ 2.1 Do you have a strong perception that you always know the reason why you are executing that specific gesture/action, at any time? Is there any moment in which you are in a position of confusion and so you question yourself this way *"What am I exactly doing now? Why am I acting this way? What should I do, now, and why?"*.

✓ *The lack of consciousness and awareness is quite often connected to a lack of strategy. You cannot afford such a mental state in a crucial competition.*

❑

➢ 2.2 Explain and detail your favorite/usual strategy during your performance. Something that you're quite familiar with. Explain this strategy and why and how you're good at executing such an approach.

✓ *Start stigmatizing your best and most effective strategies. You need to list them precisely, to define the way they work, which kind of situation they specifically fit, and how they require to be driven until the end of the competition. Secure such a scheme in your mind for the future.*

❑

➢ 2.3 Did this strategy reveal to be always effective and successful? Explain and present some circumstances in which you lost your match and why.

✓ *One strategy for all is never a good choice. You must accept this limitation. You can accept this limitation by going back through your past failures.*

❑

➢ 2.4 Do you always know the reason why you are making that specific action? Can you explain and detail the actual driver of any single action (or inaction)?

✓ *You must catch and understand the chain command of action: (solicitude) → emotion → belief → resource activation → decision making → action. You must isolate the drivers of your actions and decisions and you need to work on them.*

❑

➢ 2.5 List at least three tactics you are familiar with and explain the specific finalization.

✓ *Tactic #1/#2/#3 → Finalization → additional instructions. You need 3 tactics at least, to survive your opponents.*

❑

➤ 2.6 How do you make a decision, while performing? Describe your DMP (*Decision-Making Process*) and the feeling and perceptions you are connected with, before and while executing this decision.

✓ *You need to submit your DMP to a resistance test and you also need to check if you are able to make a decision according to rational aspects rather than being emotionally imprisoned.*

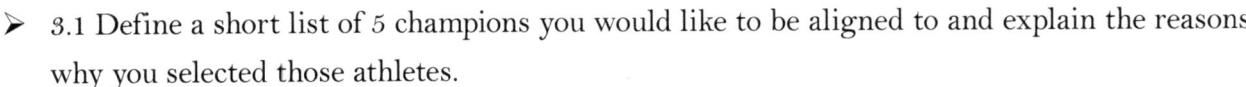

➤ 3.1 Define a short list of 5 champions you would like to be aligned to and explain the reasons why you selected those athletes.

✓ *Technical style, mental attitude, gestures elegance, fair play, strategic intelligence, attitude to success, resilience: you need to check which are the actual elements you envy because these elements are the real ones you are in lack of (unconscious incompetence).*

❐

➤ 3.2 Describe their tactics, strategies, strengths/weaknesses, and habits and explain (*your opinion*) why they are or have become the *Number-1* of their discipline.

✓ *This exercise is useful to understand your current level of awareness and the level of involvement in the sports discipline you practice: the rule of the games.*

❐

➤ 3.3 Now take 2-3 skills: what do you think you can do to fill the gaps? Is there any priority? Is there a way to quicken your enhancement?

✓ *Start planning your strategy to fill the gaps between your current version and the Ideal Performance State (IPS).*

❐

➤ 3.4 Make a plan or a program to attain that specific skill in 3-5 months and then switch to another crucial skill.

✓ *Depending on your discipline and your training rhythm/pace 12-15 weeks is the least period of time to develop and consolidate one special skill to your arsenal.*

❐

➤ 3.5 What belief does prevent you from becoming as good as one of your favorite idols currently is?

✓ *Start detecting your limiting beliefs.*

❐

➤ 4.1 Picture your career till 5-10-15 years from now: what do you see? Can you figure out yourself within this picture?

✓ *Does the clarity of your vision actually enhance your career and set your psychic and physical state to achieve a huge result?*

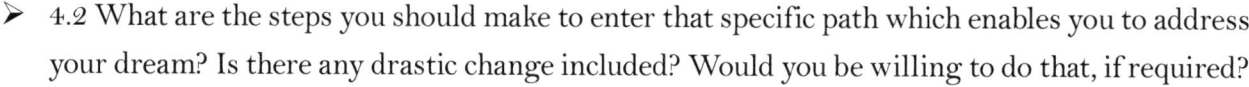

➤ 4.2 What are the steps you should make to enter that specific path which enables you to address your dream? Is there any drastic change included? Would you be willing to do that, if required?

✓ *You need to have a clear and honest awareness of the size of your commitment and devotion. A huge goal requires huge efforts and huge sacrifices. Something you voluntarily decide to neglect and something additional you decide to execute. It's up to you.*

➤ 4.3 Is there any person who might facilitate your choices? Develop an action plan to deal with such persons or clubs or entities and join.

✓ *Sometimes filling the gaps may be accelerated by making the decision to ask for help and support from other people: companions, sports clubs, associations, and elite coaches. To quicken your pathway, you need to overcome your ego (pride) and join whoever may give you pieces of advice or opportunities to learn.*

➤ 5.1 Do you think you have a kind of control over the external world or is there always something you cannot control and you are condemned to undergo?

✓ *You need to know if you are the pawn or the chess if you are the Slave (of circumstances) or the Master (of your world). Everything depends on your beliefs and on your relevant choice.*

➤ 5.2 Do you believe in luckiness? Do you believe in misfortune? Why? Describe some events in which your view has been confirmed.

✓ *Be very careful: if you believe in luckiness, you also believe in misfortune. This means that you accept the idea that you cannot control your world, your events, or your performance. Deeply and progressively explore your inner belief related to luckiness/unluckiness, because is crucial. Be informed that a champion neither believes in luckiness, nor in misfortune, but only relies on him/herself.*

➤ 5.3 How do you explain that there are champions who are capable of winning against hostile situations? Against any hurdles or issues, in any circumstances?

✓ *Self-confidence, adaptation, and resilience are other ways to name luckiness. Luckiness is preparation added to opportunity, in a sense.*

❏

➢ *5.4 Being → Knowing → Doing → Having*: how do you feel comfortable with such a theory?

✓ *People currently upheaval such a true pattern. Low-quality athletes are convinced that having leads to doing, which leads to being the champion. You need to go through such a pattern and decide what you really believe. The person you want to become depends on such an answer because you will activate your resources for being or for having. Your world will be the consequence of the decision you made.*

❏

➢ 6.1 Please describe the identity of that individual who lies inside your mind and who talks to you continuously. Who is this person? Why do you assign the whole of your trust to him/her?

✓ *You need to realize another person cohabits with your brain and your body. You need to detect his/her identity.*

❏

➢ 6.2 Tell a few examples for which the recommendations of this internal individual were revealed to be right.

✓ *Quite frequently your inner voice is right when his/her recommendations are related to non-significant challenges or events. Just realize that personally.*

❏

➢ 6.3 Shortlist a few sentences which make you feel great, successful, excited, and full of energy. These sentences ought to become your personal mantra and you have to teach your internal host narrating to you any day, any time, before and after your training sessions.

✓ *Exercise useful sentences to enter your motivational mantra-daily-routine.*

❏

➢ 6.4 Develop a narrative plan finalized to confront your inner voice and overcome your fears, worries, concerns, laziness, and sense of inferiority. You have to win against him.

✓ *SAME. Develop a script to rationally contrast your inner enemy.*

❏

➢ 6.5 Henry Ford once said: *"If you think you can do a thing or think you can't do a thing, you're right"* How do you resonate with such a statement?

✓ *This quote exactly summarizes the "Cycle of Action": Solicitation → Beliefs → Decision → Resources Activation → Action → results.*

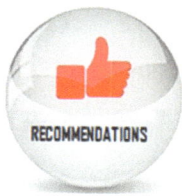

23 – Instructions & Recommendations

Develop and strengthen a plan which instructs you on *"what to do when"* and train yourself to activate such an action subconsciously. Define and use specific circumstances as *"mental triggers"* to activate actions and reactions while competing. Define your strategic approach based on your characteristics. If you are driven by a strong and unstoppable desire, just take action, be aggressive in your attack, astonish and surprise your opponent, and create and manage your advantage. If you can easily control your emotion and you can observe the situation clearly, then strengthen your defensive patterns and bet whatever you have on defense. If you're an evolved strategist, you can exploit more sophisticated techniques. Start mastering both defense and attack, then mix the tactics and apply the finest art of counterattack. Fine-tune your defense, nullify your opponent's attack, and assault him/her aggressively. Affirm your superiority through the counterattack.

After choosing your model, start a process of psycho/technical identification with him/her. Nobody needs to know your secret either because you might be misunderstood and also you don't need to extend your strategies to others but yourself. Start connecting mentally and emotionally with your idol and use his/her energy to enhance your motivation and progressively set your targets to a higher level. Become a *copycat* and use your model as a driver, but keep yourself balanced.

Nobody wants you to become the champion, if you don't want to: nobody is interested but you. Push your dreams to their max: what you can visualize defines the limitations of your goals and depend on your current beliefs. If you want to overcome such a constraint you need to go back to your beliefs and understand what the real cause lies behind. Then you have to work on it. Your dream comes through only when you take the responsibility to become the champion. No one can help you become a responsible athlete: you must take this weight upon your shoulders by yourself. You ought to make your solitary through the black valley of your monsters and your demons. You ought to go alone and survive. Then you come back and nothing would even haunt you anymore. Win the game inside, then you come out and take what you finally desire: nobody would stop you.

According to a psychological approach, Vision also performs an additional task. Vision requires that you have developed the *Big-Picture* of your sports achievements and career. Vision, in fact, *is* the big-picture. Whenever an issue or a huge problem occurs, you need to put it into perspective: everything ought to be put in total perspective because everything which happens is competing in working for this total perspective. The truth is that *your problem is never your problem*: your reaction to this problem is your problem. You cannot control the events, but you can (and you need) control your reaction to these events. *Something bad occurs, which may strongly affect your training routine → you have to take an emotional step back from this situation → you have to analyze the situation → you have to put the occurrence in the total perspective → you have to decide your reaction → you have to apply your decision.* Finally what you have to understand is that when you change the way you look at things, the things you're looking at, suddenly change. Such kind of truth is a precise corollary of the *Law of Resonance*: the world is such because I am such (like attracts like). Any occurrence always hides a specific reason why it happens to you that way, that time, that intensity. You have to understand the real reason which generated that event and which might be the lesson you still have to learn from that. Meantime you need to put everything into perspective: if you see this event in the big-picture you will both be provided with the energy to go through that and with a deep understanding of the benefit of your action/reaction. Then you make your appropriate decision and keep on going on the right track.

Material possessions, wealth, luxury, money, awards, and public reputation are kind of *extrinsic motivators*: masses, average people, and low-class athletes are motivated by such extrinsic features. The typical mental pattern through which they interpret external environment impact on their own is *Having → Knowing → Being (I need to have, to learn how to be)*. They want to have, rather being, according to the old classic principle of reward. The world-class performers and the champions are intrinsically motivated by their dreams, desires, and inner passions. They act according to a completely opposite mental pattern: *Being → Knowing → Doing → Having (If I have a high quality of being, I can know and understand things accordingly, then I know what to do, and wealth and possessions will follow)*. In fact, champions know the inner secret of motivating themselves and others, discovering what they will fight for when the going gets tough. Such a psychic attitude comes from a mental switch: they move from *"logic-bases-motivations"* (extrinsic motivators) to *"emotions-based-motivations"* (intrinsic motivators). So if you want to become a champion you ought to find and empower your intrinsic motivators. A coaching or self-coaching session may help you discover such a precious resource: (a) what am I fighting for? which is my ultimate goal. – (b) which are the strongest values I keep holding onto my heart, regardless of the adversities? – (c) what ethical values would I be willing to die for?

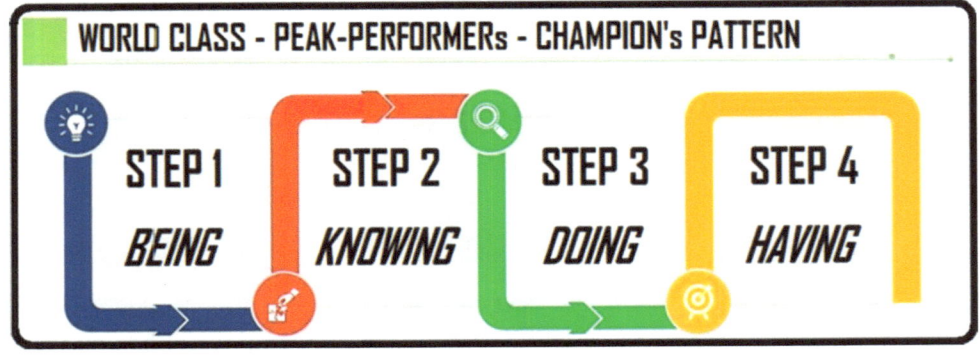

Champions and Peak Performers operate according to a 4-step pattern which is funded on being, ethical code, inner skills qualities, vision, and integrity.

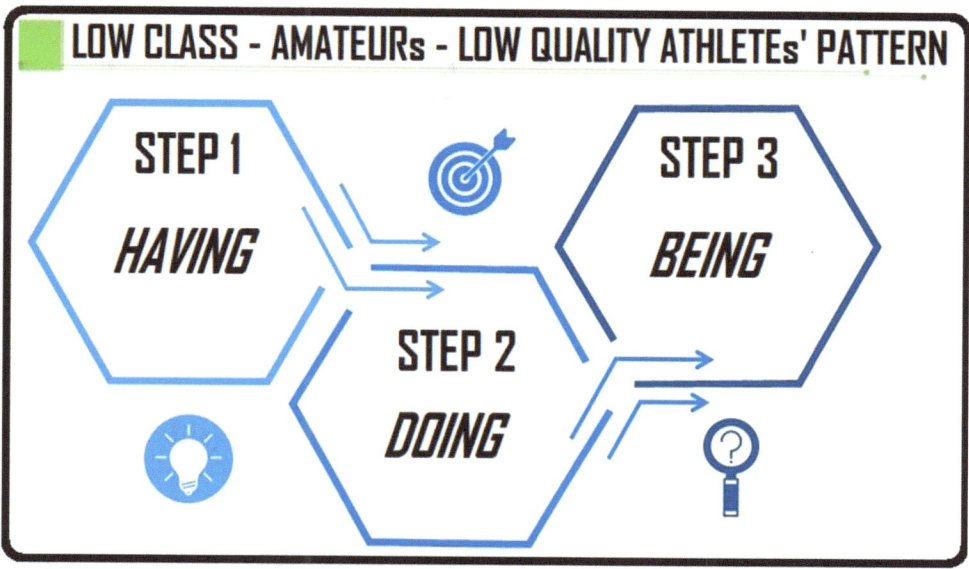

Low-quality Athletes, Amateurs, and Semi-PRO operate according to a 3-step pattern that is funded on having, possessions and expectations of material rewards.

## CHAPTER 4

Sports Code of Ethics

24 – Definition

Results are the consequences of one's inner quality because there is a particular resonance between the ethics of a man/woman and what he/she actually deserves (*Law of Resonance* mixed with the *Principle of Strong Internal LOC*). In Sports, just like in any other area of human life, the result is the projection of your state, through time (*Law of Responsibility*). According to such a psychological and psychodynamic definition, there is no technical difference between failure and victory: both events score a specific degree on a scale of quality of being. If you want to switch to a higher level, you only have to become better in your sports and higher in the quality of being. The Sports Code of Ethics defines the pattern and the minimum standards to be a good, smart, and fair athlete. Which is the starting point to becoming a PRO and a Peak Performer.

Sports Code of Ethics: A code of ethics is a guide of principles designed to help professionals conduct business and sports honestly and with integrity. Ethics in sports requires four key virtues: *fairness, integrity, responsibility*, and *respect*.

> WE PLAY AND WE PLAY HARD. IF WE WIN THE GAME, WE WIN, IF WE LOSE THE GAME, WE LOSE.
>
> [JASON WILLIAMS – AMERICAN WORLD CLASS BASKETBALL PLAYER]

25 – Contextualization

The Sports Code of Ethics affects the mind of the athlete because both solicits the ethics and the moral code. At the same time also the spirit of an athlete is strongly influenced. The ambition, the desire for affirmation, and the aim to succeed ought to be addressed toward the final goal with respect to the rules, regulations, and code of ethics, necessarily. So even though the Code of Ethics primarily affects spirit and mind, it also influences the body of the athlete, because it defines the standards which have to be achieved to compete. The obedience to this Code gives the athlete the legitimation to compete, in a sense, and competition is a means to become a Champion.

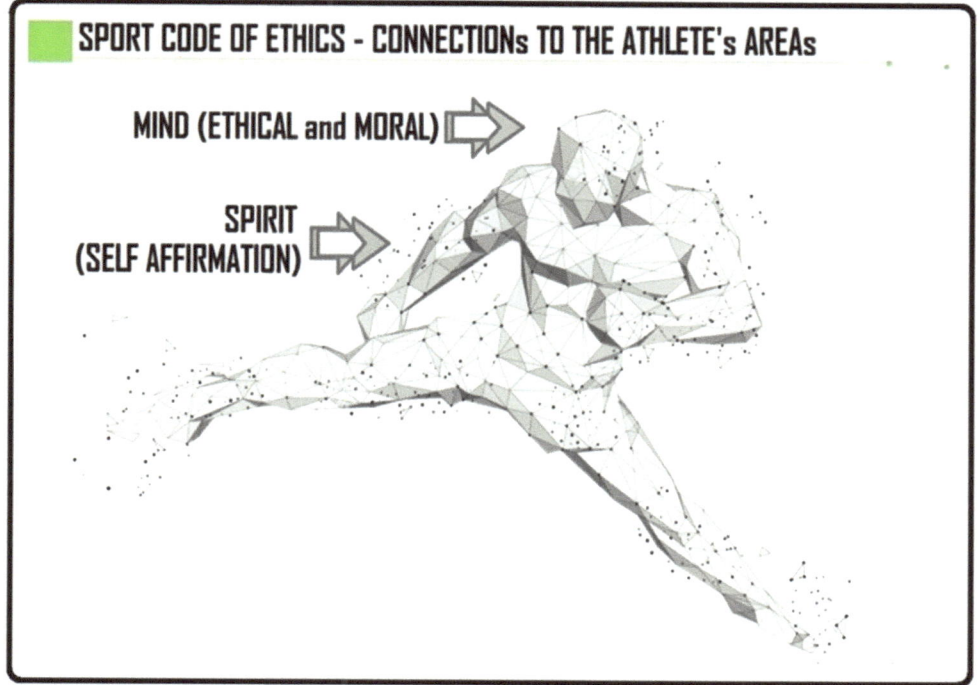

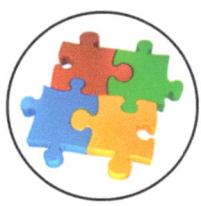

26 – Factors

Sports Code of Ethics features, which are significant for the development of the Champion's Mindset, are 6: (1) Honesty – (2) Fair play – (3) Integrity – (4) Coherence – (5) Programming – (6) Diversion.

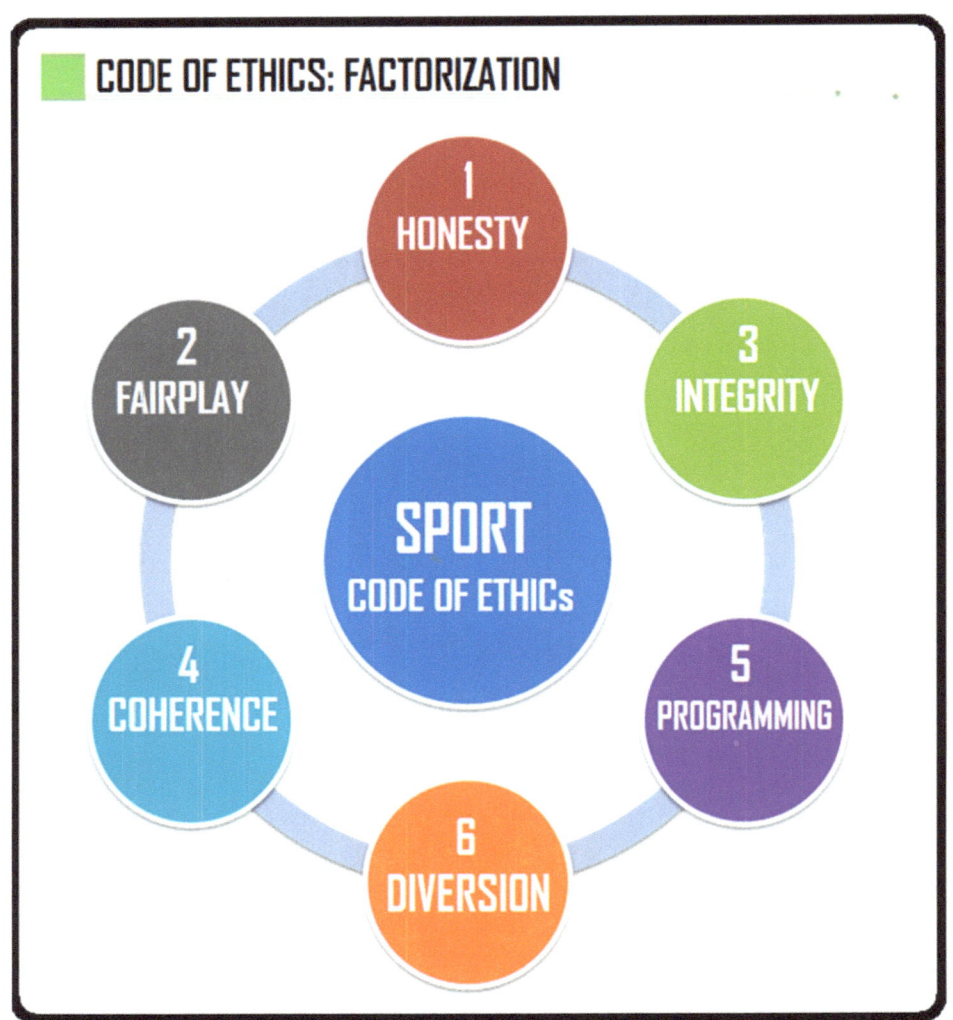

1) **Honesty**: *is a facet of moral character that connotes positive and virtuous attributes such as integrity, truthfulness, and straightforwardness, including straightforwardness of conduct, along with the absence of lying, cheating, and theft. Honesty also involves being trustworthy, loyal, fair, and sincere.*
Honesty is one of the central virtues of a global ethical code. Nevertheless, we are used to looking at honesty only *one way*: we only consider the external dimension: being true, fair, and smart with

other people. According to an inside-out perspective (Strong Internal LOC), we must consider honesty as the quality of being true to ourselves and, as a consequence, coherent with others. Such a kind of virtue is hugely important for any ambitious athlete because is the origin of *Self-Image*. Self-Image is connected to consciousness, awareness of one's strengths and weaknesses, self-improvement, and resilience. So, honesty is preliminary to a deep knowledge of yourself, which leads to enhancement in any dimension of human life.

> HONESTY IS THE FASTEST WAY TO PREVENT A MISTAKE FROM TURNING INTO A FAILURE.
>
> [JAMES ALTUCHER – ENGLISH BESTSELLING AUTHOR AND SPORT COACH]

2) **Fair play**: *the properly conducted conditions for a game, giving all participants an equal chance. The expression is also used more widely to mean fairness and justice in contexts other than games.*
Like attracts like. Kindness attracts kindness. Fair play attracts Fair play. There is not any reason which recommend you to be unfair. The rules of your discipline define a direction and drive your training strategy, your kindness will attract appreciation and you will be given back referees', sponsors', and coaches' appraisal and interest.
You cannot be selected to represent your country unless you behave unfairly, both during the competition and in other special situations.

> BE FAIR, PLAY HARD.
>
> [DAN VENEZIA – AUSTRALIAN WORLD CLASS FOOTBALL PLAYER]

3) **Integrity**: *firm adherence to a code of especially moral or ethical values. Same for human behaviors.*
Integrity is that peculiar virtue that recommends you make decisions coherent with your internal principles and beliefs. Integrity, therefore, is action. You have to protect your principles from any threat which may occur. Even in a time of crisis (injuries, suspension, crisis coming from lack of results), integrity is the mental resource that may provide you with the energy to start over and stand up back. Is the source of your rise. From another perspective, integrity is that native virtue which facilitates a strong attitude to physical training and sacrifice, because it intrinsically includes both.

> INTEGRITY IS TELLING MYSELF THE TRUTH AND HONESTY IS TELLING THE TRUTH TO OTHER PEOPLE.
>
> [SPENCER JOHNSON – AMERICAN BESTSELLING AUTHOR]

4) **Coherence**: *This is the systematic or logical connection or consistency amongst a set of similar/ homogeneous things.*

A sports career is made up of trials, experiments, changes of direction, failures, and victories, attempts. The only way to keep you in the right direction toward your goals is determined by your will to continue, in spite of apparent chaos. Coherence empowers will and internal power. Coherence facilitates self-study and leads to a truer self-image, which is necessary to expand one's personal power and support self-improvement.

> THE GOAL IS NOTHING OTHER THAN THE COHERENCE AND COMPLETENESS OF THE SYSTEM NOT ONLY IN RESPECT OF ALL DETAILS, BUT ALSO IN RESPECT OF ALL PHYSICISTS OF ALL PLACES, ALL TIMES, ALL PEOPLES AND ALL CULTURES.
>
> [MAX PLANCK – GERMAN PHYSICIAN, NOBEL PRIZE IN PHYSICS]

5) **Programming**: *The planning, scheduling, or performing of a program.*

In case of mental fatigue, stress, and demotivation, the program can facilitate your training session and your daily mission, because it contains a short list of tasks to be completed and instructions to complete these tasks. It basically allows you to neglect additional efforts (psychic) and prevent you from undoing (inertia). In addition to that, programming is a crucial activity in the process of achieving any kind of goal. *Vision → Planning → Programming → Instructions → Goal.* There is no other way to hit the target but programming is the best and most effective way to get closer. Your mental attitude must be familiar with programming. You need to know in advance the time, targets, activities, and tasks for any training session. You have to learn how to refuse to attend any session which is not provided by a plan or by a program when you do not feel motivated enough, otherwise, you will only lose time and energy.

Apart from *technical programming, mental programming* consists of conditioning beliefs and being *"set in your ways"*. This means that your brain (*hardware*) is executing your programs and beliefs (*software*) just like they have been installed and consolidated so far. The degree to which mental programming constricts your life and creativity is the extent to which you are unaware of its control over you, or unwilling to change it. Freedom begins with the awareness to probe and question your indoctrinations. Be they religious, political, societal, financial, or about your perception of your health and personal abilities. To break free is to first become aware that we are a *product of our environment*; that much of what we think — our construct of reality — is the result of outer input imprinted into our psyche. Becoming aware begins with questioning our assumptions.

> SPECTACULAR ACHIEVEMENTS ARE ALWAYS PRECEDED BY UNSPECTACULAR PROGRAMMING AND PHYSICAL EXECUTION OF THOSE PROGRAMS.
>
> [ROGER STAUBACH – AMERICAN WORLD CLASS FOOTBALL PLAYER]

6) **Diversion**: *The act of diverting or turning aside, from a course or purpose.*

The threat of diversion from the right direction is infrequent, but is constant and accompanies any athlete until his/her resignation and retirement. That's the reason why you must know such a risk in the very advance and need a strategy to handle bad times when arriving. Even though the best would be to ensure training process continuity through the years, we need to be ready to manage diversion: unpredictable events will turn your focus elsewhere and if you're not prepared to handle them, you may run the risk to quit. One good hack to ensure you will be keeping on track consists of planning some periods of complete vacation from your discipline, both physically and mentally.

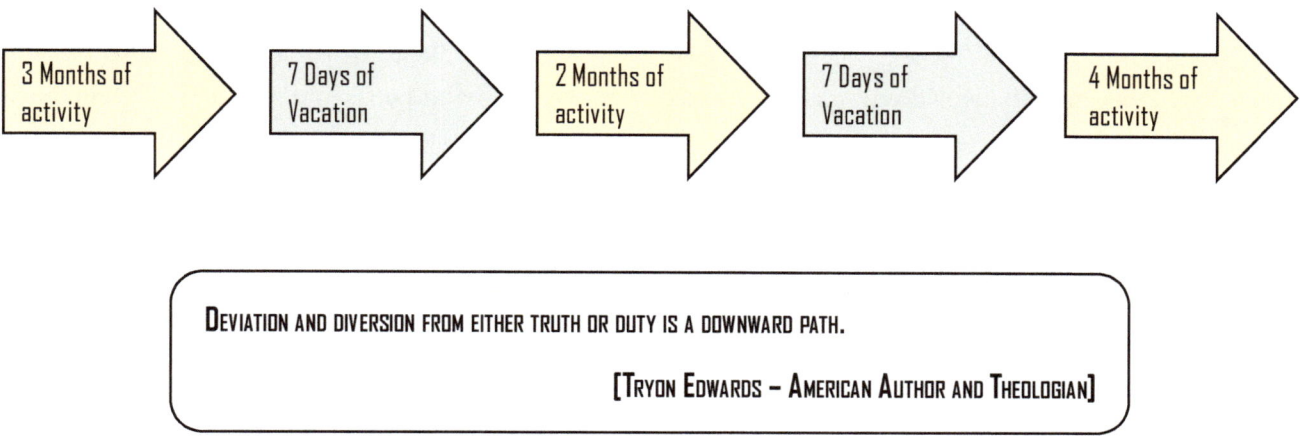

DEVIATION AND DIVERSION FROM EITHER TRUTH OR DUTY IS A DOWNWARD PATH.

[TRYON EDWARDS – AMERICAN AUTHOR AND THEOLOGIAN]

27 – Threats

According to the *Law of Resonance*, if you want something, you need to give something back. The quickest you pay, the better. If you are given something for free, this means you're actually stealing something, you are creating a debt with your future. Learn how to be fair, polite, generous, honest, clear, and coherent. The world will quickly realize your attitudes and behaviors and will give you back chances. Otherwise, you will only earn a free ticket to hell: debts, confusion, hate, low profile chances. Nothing really good happens to you, in spite of your efforts. This is what may happen if you do not respect these factors:

#	FACTOR	POSSIBLE THREAT
1	HONESTY	• Debts creation with Sports Community • Debts creation with Fate
2	FAIRPLAY	• Attracting bad reactions • National Team exclusion
3	INTEGRITY	• Inconsistency • Inner brake
4	COEHERENCE	• Inconsistency • Internal fracture • Targetless-ness
5	PROGRAMMING	• Improvisation in training • Amateur approach • Routine victim
6	DIVERSION	• Discontinuity • Quitting

1 Honesty is a spiritual and ethical virtue that drives you to integrity, which is a tangible attitude to make the right decisions. If you fail to be honest you will incur long-term debts with your fate and the sports community. A dishonest athlete cannot become a Champion, ever, because the world will balance everything, in the long term, and you will always be in need of extra time to achieve.

2 Being unfair will equally lead you to get back disillusions and bad reactions from your sports community, from the media, and your same companions. Will turn you into an impolite athlete, at least, and, with very few exceptions, no real Champion has ever been an impolite, but inspirational person.

3 If you fail to be honest and fair, you cannot be intact, as a human being and an athlete. This will cause a fracture inside your inner being. Such an inner break will create problems in relationships, disillusions, and disappointments, discontinuity in executing your training program. Your sports career cannot be pushed to its higher level.

4 The lack of coherence will generate confusion, inside and outside. The lack of the whole of these 4 main virtues/attitudes will create an inner mix that will actually weaken your character and sporty temperament.

5 If you are not familiar with planning and programming you are condemned to improvise everything, in life. Huge goals, as much as any kind of achievement, require a strong attitude to the program and a strong will to execute the program. The amateur and the low-profile athlete don't ever care about that, because they are victims of routine, and routine and ordinary goals are what they definitely deserve.

6 Diversion may lead you to even quit your practice. The best option is discontinuity, which condemns you not to find your talent, ever. You are condemned to be an amateur and a low-profile athlete.

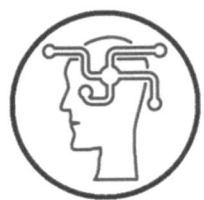

28 – Opportunities

Any of us has *something unique* to give to others. We can start giving while practicing our sports discipline and we can do this for free. We will inspire other athletes, we will create strong and loyal relationships with companions, coaches, and even competitors. We will create a credit towards our sports community, from one side, and with our fate, for another hand. If we act this way and we will continue to *train like hell*, one day we will be awarded, and we will be given back the whole that we gave for free, so far.

#	FACTOR	STRATEGIC ADVANTAGE
1	HONESTY	• Credits creation • Fair play attraction
2	FAIRPLAY	• Polite and fair athlete • National Team appreciation • Possible sponsorship
3	INTEGRITY	• Consistency • Strength • Strong Psychology
4	COEHERENCE	• Extra push of internal energy • Coherent targets
5	PROGRAMMING	• Progressive improvement • Enhancement • Self confidence
6	DIVERSION	• Persistence

1 Honesty will create resonance with loyal companions and coaches. Will also grant you a huge credit with fortune and fate.

2 A fair-play passionate and serious athlete becomes inspirational. Such a quality attracts trust and loyalty from both your community and the national team coaches. Such an attitude, which is cogent for a PRO, may surely quicken your sports career.

3 An athlete who makes decisions according to his/her own inner ethics is provided with strong psychology, in the medium/long term. The secret consists of being strong and determined to make decisions that are compliant with your principles, even if the impacts may affect your personal interest. Such a kind of coherence creates credits with the future.

4 Same, with the additional result that the mix of the 3 abovementioned virtue, will create gratitude and will also give you back lots of additional energy.

5 When you become good at planning and programming you will also achieve your targets, which are "*included*" in such programs. Your actual enhancement starts here.

6 Being persistent prevents you from diverting to alternative options and activities which may jeopardize your plan. At the same time, the commitment to avoid diversions makes you more and more persistent. You must find a sense of satisfaction to be stubborn, then you will become more and more persistent.

29 – Methodologies

The primary psychic factors related to the Code of Ethics are the following:

- Coherence —
- Programming —
- Diversion —

The methodologies for empowering these factors are based on psychic and motivational skills and competencies.

Coherence is achieved thanks to a retrospective analysis of your residual goals and of the match between these goals and your sport's final purpose. You need an ecologic consistency to achieve, which you need to resist flattery and facilitators. Your ethics and your principles need to overcome false and quicker chances.

Programming attitude may only be achieved through programming anything in advance and executing the programs. It's another self-referential attitude: you cannot escape programming, to learn programming attitude.

To manage diversion threats you must become familiar with check and monitoring, but you also need to learn how to precisely isolate the real causes of diversions, to work on them specifically.

PILLAR # 03 - CODE OF ETHICS

	TOPIC	GOAL	ACTION	EXERCISE	REPETITION
1	COHERENCE	Ecologically systematize your decisions and goals - Integrity and strength	Resistance to flattery and facilitations	Set your goals according to an ecologic criterion Test your commitment	Twice per year
2	PROGRAMMING	Plan and program schemes Being consequent	Goals Plan Program and relevant actions	Peculiar exercises	Once per month According to periodization
3	DIVERSION	Control the possible diversion Getting back to your pathway and direction	Cogent prevention Understanding reasons Isolating	Test your ambition and aspiration	

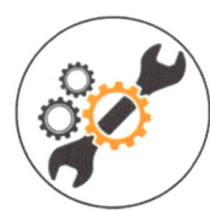

30 – Practical Techniques

Honesty is directly related to your self-image, which may strongly impact your attitude, your training sessions, your behaviors, and, finally, your performance. (1) Be honest with yourself – (2) pay attention to your feelings and sensations – (3) don't say *yes* when you mean *no*: start to be as clear as water – (4) accept the fact that truth changes – (5) be willing to transform your beliefs and to change your Self-Image – (6) be honest with others about how you are feeling – (7) be 100% responsible for your words and actions.

Hard work, patience, success, and calmness actually facilitate Fair play: they magically enable the emersion of politeness and kindness in any contest. If you're not enough familiar with that, try applying fair play and evaluate the rewards you're given back: respect, gratitude, and resonance. Become familiar with Fair play offering to others your kindness and courtesy. So, start forcing yourself until this becomes your second nature. Learn to deeply reflect and think it over before making crucial decisions and start adopting those decisions which resonate with your principles and internal criteria. Maybe these decisions might influence your personal interest, but you have to follow them. Try to catch the inner benefit coming from such an approach: *becoming an intact human being.* Such an approach turns ordinary behavior into Integrity, in the long term.

Coherence is both related to integrity (whose is the original cause) and with the *"Sense of coherence"* (*SOC*), which reflects a coping capacity of people to deal with everyday life stressors The *Sense of Coherence* consists of three main elements: *comprehensibility*, *manageability*, and *meaningfulness*. To empower your coherence, you need to go through your ultimate goal (which needs to be set), your ethics (whose principles need to be clear), and your self-image (which ought to include self-love and respect for yourself). So, work on these three elements, mix it all, and commit your heart to follow coherence.

Become aware of the Principles and Methodologies of training, and learn how precisely exercises ought to be executed. Then start periodizing your training program, planning and programming your training sessions, events, and sports trips, and apply. Start writing your *"Athlete's Log-book"* and enrich your journal with specific checklists: equipment, diet, schedules, and vacations. Update, track and monitor it all. Programming is a *"cannot-escape"* tool for achieving.

Explore the real motivations which lie behind your decisions: your feeling, sensations, emotions, and pulsions which generate that temporary abandonment of your training routine. Try understanding *"why?"* and evaluate the real severity of such a diversion. Prepare to live with upcoming occurrences: when Diversion is coming, you must be prepared and know in advance that such a suspension will come and go fast.

31 – Powerful Questions

Use these questions to force yourself (as an athlete) or your coachees to switch to a higher mental perspective and unlock additional energy to keep being in the right direction. All the questions require specific and honest answers which may also take a few minutes or more, to be developed.

➢ 1.1 Describe your conception of honesty. How does this attitude deal with your sport discipline, your experience, and your practice?

✓ *Honesty is preliminary to getting a true Self-Image, which is necessary to achieve consciousness and awareness. Consciousness is the key to improvement and enhancement, so you cannot escape being honest in all your exteriorizations.*

❒

➢ 1.2 Is there any circumstance in which you saw or experienced an absence or a violation of honesty, during a sports competition?

✓ *Is much significant that you strive to catch the concept of honesty "applied" in the contest of your sports discipline. You must see it in action, to better understand its crucial importance. Is a global and all-encompassing virtue that determines lots of positive consequences in your personal life.*

❒

➢ 1.3 (If any) How do you decline "being honest" in your sports practice?

✓ *Try to define honesty in your contest. Then plan how to consolidate this virtue into your personality.*

❒

➢ 2.1 Describe the way you would like to win a great and prestigious tournament. Is there any space for "fair play"? Which is the way *fair play* is manifesting?

✓ *Dreaming of your goal accomplished is crucial: you need to figure out whether the fair play is included in the movie or it is not. In this second option, try to understand why you cannot escape fair play.*

❒

➢ 2.2 How do you really feel when something wrong is happening to you, while performing? Which is your self-talk related to that experience?

✓ *When any unpredictable event is reversing the final outcome of your competition, a special self-talk is activated: strive to remember and report this peculiar dialogue. Your internal enemy is talking to you, then.*

❑

➤ 2.3 How do your champions and models use to *"win their game"*? How their fair play attitude is actually revealed to the audience?

✓ *Observation of huge skills, competencies, and ethics in action facilitates a crucial lesson-learning process you won't escape.*

❑

➤ 2.4 Which occasion do you think fair play might be overcome or violated during an official tournament and why?

✓ *You're forced to understand and declare the limits of your Code of Ethics. There's no correct answer: you are exploring your final price: you have to know that.*

❑

➤ 3.1 Explain your theory *(concept of integrity)*. How do you judge your behavior: do you believe you are a person of integrity? Why? How is such a quality expressed in your approach to sport? Which is its influence upon it?

✓ *What you have to accept is that only an "intact person" is really free. And only a free person can become a Champion. Free from vanity, free from fear, free from the Ego. Once you have accepted this, life starts significantly changing.*

❑

➤ 3.2 Factorize your areas of capabilities related to sports performance, then understand which of these skills are oriented towards the same final goal and direction.

✓ *A stress test to check how much coherent your approach is and how much sustainable your efforts will be, in the long run.*

❑

➤ 3.3 What are the gaps you believe you currently have? How do you think you can fill them and integrate them into other skills? Develop an action plan to fill these gaps and attain proper integration.

✓ *Gaps-Checking is the result of a benchmark analysis that you have to execute between your current (known) skills and your best opponents' (or sports models). As a result, you can easily catch the gaps which separate you from your Ideal Performance State (IPS). Knowledge is the first step: actions follow.*

❑

➤ 4.1 Analyze the consequences of the attainment of your sports goal and try to catch if such consequences are coherent with your current/future priorities and residual desires and goals.

✓ *Ecologic Stress-Test to check how solid and sustainable your final goal is if viewed with the perspective of your future eyes. The whole of your crucial activities must be coherent amongst themselves, otherwise, one of them (at least) will be rejected.*

☐

➤ 4.2 You say you want to accomplish your (big) sports goals, to realize your dream: are these activities you mix in your current routine coherent amongst them (or not) and congruent to the ultimate finalization? How can you re-plan everything to be consistent?

✓ *Are your goals coherent (for future consistency) as much as your current efforts should be, to achieve your sports goal? Sometimes a few activities are challenging your efforts even though you are not aware.*

☐

➤ 4.3 Coherence and Integrity are a matter of practical and pragmatic behavior: how do you think you have to re-plan your routine to keep all your activities consistent?

✓ *Start with defining your ethics, questioning yourself which is your Decision-Making Process (if any), and striving to understand if your usual and ordinary decisions are coherent with your ethics. In case they are not, you have a problem.*

☐

➤ 5.1 How much of your current routine workout is based on plan and programming and how much is actually based on improvisation? Explain in percentage. Why so much is not programmed?

✓ *70% is a good figure. Do not accept starting a training session if this figure is lower. You run the risk of deceiving yourself and of settling yourself for further ineffective sessions being unaware,*

☐

➤ 5.2 Explain how you program your *"extra-training sessions"* – if any. Which criterion did you use to do that, which goals, which kind of methodology, KPIs, and systematic monitoring?

✓ *Start programming your additional Training Sessions to achieve additional skills, which you cannot in any ordinary and conventional training program with your club.*

☐

➤ 6.1 Is there any kind of *alternative activity*, hobby, sport, game, or interest, which you think may divert you from the right direction? Which kind of risk, threat, or simply unproductive effects may this activity bring to your sports career?

✓ *Just explore the analytics related to sports injuries of other disciplines (ex: soccer, volleyball, skiing) and think it over a bit: is that risk worth it? What can you additionally gain from those experiences?*

❑

➤ 6.2 How many years of commitment do you plan to dedicate to your sport until you reach your final goal? Would you divert from it, in case you did not achieve it, or would you be willing to push inside additional time?

✓ *Did you already make the decision to devote at least 10 years to your sports discipline, before developing your dream of glory? 10 years might not be enough. What if additional years are required?*

❑

➤ 6.3 You spoke about years and figures: do you think that this sounds reasonable, that your greatest goal may be influenced by a limitation? If your training and chances required extra time and energy, would you find it or not? What commitment do you really think your goal would really deserve, to be accomplished?

✓ *If you define a time limit, you're making three errors: (1) you're offending your sport discipline – (2) you're affirming your arrogance – (3) you are thinking (today) that you can nullify (tomorrow) the time that has elapsed until then.*

❑

➤ 6.4 Each time you feel close to quitting, are you thinking about your inability, the pain required, the sacrifices and the possibility to enjoy in a different way? Explain your alternatives.

✓ *A fixed Mindset doesn't like setbacks so an athlete which is provided with a fixed mindset will be close to quitting after a frustrating failure. Which is the alternative? What about the whole time and efforts that you have devoted to your sports discipline till then? You have any alternative, have not you?*

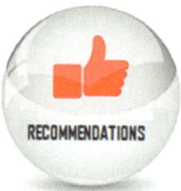

32 – Instructions & Recommendations

Your global approach requires a strong revisiting. Choose ethics and transform your principles until they are aligned with fair play. Bet all your chances on being an ethically strong committed contender.

Effective emulation requires intelligence and humility: first, you have to understand you are in lack a specific element that you have isolated, and then you need to strive with all your energy to attain a result. You need to be balanced: no identification process can push you forward, but only technical emulation. One thing at a time. You must think *"I can do that, I can learn how to do it"*, and then you start working.

Whenever you become familiar with programming, you will instinctively entrust only programs and plans and then you will always require a methodological approach to everything. Your mental pattern will be based on the following: a) time – (b) resources – (c) tools – (d) methodology – (e) intensity – (f) series. Switch up your pattern and transform it into a mantra: *targets – tools – methodology, targets – tools – methodology*. Become more than a fanatic of programming.

Being a champion is a matter of *"being"*. A champion is such because of his/her level of expressing such a quality. For this reason, champions pride themselves on being honest, open, and straightforward: they have already realized so far that real success consists of who you are and become, not of what you acquire. You need to accept and bear in your mind that you cannot achieve the world title until you do not deserve it. It's a matter of getting something that is aligned with your inner qualities as a human being: *like-attracts-like*, according to the *Law of Resonance*. For such a reason being honest is not only a fair rule to observe, but a recommendation that will quicken your pathway to success. You need to learn *"how to be"*, not *"how to have"* or *"how to achieve"*. The achievements are nothing but a consequence of who you are.

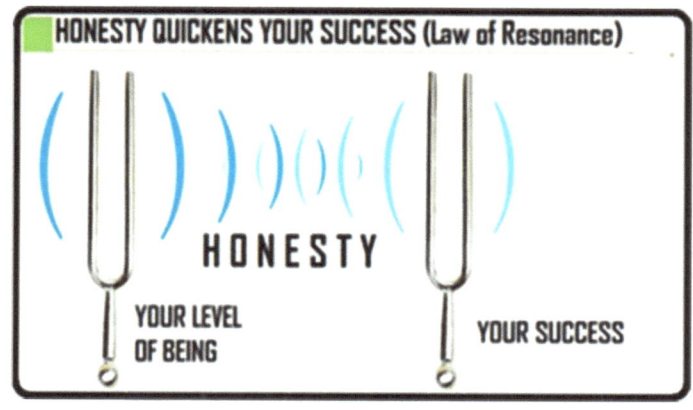

Integrity is a world-class attitude, is the primary habit of the PROs, not because it actually succeeds, but because it's the right thing to do. Average athletes are convinced that being honest and intact as a person is a luxury, in a sense, but this belief is completely wrong. They think that is none of their business, that there is no connection between the performance and the ethical virtues because they do not believe in the *Law of Resonance* and they have no interest in investigating. As a consequence, they do not engage any of their resources to pursue honesty and integrity: they simply don't understand the sense. *Being* is the ultimate state of a human being, no matter whether you are an athlete, a businessman, or a professional: your level of being will push you to achieve what you deserve, always. Total integrity is the rule number one amongst top players, not only in their community but in any case.

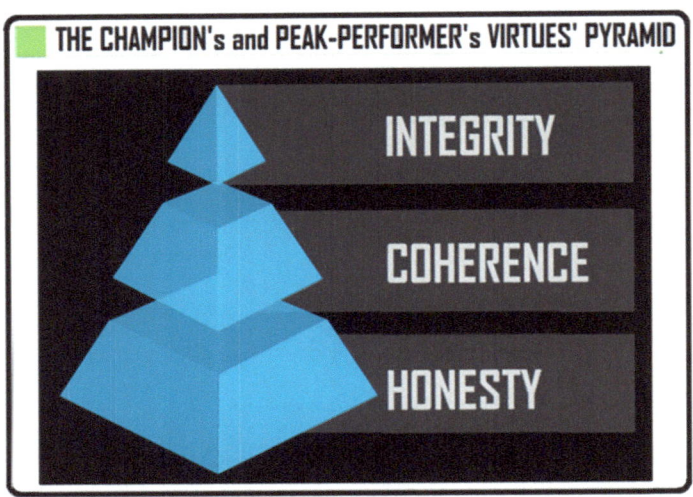

## CHAPTER FIVE

Goal Setting

33 – Definition

As a general recommendation, *you have to start with the end in your mind*. This means that you have to know why are you behaving that way and which goals you are striving for. From a sports and competitive perspective, you need to understand who you are (*current state*), and who you want to become (*ideal state*) and then you have to define the correct pathway to get there the quicker you can.

Very often, individuals, sports professionals, or business-men settle themselves up for failure by setting general and unrealistic goals such as "*I want to be the best at X*", but this goal is vague, with no sense of direction. SMART goals set you up for success by making goals specific, measurable, achievable, realistic, and timely. The SMART method helps push you further, gives you a sense of direction, and helps you organize and reach your goals.

Goal Setting: The definition of goals as an aim of action serves to portray goals as the drivers (or cognitive regulators) behind goal-directed behaviors.

> SUCCESS IS STEADY PROGRESS TOWARDS ONE'S PERSONAL GOAL.
>
> [JIM ROHN - AMERICAN BESTSELLING AUTHOR, MOTIVATIONAL SPEAKER

34 – Contextualization

Goal Setting affects both the logic and the strategic mind of the athlete: it is connected to analytics, rationality, and conscious actions. It also influences the spirit of the athlete, because it speaks directly to his/her heart: the language of triumph, podium, and success touches the spirit and the passion. Finally, Goal Setting strongly affects the body. The training sessions, the sense of sacrifice and responsibility, the call to action, and the whole of the activities which are activated as direct consequences, require a healthy and strong-shaped body to strive.

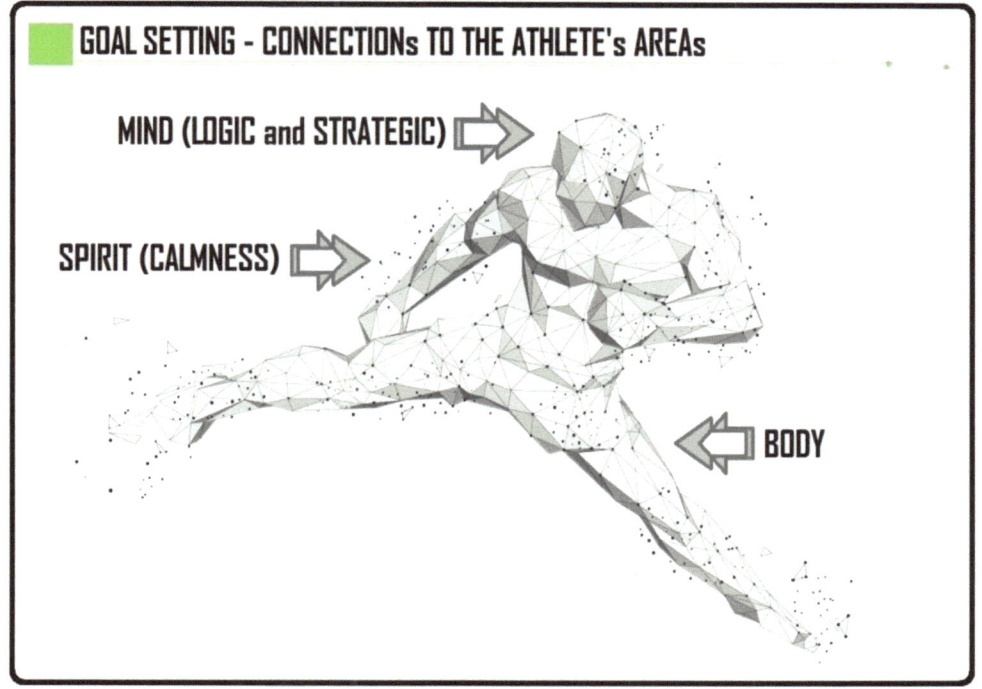

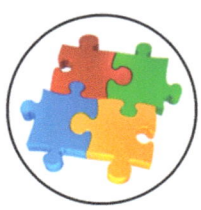

35 – Factors

Goal Setting features, which are significant for the development of the Champion's Mindset, are 9: (1) Sports Goal – (2) Monitoring – (3) Motivation – (4) Self-Improvement – (5) Excellence – (6) Programming – (7) Periodization – (8) Performance Deviation – (9) Methodology.

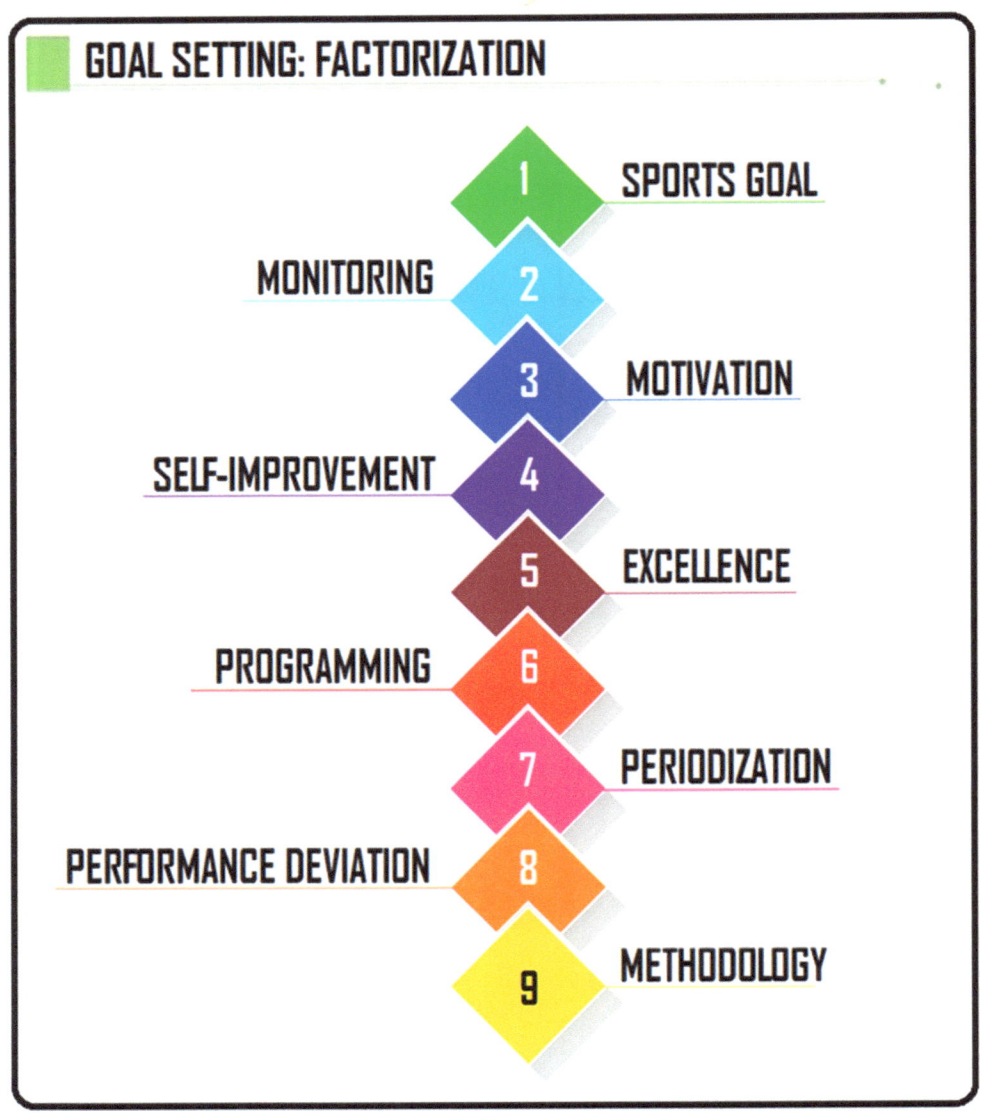

1) **Goal**: *An objective is something that our efforts or actions are intended to attain or accomplish. Objectives are measurable and tangible, while goals usually are not. Goals generally look at the long-term while objectives are either mid-term or short-term.*

Goals are part of every aspect of business/life and provide a sense of direction, motivation, a clear focus, and clarity of importance. By setting goals, you are providing yourself with a target to aim for. A SMART goal is used to help guide goal setting. SMART is an acronym that stands for *Specific, Measurable, Achievable, Realistic,* and *Timely.* Therefore, a SMART goal incorporates all of these criteria to help focus your efforts and increase the chances of achieving your goal.

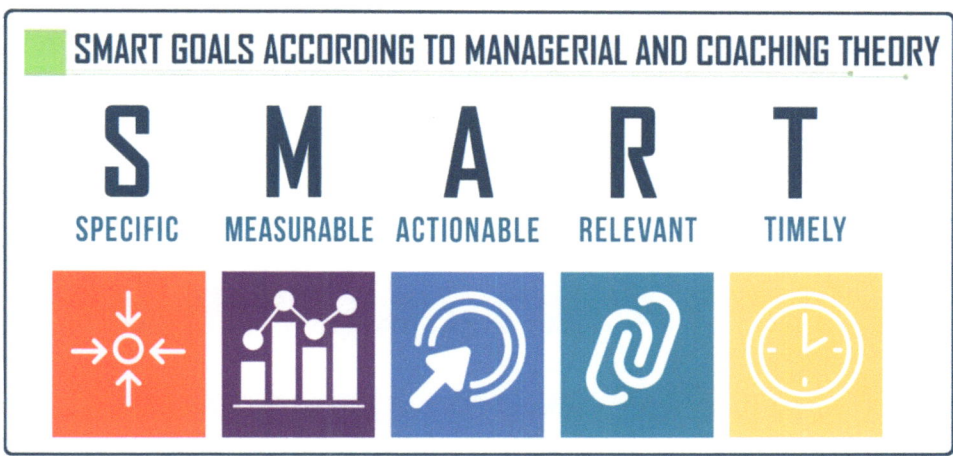

SMART goals are:

- *Specific*: Well-defined, clear, and unambiguous.
- *Measurable*: With specific criteria that measure your progress toward the accomplishment of the goal.
- *Achievable*: Attainable and not impossible to achieve.
- *Realistic*: Within reach, realistic, and relevant to your life purpose.
- *Timely*: With a clearly defined timeline, including a starting date and a target date. The purpose is to create urgency.

Specific SMART Goals questions: (1): Who is involved in this goal? (2) *What*: What do I want to accomplish? (3) *Where*: Where is this goal to be achieved? (4) *When*: When do I want to achieve this goal? (5) *Why*: Why do I want to achieve this goal?

Measurability of SMART Goals questions: (1) How many/much? (2) How do I know if I have reached my goal? (3) What is my indicator of progress (Sports KPIs)?

Achievability SMART Goals questions: (1) Do I have the resources and capabilities to achieve the goal? If not, what am I missing? (2) Have others done it successfully before?

Realistic SMART Goals questions: (1) Is the goal realistic and within reach? (2) Is the goal reachable, given the time and resources? (3) Are you able to commit to achieving the goal?

Timing SMART Goals questions: (1) Does my goal have a deadline? (2) By when do you want to achieve your goal?

In addition to that, you must consider that the GOAL you want to plan needs also to be coherent with your current state (who you currently are, your current state, and sports arsenal) and with your residual goals: your goal ought to be *ecologic*, in a sense. Apart from the view of your coach, which is not significant and may impact the quality of your dreams and your goal, such an exercise allows you to catch the size of the efforts and the seriousness of your promise and commitment. So, define your goal and let it become your Boss and your Master. Prepare yourself (and your social proximity) to fulfill your dream's requirements.

> WHAT KEEPS ME GOING IS GOALS.
>
> [MOHAMMED ALÌ – AMERICAN BOXE HEAVYWEIGHT WORLD CHAMPION]

2) **Monitoring**: *Monitoring of a program or intervention involves the collection of routine data that measure progress toward achieving program objectives.*

Knowledge without action is nothing, but a goal without monitoring is completely useless and becomes unattainable. There is a bundle of specific time to attain a result: if you overcome this amount of time, your focus will get weaker and weaker, so you need to keep track and complete the tasks at the right time, otherwise, the efforts you made would vanish fast. So monitoring is crucial to correct your behavior or even the direction you choose for your pathway. You have to check your state systematically and detect the gaps between your current condition (what you did till now) and the ideal (what you still have to do).

> SPEND TIME ALL DAY AND ALL NIGHT MONITORING YOUR THOUGHTS, CONSTANTLY KEEPING THEM IN A HIGH PLATEAU.
> AVOID PLACES AND PEOPLE THAT PULL YOUR ENERGY DOWN. APPLY SUCH MONITORING IN A ROBUST WAY.
>
> [FREDERICK LINDEMANN, ENGLISH POLITICIAN, 1ST VISCOUNT CHERWELL]

3) **Motivation**: *Motivation is defined as the process that initiates, guides, and maintains goal-oriented behaviors.*

There are 7 kinds of motivation, in sports as in any other competitive contest (ex: politics and business): *Achievement* Motivation, *Affiliation* Motivation, *Competence* Motivation, *Power* Motivation, *Attitude* Motivation, *Incentive* Motivation, *and Fear* Motivation. To better manage your motivation and keep it high when needed, you first need to know exactly which is the declination of motivation(s) that better fits you and, in the second instance, which is the real origin of such motivation(s). Knowing your motivation(s) means that you know a deep part of yourself.

As an athlete who wants to become a champion, you need to develop a strong, hot, and unstoppable desire to take control of your programs. *You need to reprogram yourself:* you need to select and install new habits, philosophies, ethical codes, traits, and beliefs finalized to empower your skills and competencies. Do not ever settle for being programmed by others, no matter if is your coach, your teacher, or your elder companions. You need to develop a technical and psychic awareness of who you are (*psychic programs*) and to switch to whom you want to be (re-programming your psyche) through a step-by-step process. This will take time, but your new consciousness and your responsibility will quicken the process and will give you back results. Technicalities need training plans and programs, which you need to develop, check and apply with perseverance. Psychic skills need a process of empowerment, as well. You need to accept that your beliefs influence your performance and that you are currently the result of those sets of beliefs which you did not ever doubt, so far. As a recommendation you ought to follow these steps: (1) detect the old programs which were installed in your psyche – (b) pick those programs which have limited your performance and your life (till now, according to your view) – (c) cancel these programs (beliefs/habits) and replace them with new, powerful programs – (d) suspend your innate disbelief and apply your new set of powerful programs – (e) strive hard and try reaching the target – (f) check the connection (programs ↔ results) – (g) secure to your arsenal – (h) consolidate your new program.

> MOTIVATION IS A FIRE FROM WITHIN. IF SOMEONE ELSE TRIES TO LIGHT THAT FIRE UNDER YOU, CHANCES ARE IT WILL BURN VERY BRIEFLY.
>
> [BENNY *"THE JET"* URQUIDEZ – KICKBOXING WORLD CHAMPION]

4) **Self-Improvement:** *The activity of learning new things on your own that make you a more skilled or able person.*

The Peak-Performance attitude is a dynamic state of the spirit: you cannot achieve this condition once and for all. The actual challenge is with yourself, with your ego: a champion doesn't ever settle for being second to anyone, even to him/herself. A champion doesn't ever settle to win by chance, or to win easily: he/she is always pushed to perform at his/her possible best until retirement. Such a kind of attitude is directly related to the inner spirit of self-improvement: continuously longing to learn new skills, techniques, and competencies which may enhance global performance. Self-Improvement is an instinct, but not a natural skill: you have to develop it and you have to drive it towards positive and useful targets.

> THE WILL TO WIN, THE DESIRE TO SUCCEED, THE URGE TO REACH YOUR FULL POTENTIAL. THESE ARE THE KEYS THAT WILL UNLOCK THE DOOR TO PERSONAL EXCELLENCE.
>
> [CONFUCIUS – ANCIENT CHINESE PHILOSOPHER AND FOUNDER OF CONFUCIANISM]

5) **Excellence**: *The fact or state of excelling; superiority, eminence.*
The Champion's mindset is primarily focused to achieve the target, whilst the Peak-Performer's attitude is aimed at expressing the arsenal at its possible best. The concept of excellence needs to be framed within these two different but similar approaches. The will to win and the determination to perform at your best are both connected to a special sensitivity to excellence. I am not talking about technicalities or sports gestures. I'm rather talking about procedures, processes, and patterns. You can have *"the job done"* in many ways, but the most effective is the one that is compliant with the best practice. This means that if you want to hit the target performing at your best, you got to be used to proceeding based on precise procedures and correct patterns and models. You choose to do something only that way, otherwise, you give up, this is the starting point of the attitude to excellence. Is a slow and intensive process that leads you to become an excellent athlete.

> EXCELLENCE IS NOT A DESTINATION, IT IS A CONTINUOUS JOURNEY THAT NEVER ENDS.
>
> [BRIAN TRACEY – WORLD CLASS PROFESSIONAL, RUGBY LEAGUE]

6) **Program**: *A series of subroutines organized into the correct sequence to perform a movement.*
The most important advice is that you need to take a specific commitment to yourself: never more training sessions that have not been programmed (at least 70%). You need a program because you need the plan to achieve a specific result. Training is not having fun, is forcing your body to adapt to a load (exercise). So you stay on track by following 5 easy rules: (1) assess your training needs – (2) set smart training objectives – (3) create a training action plan – (4) implement training sessions based on specific exercises – (5) evaluate & revise your training.

> BUILD A BRIDGE AND GET OVER IT.
>
> [RAFAEL AGHAYEV – WORLD CLASS PROFESSIONAL, KARATE LEAGUE]

7) **Periodization**: *The systematic manipulation of the acute variables of training over a period that may range from days to years.*
You have to accept that you cannot achieve a steady state of physical and mental shape. Sport Psychology and the Science of Performance affirm that skills, competencies, and capabilities need

to be developed and improved according to a precise plan, which is based on both psychology and physiology. A Peak-Performer is frequently aware of such a peculiarity and then he/she plans the agonistic season after the primary tournaments have been selected. Motor skills have to be activated or developed at the first stage of the training season, whilst technical skills have to be attained as a second target. In the third period of the season, the strategic and psychic skills ought to be pushed to their max. A rational approach, then, recommends focusing on specific objectives at a specific stage to finalize the preparation for one or two competitions. The residuals do not need to be neglected but can be utilized to detect the state of your sport shape to correct the preparation when needed.

> EVERY AREA OF THE ATHLETE'S PERSONALITY OUGHT TO BE EMPOWERED ACCORDING TO SPECIFIC TIME, TOOLS, EXERCISES, PACE AND METHODOLOGY. SEPARATE, SCHEDULE AND ACCOMPLISH SPECIFIC GOALS. THEN ASSEMBLE THE RESULTS AND TARGET YOUR GOAL.
>
> [GLITTER JEAN SUDOMYO – SERBIAN WORLD CLASS SPORT COACH]

8) **Performance Deviation**: *Datum or result outside of the expected range.*

Monitoring is finalized to check the performance deviation, which is the gap between the ideal behavior and the current one (what you actually did till now). Self-improvement goes through an analytical and comparative attitude amongst a set of crucial elements which affect global performance and, from the other perspective, are evidence of the current state of your physical shape. Any tournament must be explored and detected: the performance deviation is useful to understand what is working the right way and what is not, needing corrections and amendments.

> PONDER AND DELIBERATE BEFORE YOU MAKE YOUR MOVE. HE WILL CONQUER WHO HAS LEARNED THE ARTIFICE OF DEVIATION. SUCH IS THE ART OF MANOEUVRING.
>
> [SUN TZU – CHINESE MILITARY GENERAL, AUTHOR, PHILOSOPHER]

9) **Methodology**: *A contextual framework' for research, a coherent and logical scheme based on views, beliefs, and values, that guides the choices researchers [or other users] make.*

From a generic perspective the Sport Professional approach consists of a twofold quality: (1) always being aware of what needs to be done (*knowing*) – (2) immediately being consequent (*doing*). No fear, no doubts, nothing can influence the action: the behavior straight follows the decision. From a specific perspective, we can affirm that nothing occurs by chance: any event follows its origin, and any occurrence has its specific cause. It's difficult to catch the trueness of such a process, but it actually determines its consequences even if we do not believe it or we cannot see it working. In professional sports, any activity is the output of a precise methodology. If you apply the correct instructions to the correct skills, you will cause the correct gestures and you will get back the appropriate result. This is true at all levels: gestures, tactics, strategies, focus, and concentration. After you have accepted there is a methodology to get anything, you have to become curious and you need to learn and master the relevant technicalities. Then you will integrate these new skills into your arsenal. The methodology will become second nature and will free you from consuming precious energy.

> PROFESSIONALS WHO KNOW WHAT THEY ARE DOING CAN BE COUNTED ON TO FOLLOW A WELL-THOUGHT-OUT METHODOLOGY.
>
> RAYMOND KHOURY – LEBANESE BESTSELLING AUTHOR AND SCRIPTWRITER]

36 – Threats

Consciousness is the key factor to success. You cannot become a real champion if you're in lack consciousness and awareness. Your efforts need to be programmed, sized, monitored, and driven: need to stay *"connected"*. Your motivation needs to be fed and protected. Your body needs to be respected and pushed forwards according to its specific rules and physiology. Our mindset ought to be led by a coherent leader who actually knows which are the threats, the risk, and the flattery of the outside world. If you escape setting the whole of these goals, you will fall into chaos and confusion and will be imprisoned in a false and fake version of yourself as an athlete, whilst you only are an amateur, ignoring the rules of the games of success. Fail on programming, program yourself to fail. The threats in case of violation:

#	FACTOR	POSSIBLE THREAT
1	SPORTS GOAL	• Amateur • Goals not achieved
2	MONITORING	• Unaware of improvements • Distorted self-image
3	MOTIVATION	• Resistance to suffer and pain • Boredom • Alienation
4	SELF-IMPROVEMENT	• Progressive worsening • Being stuck in your current state
5	EXCELLENCE	• Condemnation to be an average athlete • Unwilling to perfect technicalities
6	PROGRAMMING	• Improvisation • Routine
7	PERIODIZATION	• Inconsistent areas of resources • Inconsistent arsenal • Injuries

8	PERFORMANCE DEVIATION	• Failures • Unpreparedness
9	METHODOLOGY	• Injuries • Ineffectiveness • Approximation

1 Sports goal is intrinsic to desire. If you have a true, passionate desire to achieve and to become somebody in your sports discipline, you also have that huge relevant dream in your mind and your heart. The dream must be turned into a goal because a goal is nothing but a dream provided with a deadline. If you fail to define your goal with clearness, you're settling for being an amateur and a low-profile athlete. Without visualizing and defining a goal you cannot achieve anything, in sports and in life. Your achievements will be extemporary, destined to vanish. Achieving targets *"by chance"* is dangerous.

2 Monitoring your current state, according to a systematic check plan, enables you to be conscious of your improvement. Without such evidence and comparison, you will be unaware of improvements/worsening and you will strengthen a false self-image. You will never know exactly who you are and whether you are improving yourself or only wasting your time.

3 If you train yourself without the right motivation, you are only deluding yourself. Maybe you are sweating a lot, you are feeling fatigue arrival, but you're only moving muscles and alternating breathing to exhaling. Motivation focuses your efforts and drives your conditioning in the appropriate direction. When you're not motivated, you're only executing ineffective training sessions. You're losing your time and your energy and this will lead you to delusion (*first*) and to alienation (*later*).

4 Self-improvement is not an output, but a spirit-attitude. What you have to know is that if you neglect such an attitude, it will take much more time to achieve. So you'd better learn how to force yourself to invent ways to learn new solutions, new methodologies, new approaches, and new skills.

5 Excellence is not a result, but a process. *Devil is in details*: if you neglect details, you will ever, systematically, finally, have a meeting with the Devil, which means inner demons, misfortune, criticism, crucial mistakes, and failures. If you escape excellence, you settle yourself to average and mediocrity.

6 Failing in programming exposes you to being a slave of improvisation, routine sessions, and, first of all, an unconscious servant of the external world. This world has a plan for all the unconscious people: making them useful to achieve the plans and dreams of other conscious people. Programming includes the preliminary *"will to do something"* that you have in your mind and that you believe is fitting your needs. Otherwise, you only improvise and succeed, just keep in your mind, doesn't ever happen by chance.

7 You cannot enhance the whole of your skills contemporarily. If you strive to do that you will never get the appropriate physical shape to achieve (IPS: *Ideal Performance State*). You will cope with low performances and, most probably, with injuries, which depend on your training overstress.

8 Performance deviation is a useful tool that informs you of your current state. You neither have to avoid that only because you do not want to know nor even can escape it if you want to achieve. Improvement goes through the check of your current state.

9 If you want to train without a methodology then you have to know that *you don't actually want to train yourself.* No skill improved, no technicalities, no chances at all. Any sports discipline is provided with specific and generic methodologies: if you want to become a champion you have to master anything in detail. It's a huge commitment that you cannot escape.

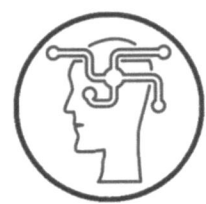

37 – Opportunities

Setting goals, defining a plan for achieving, and executing this plan seriously ensures a great physical shape, your arsenal enhancement, effectiveness, and high caliber performances. Starting over with the final purpose in your head requires a strong vision, but is the quickest way to success.

#	FACTOR	STRATEGIC ADVANTAGE
1	SPORTS GOAL	• Clear direction • Strong vision • Coherent and effective efforts
2	MONITORING	• Performance index awareness • Effective process of preparation
3	MOTIVATION	• Sacrifice skill enhancement • Resilience • Perseverance
4	SELF-IMPROVEMENT	• Contentment • Constant self-motivation • Arsenal enhancement
5	EXCELLENCE	• Technicalities perfection • Winning mental approach • Second to no one
6	PROGRAMMING	• Awareness • Right self-image
7	PERIODIZATION	• Consistent increase of all arsenal
8	PERFORMANCE DEVIATION	• Awareness • True self-image
9	METHODOLOGY	• True way of effective training

1 SMART Goals are not only a must in business. SMART-Methodology actually works better than any other, because the achiever is forced to define, measure, and to taking care of execution, according to scheduled deadlines. We normally apply such kind of methodology, even though we are unaware. Defining a Goal which is compliant with such a methodology ensures a clear direction and also protects your clear vision of the accomplishment to be respected. All the efforts you make are driven towards the right achievement.

2 When you start checking and monitoring according to a specific framework, you can take advantage of important information regarding your current state and shape and regarding your training process. This bundle of information can ensure the effectiveness of your training sessions. This will grant huge improvements.

3 If you are strongly motivated you are equally determined to sacrifice any other alternative activity which does not add usefulness to your goal. Your goal, in fact, requires you all and this means that you have fatally fallen into a new state: you have become essential, a kind of elemental, in a sense: you will only follow those actions and activities which get you closer to your goal, neglecting any other, because useless.

4 Self-improvement attitude leads to your arsenal improvement, in addition to everything else. You can see small improvements depending on your commitment. Even 1% of performance improvement per month (or per semester) can empower your final performance.

5 The PRO-Attitude is totally focused on the results, but the results require a high awareness and knowledge of the details. So, if you want to become a champion, you first need to behave like a PRO, then you must learn to love excellence in details: gestures, timing, sports personal equipment, rules of the games, and any other factor which is connected to the competition. You need this to become your second skin, then you enter the flow.

6 Programming requires awareness and leads to effectiveness. It will grant huge achievements and will progressively drive you to quick improvements and to higher and higher performances.

7 Periodization is a special declination of Programming. Gives you precise instructions to work on any aspect of your shape, both mental and physical, and prepares you for the best way for approaching a tournament.

8 When you become good at interpreting KPIs and all the other evidence of a performance deviation in the very advance (training) or during and after an official competition (contest), then you can easily schedule/reschedule your agenda and take part in those tournaments which match your physical shape. From a strategic perspective, such a hack is really significant, because prevents you from bad and predictable failures or even from physical injuries.

9 Methodology is the set of rational and empiric instructions (*Rules of Thumb*) which are simply required to be followed to get the job done. Do not accept to approach any activity, target, or even training sessions that are not supported by a clear methodology. The use of methodology will ensure your physical shape enhancement.

38 – Methodologies

The primary psychic factors related to Goal Setting are the following:

- Monitoring —
- Periodization —
- Performance Deviation —

The methodologies for empowering these factors are based on managerial and analytical skills and competencies.

Monitoring is actually related to Performance Deviation. You need to develop KPIs (*Key Performance Indicators*) and additional EIs (*Emotional Indicators*) to precisely define your physical shape and your current performance state. While KPIs specifically belong to your sports discipline and thus depend on peculiar standards, EIs are generic and transversal and can be used to check the level of calmness, focus, physical relaxation, re-absorption, rage, and other emotions which can (and actually do) affect the performance. *Definition of the KPIs and EIs → Definition of the criteria to detect the KPIs/EIs → Schedule check/monitoring → Detection → Interpretation → Back to training* (inclusion of this information to correct/enhance the training program).

Periodization is applied through a kind of break-down of the whole period (the sports season of the athlete) into *macro-cycles* (2-3, each for 6-4 months), *mesocycles* (7-10, each for 2-1,5 months) and *micro-cycles* (52, each for 7 days). Once you break down your program, you can define the relevant goals and exercises and act accordingly.

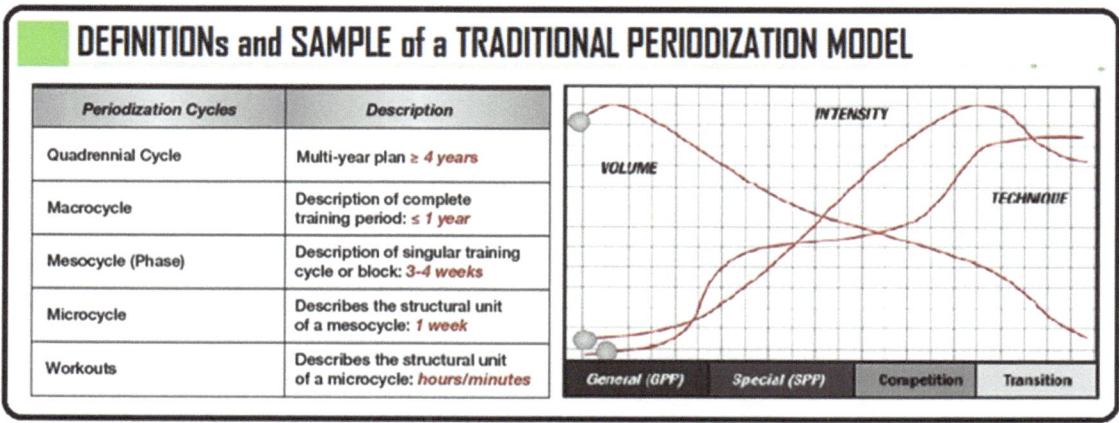

PILLAR # 04 - GOAL SETTING

	TOPIC	GOAL	ACTION	EXERCISE	REPETITION
1	MONITORING	Size, check and control Action based on plans and programs	Check KPIs and compare with previous	Revisit plan and programs: Confirmation Reduction Intensification	Twice per month
2	PERIODIZATION	Separate periods and relevant goals and apply methodologies	Understand and isolate an escalation Goals → Periodization Define KPIs for PHY/TECH	Execute the program relevant to the current period of season (seasonal plan)	1 x Year 3 Macro-cycles 9 Meso-cycles
3	PERFORMANCE DEVIATION	Define KPIs and Check deviation Draft down graphs Write a Log-Journal	Plan checks Evaluate deviations and Gaps Evaluate progression	Work on weaknesses Reinforce strengths	2 times per month

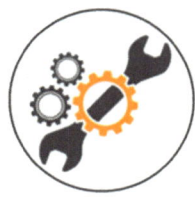

39 – Practical Techniques

Define your Ultimate Goal. Then impose such a Goal on the SMART-Approach and store the outputs. Then break down the Ultimate Goal into micro and preliminary targets and goals and proceed on monitoring (*measurability*) whether these targets are achieved within the appropriate deadlines (*time-related*).

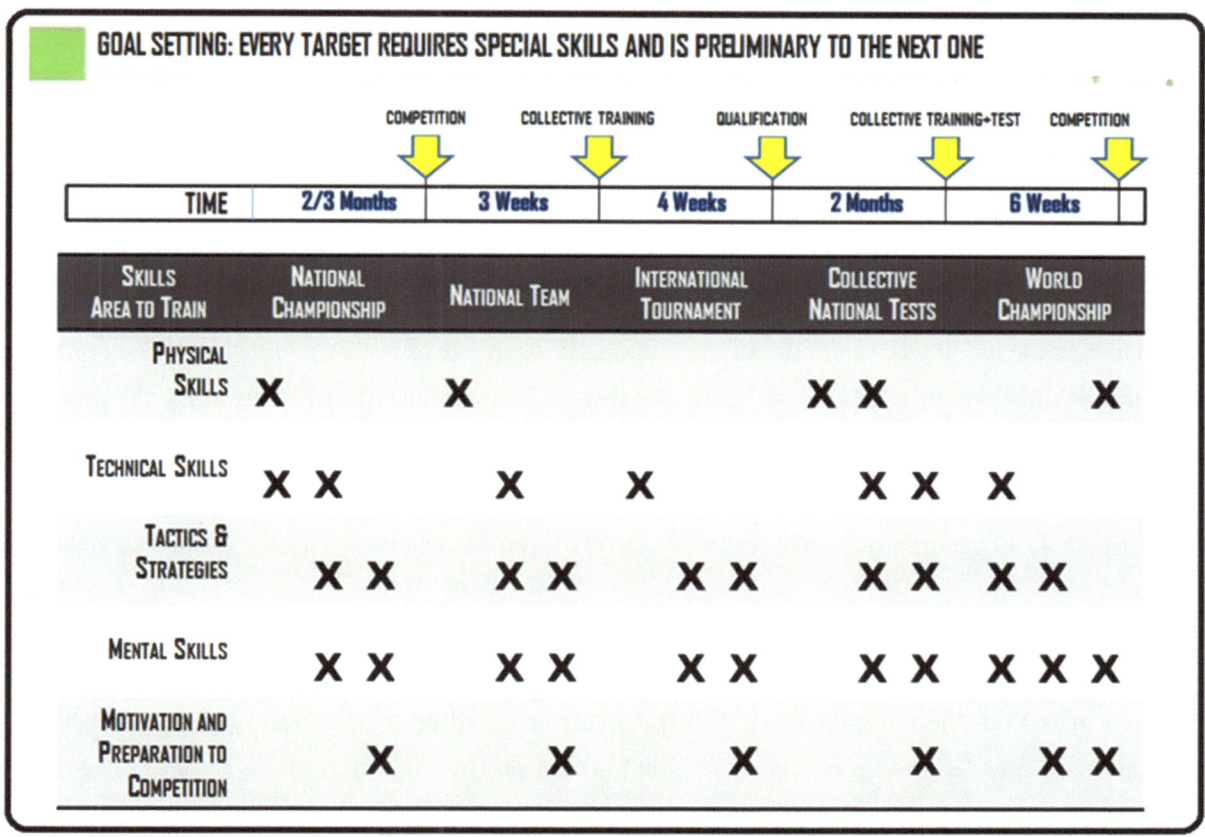

GOAL SETTING: EVERY TARGET REQUIRES SPECIAL SKILLS AND IS PRELIMINARY TO THE NEXT ONE

		COMPETITION	COLLECTIVE TRAINING	QUALIFICATION	COLLECTIVE TRAINING+TEST	COMPETITION
TIME		2/3 Months	3 Weeks	4 Weeks	2 Months	6 Weeks

SKILLS AREA TO TRAIN	NATIONAL CHAMPIONSHIP	NATIONAL TEAM	INTERNATIONAL TOURNAMENT	COLLECTIVE NATIONAL TESTS	WORLD CHAMPIONSHIP
PHYSICAL SKILLS	X	X		X X	X
TECHNICAL SKILLS	X X	X	X	X X X	
TACTICS & STRATEGIES	X X	X X	X X	X X	X X
MENTAL SKILLS	X X	X X	X X	X X	X X X
MOTIVATION AND PREPARATION TO COMPETITION	X	X	X	X	X X

Monitoring is related to Goal Setting and to Periodization. (1) Define generic KPIs (condition), weight/pace, specific KPIs (gestures), and EIs (emotional indexes) – (2) define and schedule cogent deadlines for monitoring the data – (3) analyze and interpret the data – (4) correct your training program accordingly.

Most people want to change at least one thing in their life. But it can be challenging to find the motivation just to make a start. It helps to understand what motivation means to you so you can find your own ways to get motivated. To enhance or heighten your Motivation as an athlete you should do the following: (1) set yourself one specific, achievable goal – (2) think about how to include that goal in your life, what you need to do to make it happen, and then put a timeframe on it – (3) break your goal into small, easy tasks and set regular reminders – (4) make your goal part of your routine by using a diary (log-journal) – (5) positive self-talk is important and effective in managing depression or anxiety – (6) mindfulness helps keep you relaxed and focused – (7) reward yourself when you have completed a step or goal – (8) regularly review your goals and progress. Seeing progress is a great motivator in itself, and also improves your self-esteem – (9) continue to set new goals – (10) keep the momentum up. It takes up to 2/3 months to develop a new habit (21 continuous repetitions, at least), so keeping the momentum and routine helps a lot, because it feels more automatic over time – (11) find mentors and start emulating him/her – (12) surround yourself with positive people, Champions and Peak-Performers – (13) use exercise as one of your daily goals to improve your mental health – (14) review your goals and see if they are realistic in the timeframe you have set. You may need to break your goal down further into smaller and more achievable goals – (15) remember why you wanted to get motivated or reach that goal in the first place – (16) take motivation from others, when needed.

To strengthen your Self-Improvement attitude, you need to define avulse or adjacent activities, select a couple of them and start learning/practicing periodically: swimming, gardening, biking, and listening to opera. Your self-improvement skills would increase as much as you love your side activity. This skill will generate benefits for your main activity.

You need to become passionate about details, precision, the elegance of gestures and solutions, of procedures. Learn and keep in your mind the ideal action (gesture) and compare it with your current (your current performance). Then isolate the stage of everything (dissection) and repeat thousands of times the gesture in the most appropriate way you can. You must keep in your mind that the *"Devil is in the details"* and that Excellence is a dynamic process that needs to be driven by a strong will, focus, and consciousness.

Periodization is related to both monitoring and sports goal setting. Start from who you (currently) are as a man/woman and an athlete. Then develop a training program that fits your current features and then break down this program according to the periodization methodology: *macrocycles* → *mesocycles* → *microcycles* → *sessions* and define the related goals to achieve. Then execute the periodization plan as the supervisor of your training program.

The Performance Deviation assessment is related to periodization, programming, and monitoring. (1) Analyze the deviation – (2) start finding the real causes – (3) isolate each of the causes – (4) work on them: empower/nullify/reduce the cause – (5) prepare for the next competition.

Always utilize the most appropriate Methodology to apply any exercise or technical gesture/solution. Do not repeat anything, unless you perfectly know the details of any procedures. Otherwise, you will learn the incorrect gesture. *Once you do great, then do lots.*

40 – Powerful Questions

Use these questions to force yourself (as an athlete) or your coachees to switch to a higher mental perspective and unlock additional energy to keep being in the right direction. All the questions require specific and honest answers which may also take a few minutes or more, to be developed.

> ➢ 1.1 Which is the genuine, true goal you have in your mind and in your heart so far? Which are the natural pre-goals which may enable you to accomplish your final target? Which are the methodologies to accomplish these (sub)goals? Have you got any strategy? Are your goals *SMART*?
>
> ✓ *First you have to catch the original, ancestral motivation which drives you as a human being and as an athlete. Then you start planning your goal according to a specific pattern.*

❒

> ➢ 1.2 Apply the SMART model to your final goal then proceed backward and list all the other "*preliminary goals*".
>
> ✓ *Define the final goal then define all the sub-objectives which ought to be achieved as preliminary to your final goal. Proceed through an "end-2-end" approach till your current state (today).*

❒

> ➢ 1.3 How much your final target is important for you? Are you already able: (1) to describe it in detail? (2) to summarize and declare it in a small sentence? (3) to feel the sensations of having it accomplished? (4) to figure out you while accomplishing?
>
> ✓ *Visualization and Imagery are two of the most important tools for Sports Self Autogenic Training (SSAT). You cannot achieve what you cannot imagine and visualize. You cannot achieve what you cannot explain. The clearer your final goal, the better.*

❒

> ➢ 1.4 Which are the skills and capabilities you are still in need of, to accomplish your final goal?
>
> ✓ *Start checking out and listing your gaps: the skill you are in lack if compared to your Ideal Performance State.*

❒

➢ 2.1 How are you familiar with KPIs? Have you already developed a few generic and a couple of specific KPIs for you, and your discipline? Just simply brainstorm and develop a plan for KPIs, monitoring each week, for evaluating your progress.

✓ *Define generic KPIs (conditional competencies), specific KPIs (relevant to your specific discipline and related to peculiar gestures or phases of the competition), and EI (emotional indexes). Then define some practical criteria to detect these KPIs periodically and store them in a Log-Journal.*

❒

➢ 2.2 How do you feel you're having a good week workout? Your feeling? Your coach's recommendations and appreciation? Do you think that this is enough? Do you believe this will push you to win the world championship, one day?

✓ *You must realize that analytics is the primary tool for checking the quality of a training session and your physical shape. Then you have to accept it. As a lesson learned you will become a fanatic for checking and monitoring.*

❒

➢ 2.3 Develop a plan for your sub-goals and micro accomplishments for 2-weeks/3-months/6-months and act accordingly and start monitoring your progress through the KPIs.

✓ *Sub Goals Plan definition and relevant KPIs for each of these goals.*

❒

➢ 3.1 What is your true and genuine motivation? What is the real reason why you started and what is after so many years that moves your body towards several sets of hard training sessions? What kind of internal aspect really burns you from within?

✓ *You must turn yourself to your inner and original state. You need to know yourself better and better. You also need to test your motivation.*

❒

➢ 3.2 Is there anything stronger than this motivation? Is money stronger than that, which may stop you from training? How much time can this motivation take you to awaken and commit and connect to your dream?

✓ *Stress and Resistance test to your motivation.*

❒

➢ 3.3 Which kind of sensations and vibrations do you feel inside when you got motivated by this inner cause? What do you really feel? Describe with details.

✓ *You must become aware of the feeling, emotions, and sensations that your original motivation determines on yourself when appropriately solicited.*

❐

➤ 3.4 Is there any space for (1) self-improvement, (2) creativity, or (3) revenge, included in your original motivation?

✓ *As a right answer, there obviously must be included.*

❐

➤ 4.1 What do you really mean by *"Self-Improvement"*? Do you think that this attitude is important for reaching your goals or can you really just train hard and listen to your coach's recommendations and instructions?

✓ *Your curiosity and attitude to self-improvement are tested.*

❐

➤ 4.2 What about *Self-Coaching*? Do you think you might already be able to perform such an activity? Why? What do you still lack?

✓ *Your ability as a Coach (of yourself) is additionally tested.*

❐

➤ 4.3 How *Self-Improvement* is connected with accomplishing the hugest goal you can? Explain with details. What may prevent you from improving yourself continuously? Speak about this.

✓ *Your convictions about self-improvement methodology and size of results are tested.*

❐

➤ 5.1 What is your definition of *"Excellence"*? Why is excellent, in your imagination? Why?

✓ *Your awareness of the rules of the game is tested. Your current definition of excellence is crucial because the gap between yours and the right one defines what you still lack.*

❐

➤ 5.2 How far is your current performance of yours, from excellence? (1-10). Why? How can you bite 1 point of this gap?

✓ *You are required to check if you see a way to gain 1% more, by yourself, to progressively increase your Current Performance Index (CPI).*

❐

➤ 5.3 What kind of commitment do you give to technical gestures, to improve them to excellence? Which is your strategy to do that?

✓ *Your level of knowledge of specific methods, models, and instructions is tested.*

❐

➤ 5.4 Details: What is your relationship with details? What about a champion's approach? Differences? Why?

✓ *You should experience a global overview of the action (and be able to perform it), but also an analytical competence of any single gesture. Analysis and Synthesis are both crucial for a professional. Experience and mindset will drive your focus on one of the twos, from time to time.*

❐

➤ 6 (Programming – see above)

✓ *Already extensively treated.*

❐

➤ 7.1 How do you isolate (and periodize) goals belonging to different segments? Which are your matrix and breakdown?

#	SEGMENT	WHAT	WHEN
1	PHYSICAL		
2	TACTICAL		
3	MOTIVATIONAL		
4	PSYCHIC		

✓ *Start planning a correct Periodization for empowering your physical shape according to physiological rules and your mindset, according to the tournaments' season timeline.*

❐

➤ 7.2 Develop a plan to periodize your activities, according to your seasonal goals, considering the following: (1) competition – (2) training sessions – (3) current physical shape – (4) physical skills (strengths/resistance) – (5) physical skills (speed/power) – (6) motivational.

✓ *SAME.*

❐

➤ 8.1 Define a date on which monitoring of KPIs is mandatory (twice per month). KPIs check, monitoring, and evaluation.

✓ *Start planning a KPI monitoring program.*

❐

➤ 8.2 How do you handle your performance deviations (from expected)? Is there any strategy?

✓ *Neglecting performance deviations, when detected, nullifies checking and monitoring.*

❒

➤ 8.3 Excellence and Peak-Performance are a matter of progressive alignment between a nominal model (*Performance*) and the current one (*Actual*). Insert a kind of Performance Deviation Control (*PDC*) between the two, which includes the reasons (emotional/technical) for such deviations. Size it somehow and archive all of that, systematically.

✓ *Find indexes and others indicators to take into account the deviations between IPS and your Current Performance. You must consider both technical and emotional causes and the origins of these deviations.*

❒

➤ 9.1 Does your methodology enhance your performance, month after month? How do you monitor the performance indicators? When? What kind of evaluation of the progress, the performance deviation?

✓ *Performance Deviation Control (PDC) Program is needed.*

❒

➤ 9.2 Do you alternate kinds of exercises? The segments of the body, sessions after sessions, during the week? Please design your weekly workout routine and break down the items of each model of each session.

✓ *Start re-designing your Weekly Workout Routine according to these principles and patterns.*

❒

➤ 9.3 How do you customize your methodology on your specific qualities, competencies, and attitudes? How do you invest in a systematic activity to work on the strengths, weaknesses, and natural talents you are provided with?

✓ *You must realize that you have to feed your specific talents parallel to the rest of your training program. If something seems to be too hard for you, do not hesitate to ask for help from an additional coach.*

❒

➤ 9.4 Is there any space and time to focus on your mental dimension in your methodology? Please design a program that includes at least 10 minutes per session, focused on mental enhancement (exercises + methodology).

✓ *Relaxation, meditation, special breathing, imagery, and visualization are a few tools for enhancing your brain and your mindset. Include such self-autogenic training in your additional training sessions systematically.*

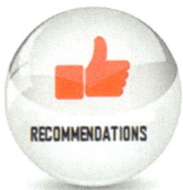

41 – Instructions & Recommendations

Define your goals and develop a detailed seasonal program (periodization). Define specific sub-goals and relevant scheduling/timelines coherent with the program. Define the most appropriate methodologies to train and bundles of training sessions segmented per specific targets and skills. Then define appropriate KPIs and start executing the plan. Check and monitor *KPIs* and *EIs* according to a mandatory schedule, then interpret the performance deviations and correct your program (and methodology) accordingly. Continue such kind of activity until you succeed. It may take 1 month, 6 months, one, or a few years: *do not quit*. Take ownership of your failures and mistakes and push towards excellence: take care of details, act precisely, and be passionate about gestures and solutions elegance. Keep your motivation strong and definitely give your future passion.

In short words: your final goal consists of becoming the champion, while sub-goals, declined and segmented in harmony with a seasonal plan and a growth plan, are preliminary targets you have to achieve, before switching to the next level. You'd better start with the end in your mind, but you have to keep your sub-goals always aligned to a set of mindset aspects: *self-confidence, self-image, self-efficacy, ambition, aim,* and *self-consciousness.* You need to periodically assess this mix, for you need to feel and understand when you're actually ready for the next step. Based on your results and your inner sensations, you should periodically detect what's in, what you have achieved, and what you're ready for.

Observe others: their habits, attitudes, mental approach to gym training sessions, schedule, and intensity. Companions, coaches, opponents: it does not matter. Observe them when achieving. Look at their faces, their emotions, the words spelled, the words unsaid. Start stealing as much as you can. Steal and personalize, steal and improve. Join champions when training, when giving an interview, and when receiving a reward. Steal as much as possible. Look for opportunities to learn something new: a gesture, a habit, an attitude. Open your mind for a different view: every day for you something new to secure to your arsenal. Select these items periodically and decide what to secure for your UPP.

Stop your routine and go deep inside: your original and genuine motivation must be haunted and found. Dig hard, go deeper and deeper until you realize you cannot go forward anymore. Be honest with yourself: catch that emotion and observe its source. That's your real motivation: rage, revenge, will affirm yourself, will prove your superiority. It doesn't matter head-on and take your motivation into your hands. Now close your hands. You are the bodyguard of your motivation: do not allow any person, any adversity, or any danger to harm your motivation. Keep protecting your motivation until it finds its way to affirm itself on the battlefield. Strive on like hell and train to make it happen.

CHAPTER SIX

Clarity

42 – Definition

A Clear Vision enables you to make the right decision in times of trouble or whenever you are haunted by doubts. If you have a clear destination in your mind, you always know what to do: you just follow your dream, your goal, and your destination. The Champion does not make a decision anymore so far: it's enough to obey the golden dream.

Clarity: Clearness or lucidity as to perception or understanding; freedom from indistinctness or ambiguity.

> AFTER YOU RUN, THERE'S A SENSE OF ACCOMPLISHMENT. YOU FEEL LIKE YOUR LIFE IS MEANINGFUL. IT'S A MOMENT OF CLARITY. EVERY TIME YOUR MIND SHIFTS, YOUR WORLD SHIFTS.
>
> [SAKYONG JAMGON MIPHAM RINPOCHE – SHAMBALA BUDDHIST AND AUTHOR]

43 – Contextualization

Clarity of destination is the light that illuminates your sports pathway, even on the darkest nights. If you have a clear mind, you always know which is the right direction, which is the right way to choose, in case you find yourself in front of a crossroads. Clarity of destination affects both your mind, from which actually emerges, and your body, which may be easily driven and led during the training programs and during the competition. Your body is the vehicle and your vision is the destination. Your brain is the driver.

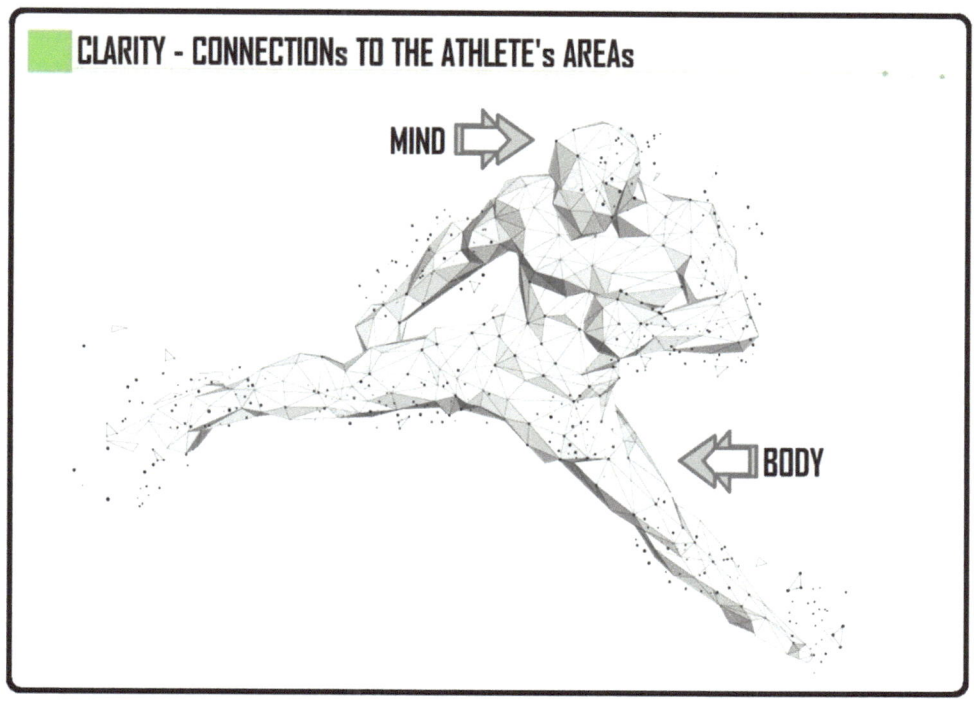

44 – Factors

Clarity features, which are significant for the development of the Champion's Mindset, are 8: (1) Situation Definition – (2) Expectations Management – (3) Be Here and Now – (4) Sensations Monitoring – (5) Concentration – (6) SW-Analysis – (7) Emotions Control – (8) B-PLAN Attitude.

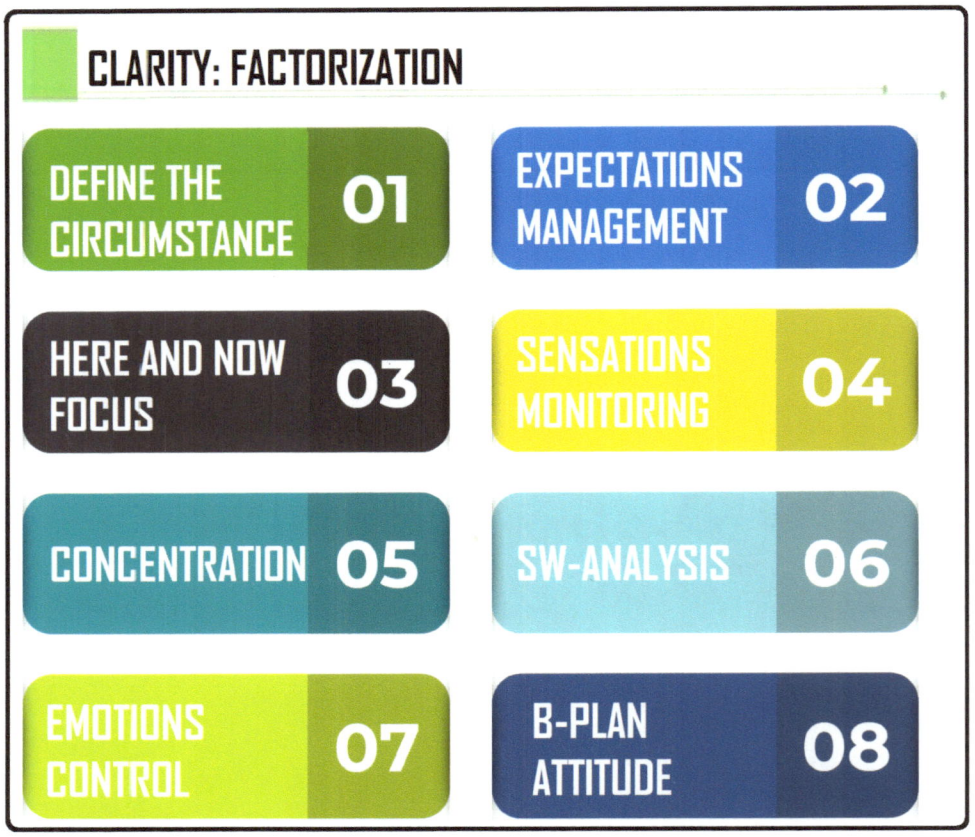

1. **Situation Definition**: *A condition or position in which you find yourself; the way in which something is placed in relation to its surroundings.*

   According to a basic principle of *Security Science*, every situation can always be segmented in one peculiar attribute: (1) *Routine* – (2) *Disturb* – (3) *Emergency*. Each of these options presents peculiar characteristics and can be considered preliminary to the next: *Routine → Disturb → Emergency*. Apart from the sports discipline you practice, the awareness of the specific stage you're in becomes crucial for planning the next move, because each option presents peculiar threats and risks, and requires specific actions to switch to the next stage (*Disturb → Emergency*) or to overturn back

(*Emergency → Disturb → Routine*). A Peak-Performer has developed an inner intuition that naturally drives him/her to activate special actions to solve a problem or to move on, in a competition. This is a very crucial skill that enables the athlete to fix an issue effectively, but unfortunately, it is not natural: you have to understand it and develop it until it is consolidated into the arsenal. The evidence you have matured such a skill is that you are perfectly aware of what's running and of the reasons why it is happening. The second level skill is that you learn what to do in any of these cases.

> LIFE IS A BALANCED SYSTEM OF LEARNING AND EVOLUTION. WHETHER PLEASURE OR PAIN. EVERY SITUATION IN YOUR LIFE SERVES A PURPOSE. IT IS UP TO US TO RECOGNIZE WHAT THAT PURPOSE COULD BE.
>
> [STEVE MARABOLI – AMERICAN AUTHOR AND LIFE COACH]

2. **Expectations Management**: *The state of looking forward to a specific result and the capability to manage and fulfill others' expectations.*

In some cases, most of the stress is caused by others' expectations. This creates bad emotions, impostor's syndrome, and other psychic issues which affect the final performance. For many athletes is very difficult to manage this occurrence. What we have to understand first is that others' expectations do not need to be managed: they only need to be ignored or even erased. Others' expectations neither add anything to your training nor to your success. You practice your sport discipline and you want to achieve because you are passionate: you do what you do for yourself. So the only expectations we need to fulfill are ours. If we fail to understand this we'd better understand that we are destined to fail, in the long term. We only respond to ourselves: we do not need the appreciation coming from outside. We must prepare ourselves to force the outside world to confirm our conviction to be the best, our mastery. There's no benefit in fulfilling others' expectations. You must convince yourself that you're alone when performing. Even if you are in an arena and 70 thousand people are observing you and shouting against you. Even if you're live on the web. You are alone, you have never been alone. There is you and there is your opponent. There is the referee and there are the rules: 4 elements. Isolate yourself from anything and go straight ahead toward your destiny. Without stress, without fear. Failure would only inform you that you're not ready, yet. So insist until even failure will surrender to your success.

> I'M NOT IN THIS WORLD TO LIVE UP TO YOUR EXPECTATIONS AND YOU'RE NOT IN THIS WORLD TO LIVE UP TO MINE.
>
> [BRUCE LEE – MARTIAL ARTIST, FOUNDER OF JKD]

3. **Here and Now Focus**: *The present, this point in time.*

Mental presence is not only being aware and conscious but also applying your internal resources to what you're currently doing at your possible best. This means awareness and action are joined together and are supported by concentration. This means voluntarily neglecting any distraction coming from inside (mind–body – emotions) and from outside (environment – the audience – expectations). *Hereandnowness* is crucial because, when applied appropriately, enables the performer to gather all the available resources and address them to hit the target. From another perspective the application of H&N is crucial because if you feel *"present"* now, you also apply yourself for the best, in your next state: the state which is close to coming will be a consequence of the previous state (mental presence). The cleaner the now, the strongest the future state. It frequently determines the success of the champion and scores the difference between the champion and the loser.

> REMEMBER YOURSELF ALWAYS AND EVERYWHERE.
>
> *HEREANDNOWNESS* MEANS PRESENCE
>
> [GEORGE IVANOVITCH GURDJIEFF – ARMENIAN PHILOSOPHER, AUTHOR]

4. **Sensations Monitoring**: *Sensation is the process that allows our brains to take in information via our five senses, which can then be experienced and interpreted by the brain.*

   If you want to achieve, you need to go through the knowledge of yourself. At any level: strengths/weaknesses, fears, limitations, worries, the origin of your motivation, emotions, sensations. You must interpret your sensations and perceptions because this information would quickly activate the most appropriate reaction; fatigue, stress, panic, fear, demotivation: any of these mental and emotional states are anticipated by specific sensations (what is called *disturb*, in *Security Sciences*). If you manage to catch it at the right time, then you are a step forward because you know what's going to happen (prediction) and you can act/react accordingly.

> LIFE IS A SERIES OF EVENTS AND SENSATIONS. EVERYTHING ELSE IS INTERPRETATION. MUCH IS LOST IN TRANSLATION AND ADDED IN ASSUMPTION/PROJECTION.
>
> SENSATION IS THE KEY.
>
> [RASHEED OGUNLARU – ENGLISH BUSINESS AND CORPORATE COACH]

5. **Concentration**: *Concentration on something involves giving all your attention to it.*

   Concentration is the queen of mental skills. The presence and the awareness of concentration actually determine a victory or a failure. No matter your preparation, no matter your professional level and qualifications, no matter your motivation: the lack or the fall of concentration can really jeopardize your performance. When you are fully concentrated you are able to recruit the resources you need, to align and engage them all against your opponent to achieve a target. Concentration is supported and endorsed by *Hereandnowness* but lies at a higher level. You need to isolate yourself from the rest, but you are also required to keep aware of what is happening and to react accordingly. Concentration includes mental presence, attention, and focus. The lack of momentary lapse of concentration would force you to improvise the competition and frequently leads you to failure.

> CONCENTRATION AND MENTAL TOUGHNESS ARE THE MARGINS OF VICTORY.
>
> [BILL RUSSELL – AMERICAN WORLD CLASS BASKETBALL PLAYER/COACH]

6. **SW-Analysis**: *Strengths are defined as character traits or skills that are considered positive. Weaknesses are the opposite.*

If you do not face a generic problem when you become aware of it and postpone to a better time, then this problem will grow and will change its size, shape, and its form. The impact of the consequences will be very high. From a sports perspective, this presents a huge consequence: if you neglect taking care of your known weaknesses, the impact that these issues will have on your performance will be very high. Your weak points must be tackled, transformed, and overcome. The Champion's attitude aims at approaching, rather than avoiding. You have to honestly detect your weaknesses, your refractoriness, and blackmail and you need to catch the consequence of passing over. Then you proceed.

> ENTER YOURSELF AND GO IN DEEP. ISOLATE YOUR WEAKNESSES AND WORK HARD ON THAT: BECOME FAMILIAR WITH HANDLING BAD TIMES. UNDERSTAND YOUR STRENGTHS AND TRANSFORM THEM INTO SPECIALS: *YOUR UNIQUENESS STARTS ON IT.*
>
> [JOE SANTANGELO – ITALIAN KICKBOXING WORLD CHAMPION AND COACH]

7. **Emotions Control**: *This is the ability to respond to the ongoing demands of experience with the range of emotions in a manner that is socially tolerable and sufficiently flexible to permit spontaneous reactions as well as the ability to delay spontaneous reactions as needed.*

In competitive sports, as far as in competitive business, hiding your intentions, potential, and emotions, is actually crucial. Managing emotions is preliminary to both feinting (simulation) and applying a specific strategy that requires the opponent to be disguised. People communicate with talk (25% of communication impact) and with gestures, moves, and body language (the residual 75% of communication impact): emotions give lots of enormous information to your opponent, giving him a cognitive advantage for free as a gift. On the other hand, if you want to give yourself a real chance at your performance you need to learn how to control your emotions, both positive and negative because emotions generate thoughts and intentions (as a *reaction*), and thoughts generate decisions and behaviors (*actions*). If you want to keep on the right track, when performing, and follow your precise plan, you have to free yourself from emotions (*Emotional Imprisonment*). Bad emotions demoralize the athlete and limit or reduce performance, whilst good emotions may reduce awareness and concentration. Emotions need to be predicted, managed, and transformed into energy, when possible. Otherwise must be erased.

> No excuses. No explanations. You don't win on emotions. You win on execution.
>
> [Anthony Kevin "*Tony*" Dungy – American World Class Baseball Player]

8. 8. **B-Plan Attitude**: *An action or set of actions for doing or achieving something that can be used if the preferred method fails.*

Even the strongest plan cannot survive enemy contact. That's why a good strategy needs to cover 95% of the pathway, at max: the last mile ought to be improvised and customized depending on what's really happening after the enemy contact. Planning is crucial never enough. Something unpredictable events may happen and always happen, which jeopardize your original plan preventing its enhancement or completion as minded. You need to be provided with a B or even a C-Plan, for such occasions. Many Peak-Performers work hard to develop a strategy that returns any occurrence to the original A-Plan: a kind of B-Plan that returns to the previous, when misplaced. But quite frequently they may rely on a strong B-Plan. A B-Plan must not be necessarily considered as a fallback: is a second options strategy you can activate whenever your primary plan becomes unfeasible for any technical or non-technical reason. B-Planning can include motivation, overturning, the arrival of fatigue, light injuries, and any other predictable or unpredictable events coming from the external environment (referee, weather, opponent's skills, cleverness, penalties, unfair play).

> Life is all about you handle your B-Plan. So brainstorm and develop your B-Plan but focus on A.
>
> [James Andrew Yorke – American Matematician]

45 – Threats

Your goal activity requires your complete focus, your presence, your efforts, and your seriousness. It's not a *democratic leader*: your goal is a *tyrant*. If you're not willing to become its servant for a long period of time, you'd better quit or you'd better settle for an average career. You need to accept that you're giving back your freedom and you're approaching the temple of your dream: your dream is becoming your boss. It's a dictator and you will become its slave. So you are neither allowed to replay nor to have a critical attitude: you have to obey. *"Where are you – What's really happening – Why this way – Who are you competing for – What are you living for – What are you striving for – Where is your focus now – What do you actually feel inside right now – Which are your current emotions – What do they tell about you – Which are your weak points and why you don't take care of them – Where are your thoughts going to right now?"*. These are only a few questions you need to be ready to answer your boss immediately when asked to do that. You must be coherent, honest, and persuasive. In case of violation:

#	FACTOR	POSSIBLE THREAT
1	**SITUATION DEFINITION**	• Improvisation • Being a pawn • Suffering others' plan
2	**EXPECTATIONS MANAGEMENT**	• Emotional stress • Weak mindset • Slow enhancement
3	**HERE AND NOW FOCUS**	• Everything difficult • Lose the chances • Failure
4	**SENSATIONS MONITORING**	• Unconsciousness • Fatigue • Unpreparedness
5	**CONCENTRATION**	• Failure • Low performance • Constantly risk running

6	SW-ANALYSIS	• Unconsciousness • Showing your weaknesses • Making mistakes • Weaknesses persistence
7	EMOTIONS CONTROL	• Stress and anxiety • (huge) Rage
8	B-PLAN ATTITUDE	• Being stuck • Suffer disadvantageous situations • Unable to overturn

1 There is neither any place for improvisers on the podium, nor for unaware performers. You cannot run a risk without being able to manage it. This will take you to failure.

2 As long as you continue to fulfill others' expectations, you will be living another one's life, not yours. Your mindset will get weaker and weaker as time passes by and you will be overwhelmed by oversized stress.

3 Mental absences do not support concentration, from one side, but even empties any of your efforts, from the other. If you fail to be "*here-and-now*", you are not present in the competition, there is "*no you*" there, completely.

4 If you don't learn to interpret your sensations and to catch your emotions in advance, you will let them take over your actions and performance. You will be emotionally kidnapped and unable to make the right decision and continue your match. Ignoring your sensations and emotions will lead you to a state of unpreparedness. You will be condemned to improvise and no certain result is possible.

5 Being "*here-and-now*" can let you enter the flow, which means that you fall into a state of huge concentration and you know what to do when doing it and why. If you are not yet skilled, then you will be the pawn and you will suffer the competition and lose your chance of succeeding. You will run any possible risk, unconsciously.

6 You need to know which are your weak points because you have to commit yourself to cope with and you need the skill to hide them in front of your opponent.

7 Emotions can push your energy to its possible size, but they can easily jeopardize any of your plans, even if yours is the best and most effective plan amongst all the competitors. The unpredictable arrival of strong emotions, both positive and negative, will kick you out of the flow, and the focus and concentration would immediately vanish. You cannot escape such emotional imprisonment and will

probably be in front of the *Instinct-Trilemma*: *Fight/Fly/Freeze*. No strategy may survive this Trilemma. The *Fight-Flight-Freeze Response*, also named *"Instinct-Trilemma"* is your body's natural reaction to danger. It's a kind of stress response that helps you react to perceived threats or unpredictable risky events. The response instantly causes hormonal and physiological changes. These changes allow you to act quickly so you can protect yourself. It's a survival instinct that our ancient ancestors developed thousands of years ago (reptilian area of the brain). Specifically, *fight-or-flight* is an active defense response where you fight (*action*) or fly (*escape*). Your heart rate gets faster, which increases oxygen flow to your major muscles. Your pain perception drops, and your hearing sharpens. These changes help you act appropriately and rapidly. Hard training can enable you to avoid freeze (which means: being still/stuck) and execute the action which best fits the circumstances and matches your purpose at the same time.

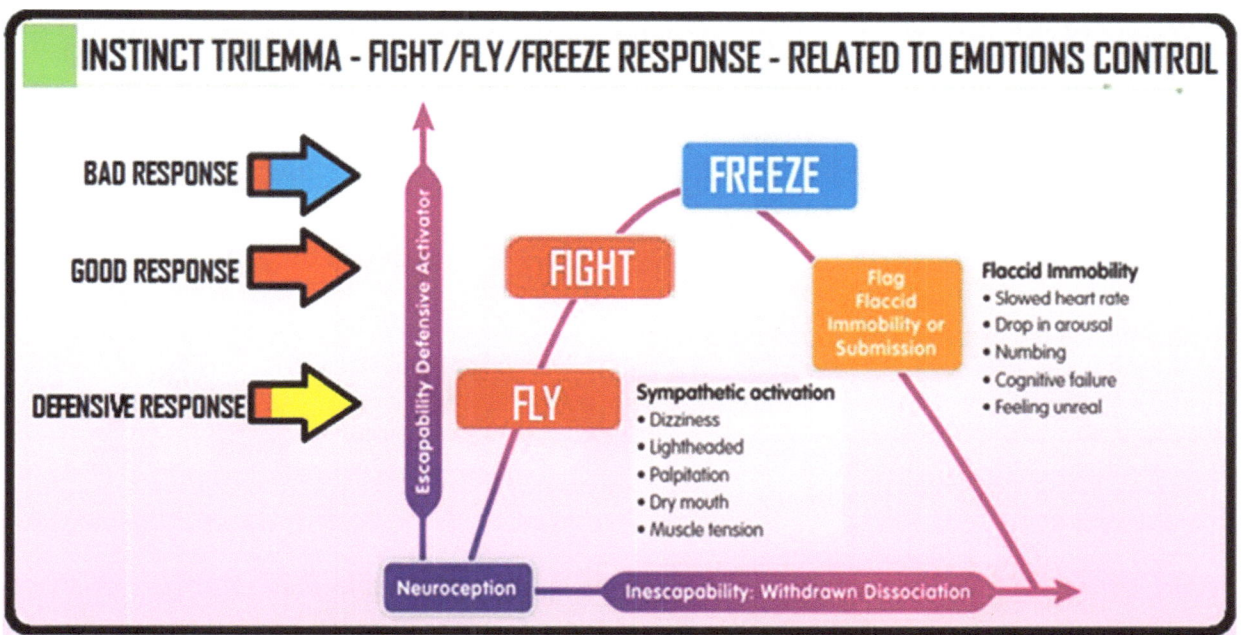

8 What are you going to do if something unpredictable affects your original plan? How will you handle the situation? Which way are you going to overturn your disadvantage? You definitely need a B-Plan and you need to develop a B-Plan attitude. As we know, no strategy can survive enemy contact, which means that even the best and most effective strategy cannot ever cover 100% of the competition, unless your opponents belong to a low-profile segment. So the absence of a B-Plan, and relevant refractoriness to such a mental attitude, will lead you to uncertain results or to failure.

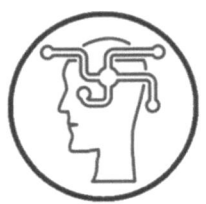

46 – Opportunities

The obedience to your boss – your goal, your dream – will make you free. Will enable you to take everything under your control. Situations, score, expectations, mental presence, feelings, emotions, concentration. Everything becomes possible if you devote yourself to your purpose. You will learn how to perform at your peak, balance and turn your bad emotions into opportunities, regain control, and overturn a bad situation.

#	FACTOR	STRATEGIC ADVANTAGE
1	SITUATION DEFINITION	• Perfect state of awareness • Effective arsenal's reaction
2	EXPECTATIONS MANAGEMENT	• Keeping the right direction • Self confidence
3	HERE AND NOW FOCUS	• Perfect timing • Performing the perfect "flow" • Attitude to sacrifice • No surprise
4	SENSATIONS MONITORING	• Emotional control • Hiding your weaknesses
5	CONCENTRATION	• Perfect timing • Performing the perfect "flow"
6	SW-ANALYSIS	• Specials • Stronger • Overturning the situation
7	EMOTIONS CONTROL	• Transforming emotions in energy • Overturning the situation
8	B-PLAN ATTITUDE	• Quickness in reactions • Regaining control

1 If you behave as a PRO you always know what's happening. If you behave like a Champion you perfectly know why is happening that special way, because you have made it happen. If you act like a Peak-Performer no matter what it's happening: you will quickly find the solution to succeed.

2 Your goal requires you to have specific expectations on both your healthy state (physical shape), and your mental state (balanced) and a set of multiple targets that will progressively get you closer and closer to your final purpose So these are the only expectations which are allowed in the game. All the other ones are only flattery, traps, and fiction movies you have to kick out away from you. Where seriousness arrives, no useless expectation is allowed.

3 *Hereandnowness* is a special state of the spirit that includes physical tension and readiness, psychic total awareness, and spiritual/strategic receptivity. This means you are totally there, focused on what's happening and on what will be happening. Such a state doesn't come easily, because is a mix of a few crucial mental tools working together in the unison. Nevertheless, you have to reach it and maybe you did. If you have ever executed something incredible, which you cannot describe or even believe you did, this means that you were in the *H&N-state* and that you were in the flow, that you were *"riding the tiger"*. H&N gives you the perfect timing (doing what the situation requires, at the right moment), and an unpredictable amount of courage to do what you have to do. A *"call to action"* catalyzer, in a sense, which contenders cannot escape to achieve and champions know very well.

4 Sensation monitoring is necessary for hiding and fainting. Is also crucial for keeping yourself on the right track: focused, concentrated, determined, and going straight to the point.

5 Concentration is crucial and keeps you away from any useless distraction and diversion. You must concentrate on what you can control 100% and you need to totally neglect what you cannot. This means being *"concentrated"* and focusing on your performance. What you can control depends on you, what you cannot, if you cope with it, turns out to be your alibi.

6 Weaknesses need to be hidden, then overcome and balanced. Strengths need to be included in your UPP (*Unique Performance Proposition*). If you create space and time for your strengths to be affirmed, you will increase your competitiveness and become capable of calmly overturning a bad situation.

7 Emotions, as far as sensations, ought to be managed. When you are capable of simulating a total absence of emotions you prevent your opponent from getting information related to your real intentions.

8 If you are provided with a strong B-Planning attitude you're equally a problem-solver. You do not only perform at your best, but your performance becomes a set of problems that have been solved. You quickly react in the most appropriate way, without any time lag and without any involvement of your rational mind.

47 – Methodologies

The primary psychic factors related to Clarity of Destination are the following:

- Situation Definition —
- Sensation Monitoring —
- Emotions Control —
- B-PLAN Attitude —

The methodologies for empowering these factors are based on emotional and psychic skills and competencies.

The RDE-Model enables you to be precisely aware of the situation which you are confronting with. The attitude of defining a situation requires a preliminary study: you need to short-list the symptoms which actually advance the arrival of a state/situation, or the switch from one state (ex: disturb) to the adjacent (ex: emergency). Once you have listed these symptoms (coming from the external environment, as far as from the internal (emotions, sensations, instincts, pulsions, desires), you need to develop a *Reaction-Plan*: each symptom informs about a state which is switching so that you need to follow specific instructions to react to this change. You define plans, you apply plans, and you consolidate such an automatic reaction to your arsenal. *Definition of the symptoms → Connections to each of the 3 states (R-D-E) → Definition of a set of actions (for each state) → Application and consolidation.*

B-Planning attitude is very likely to be such a skill/competence, but is much more generic: you ought to develop specific B-Plans which are activated on the right occurrence. *Study → Plan → Application → Consolidation.* When you do it right, you must do lots of time, so that your arsenal will subconsciously include the most appropriate reactions.

Sensations Monitoring and Emotions Control are different areas originating from the same source: *your inner being.* Sensation monitoring is useful for the right information on what you may be doing, if you follow your internal flow, while emotions control is useful to plan a feinting: creating the evidence of something, but you execute some different actions to surprise or astonish your opponent. Sensations must be caught and understood, while emotions must be controlled or even transformed into positive energy, when possible.

PILLAR # 05 - CLARITY OF DESTINATION

	TOPIC	GOAL	ACTION	EXERCISE	REPETITION
1	SITUATION DEFINITION	Self-consciousness empowerment Where are you now	Isolate RDE elements Plan-related reactions	Impose circumstances Create scenarios → Apply the RDE program	Full Time Job
2	SENSATIONS MONITORING	Physical/psychic awareness Instinctive reactions Better knowledge of yourself	Isolate your inner sensations Study the origin of your sensations	Connect sensations to specific actions	Once per training session (per week)
3	EMOTIONS CONTROL	Rage – Anger – Casualness Excitement – Positive Fear	Feinting Simulation Shadow-moving	Create scenarios and act differently Transformation of emotions into energy	Whenever emotions occur
4	B-PLAN ATTITUDE	Finding a way out Recover and overturn a situation Chuppashart: what to do Keeping control	Develop a plan → develop a B-Plan (based on occurrences)	Start applying an A-PLAN → switch to B-Plan → Finalize	Once per week

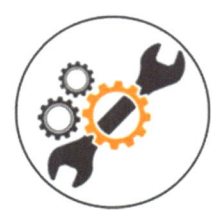

48 – Practical Techniques

You need to become familiar with understanding whether a situation represents a routine, disturbing, or emergency state, any time you are competing and even when you are only training in the gym. Then you need to understand the symptoms of each of these three states, then you need to analyze the risk/threat of each situation. Any time, any occasion, any contest you need to be aware of the Situation Definition, for any state requires specific actions and reactions to overcome a problem or to overturn a disadvantage. World-class performers are used to achieving a quick awareness of what is happening, with regard to the big-picture. Viewing any occurrence in perspective gives you back a highly competitive advantage and helps you keep on the right track and finalize your effort.

The Expectations Management can be a source of overstress and can affect your performance. You need to start hiding your habits and schedule from both your personal and public audience. Then you start declaring to your coach that you are and will always be committed to doing your best, regardless of the results (they are possibly expecting from you). That's your goal and that will be your future attitude. In case of victory, you: (1) celebrate – (2) learn the lesson – (3) forget. In case of failure: (1) become calm again – (2) analyze – (3) learn the lesson – (4) forget.

Hereandnowness attitude is really crucial for the TOP-Performer you want to become. Start challenging routine traps: (1) lies – (2) identification – (3) complains and blames – (4) expressing negative emotions – (5) noise and showing up – (6) bad language – (7) unproductive imagery. Start learning how to stop and control your thoughts and your self-talk. Make conscious activities drive your subconscious mind. Remember that *"you are always alone"* on your pathway to success.

Sensations Monitoring is crucial for getting informed regarding what is currently happening (*situation definition*) and what you may be doing (*emotional reactions*). So you need to: (1) start listing all the sensations and perceptions which (you know) actually advance the arrival of a specific emotion – (2) make the precise connections – (3) then report the instinctive reaction (or over-reaction) that emotion may generate – (4) then understand whether the sensation can activate the right or the inappropriate reaction:

Sensation Feeling	Emotion	Good Reaction	Bad Reaction
#1		X	
#2			X
#3			X

You need to empower your Concentration through both internal and external tools. As an internal tool, you must learn how to exploit the *"Anchor Capability"*, which consists of recalling in your mind something which is connected to a great performance of the past: a gesture, a peculiar noise/word, a sentence, a color. Then you have to visualize and/or mentally simulate that precise picture (anchor). You mentally enter the flow and detect the incredible actions that you made in the past: you must recall those feelings to be the focus. As soon as you do that you fall into a state of concentration. Additional external tools may be specific rituals that you are got used to executing before competing.

As an ambitious athlete, you must be aware of your Strength and Weaknesses, then you have to execute an SW-Analysis. (W) First start to assess the gaps: KPIs, EIs gaps, and technical deviations from the ideal state. Then you execute a *failure analysis*: the actual causes represent your points of weakness. Then you additionally explore all that creates problems, hurdles, and difficulties. The 3 outputs of these assessments will highlight your weaknesses: start working on them. (S) To understand your strong point, you need to list what you feel comfortable and easy doing, then you go on exploring what you can do in multiple ways (variation) and which are those actions that are always effective and are also connected to your unique features. Then you start empowering, enriching, tactically declining, turning into specials with thousands of repetitions. Your weaknesses can easily emerge if you follow these 3 rules: (1) Gaps-Detection – (2) Failure's technical causes – (3) Hurdles and difficulties.

Any Champion and Peak-Performer are familiar with a strong B-Planning Attitude. So you need to: (1) detect a crucial situation, as a starting point – (2) then decline the options and possible occurrences – (3) then you start developing the plan according to both options: *A-Option* and *B-Option* – (4) then you continue developing the two plans until the end. You should also try developing a B-Plan which overturns the situation (*B-Option*) so that you can recall the *A-Plan*.

HOW TO DEVELOP A B OR A C-PLAN AND WHEN/WHY SWITCHING FROM ONE PLAN TO THE OTHER

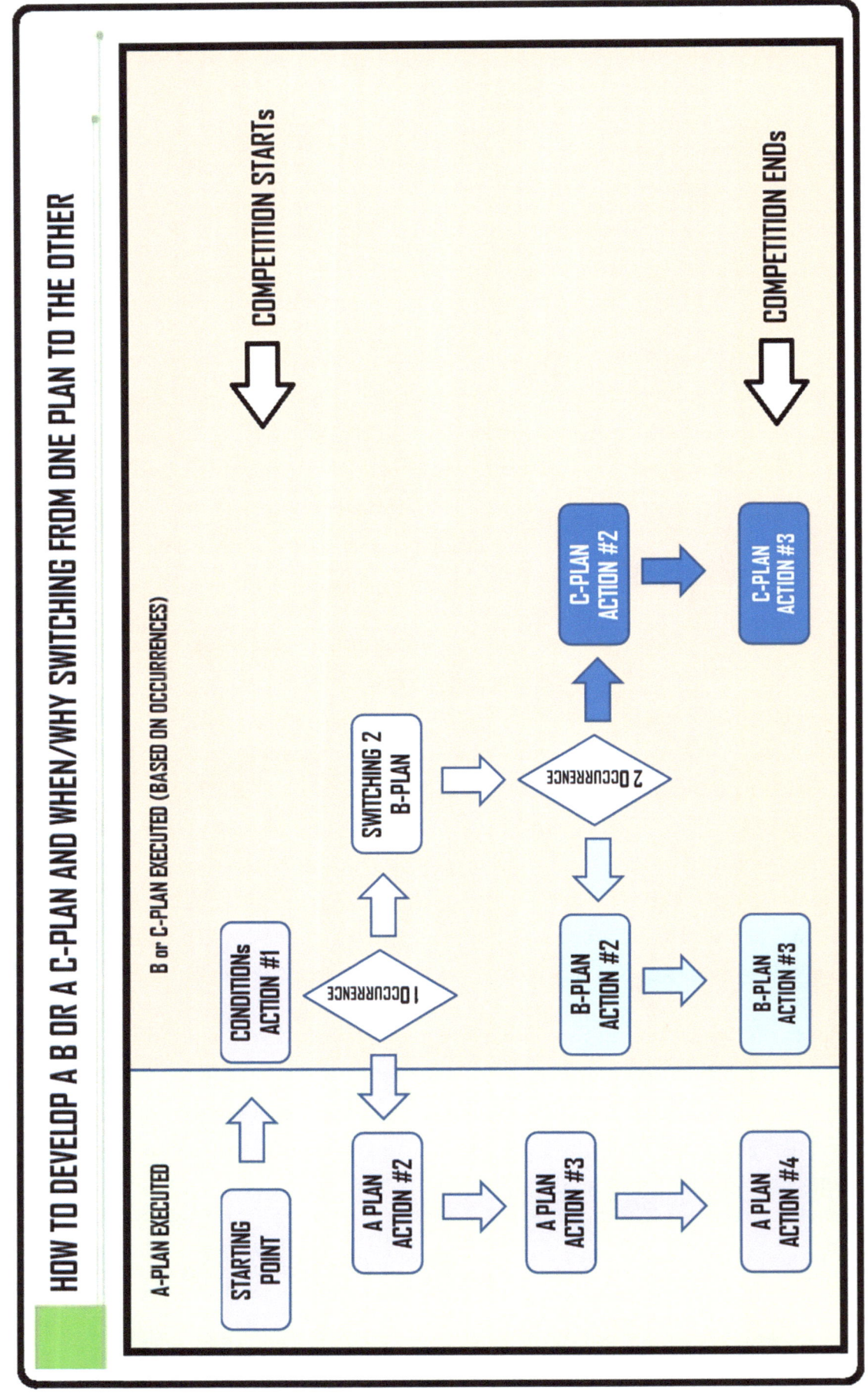

49 – Powerful Questions

Use these questions to force yourself (as an athlete) or your coachees to switch to a higher mental perspective and unlock additional energy to keep being in the right direction. All the questions require specific and honest answers which may also take a few minutes or more, to be developed.

➢ 1.1 How often do you happen to face a situation without realizing or knowing the reason why you find yourself in there? Do you always plan *"where to be"* while competing?

✓ *Rationally realizing that quite frequently you happen to find yourself in a situation, without having planned to be, in advance, means catching your strategic unawareness. This happens many times to an amateur or to a semi-pro but is never rationalized. That's why you have to do that, reversing to rationality, making it clear to yourself.*

❐

➢ 1.2 Factorize a *Routine Competition* in three different segments, depending on your emotional involvement and on the risk you are running, and then impute a sense of action for each of these three: *Routine – Disturb – Emergency.*

✓ *Regardless of the kind of discipline you practice, any situation can be framed in such a pattern. Plan and execute actions depending on the segment you're currently living in during the competition.*

❐

➢ 1.3 Do you feel confident in understanding the development of circumstances while performing during an official competition? Which are the symptoms you examine to properly frame the situation in a familiar model?

✓ *Ask yourself how you usually catch the switch of the situation. Which emotions, which perceptions, and which aspects of the external environment do you feel?*

❐

➢ 1.4 Short-List symptoms/actions related to each of the 3-4 situation-pattern: *Routine* (no-risk) – *Disturb 1* (low-risk) – *Disturb 2* (high-risk) – *Emergency* (current and actual-risk).

SITUATION # 1	SYMPTOMs	ACTIONs/INSTRUCTIONs
(NAME THE SITUATION)	(HOW DO YOU REALIZE)	(WHAT YOU HAVE TO DO) (WHICH TARGET FOR)
Routine		
Disturb type-1		
Disturb type-2		
Emergency		

✓ *If you become capable of interpreting the symptoms which advance the switch of any situation to the next, you can act consequently. If you have a plan (Security Program) you are a step forward, because you only have to follow your instructions.*

❑

➢ 2.1 Explain the reasons why you practice, the real and genuine motivation which pushes you to train hard, and the addressee of your final attainment. Whom do you want to win and become better and better for?

✓ *Fight for yourself. If your commitment is subdued to others' special expectations, then quickly become strong enough to erase them from the scenario. They're sucking your energy and you are living a life that is not yours, but theirs.*

❑

➢ 2.2 What do you think about others' judgment? Coaches, competitors, family, partner's media? How much do you feel influenced by others' judgments?

✓ *Your Self-Confidence and Criticism refractoriness is tested.*

❑

➢. 2.3 How is important that the judgment is aligned with your personal perception of truth? Who is right, in case of diversion?

✓ *SAME. The question pushes you to go deeper and better know your motivations.*

❑

➢ 2.4 Is the final result of a tournament the right decision/criterion to express a judgment? Why? What about the power of evidence? How much do you resonate with it?

✓ *Very frequently an Amateur or a Semipro is affected by the "Somebody-Nobody Syndrome", which means that you are a nobody when losing and become somebody if you win. Your affection for this is tested. A Champion is refractory to such a syndrome.*

▭

➤ 2.5 What do you expect from yourself? What do you think others expect from you?

✓ *Your awareness of others' expectations of you is tested. You need to know that, even though only your expectation is crucial.*

▭

➤ 2.6 Are you feeling comfortable in bearing a failure? How would you handle that?

✓ *Enhance your knowledge of yourself about your tolerance to failures.*

▭

➤ 2.7 Are you feeling comfortable in bearing a victory? How would you handle that?

✓ *Enhance your knowledge of yourself about your psychic balance in managing victories.*

▭

➤ 3.1 What is the most important thing on the day of the tournament? What is the most important during the competition? What may prevent you from expressing all your potential, during a competition? Which thought may jeopardize your performance?

✓ *On the day of the competition the most important thing is "the Competition" itself. It requires all your psychic and physical resources. Nothing should divert your focus from this.*

▭

➤ 3.2 Explain and detail the criterion through which you feel you are focused on *"Here and Now"*? What exactly happens in your mind/body that generates such a feeling/perception?

✓ *A good enough symptom is that you find yourself in a magic state, something which we may define as "the Flow": the sports discipline you practice "is expressing itself" through you, is just flowing through yourself. You only are an instrument of your goal, do not feel personal ego, personal desire, and personal will. You are all for your goal.*

▭

➤ 3.3 What exactly happens when you are not focused on *H&N*? Explain and detail: (1) perception – (2) self-talk – (3) body message – (4) body moves.

✓ *Answering those questions enhances your knowledge of yourself when imprisoned by chaos and confusion. The whole of these answers defines many symptoms.*

▭

➢ 3.4 When you feel you are really *"Here and Now"*, what are you able to do? What may your body and mind do?

✓ *Push yourself to your highest potential through the power of imagery and visualization, because what you can see, you can also achieve, in the future.*

➢ 3.5 Why *here and nowness* may enable you to switch to a higher level? What is really happening while you're in that special condition?

✓ *What really happens when you found yourself "in the flow"? Try to remember and describe actions, results, and relevant emotions.*

➢ 4.1 Explain and detail: what you actually feel when: (1) tired – (2) almost quitting – (3) excited – (4) depressed – (5) demotivated – (6) confused – (7) scared/frightened – (8) strong – (9) better than your opponent – (10) ready to win – (11) almost done – (12) difficulty to focus – (13) plan-less.

✓ *Sensations advance events and decisions. Sensations also advance emotions. You need to know the connections between sensations and events. In such a way you can consider those sensations as additional "symptoms" of what is close to happening and act accordingly.*

➢ 4.2 What exactly do you do, when you realize you find yourself in such a situation? (see the 13 above).

✓ *Analyze your "current" reactions, without expressing any judgment. Describe the situations and reactions "as they come".*

➢ 4.3 Draft a short plan in which you list the following: *sensations → condition → reaction*, to get back your control during competition.

TYPE OF SENSATION	CONDITION (YOUR CURRENT STATE)	REACTION (AS IS)
(NAME THE SITUATION)		
SENSATION #1		
SENSATION #2		
SENSATION #3		

✓ *Enhance the knowledge of your "reactive patterns" based on the study of your sensations and correct them, where necessary.*

❒

➤ 4.4 Explain which are the real causes that generate those (negative) sensations that you feel.

✓ *Try understanding the actual reasons which generates the pattern "(bad) sensation" → "(bad) reactions".*

❒

➤ 4.5 Explain how these sensations influence your choices and your performance, when evident.

✓ *SAME.*

❒

➤ 5.1 How do you know you are *"concentrated"* during a tournament? Which kind of sensation/perception/emotion do you impute such a preliminary and crucial accomplishment?

✓ *Which are your rituals? Is there any evidence you are actually "concentrated"? How do you realize that?*

❒

➤ 5.2 What are you able to do, in a competition, when you are really concentrated? How your performance takes advantage of such a condition?

✓ *Benchmark different states and situations which have led to different results.*

❒

➤ 5.3 How do you realize you lost your concentration? What kind of sensation or action does give you back such information?

✓ *Try understanding what really happens inside you (sensations) when you are close to losing your concentration. Try to isolate the reasons/events which determine such a switch.*

❒

➤ 5.4 What can quicken or facilitate concentration? Do you ever *"simulate"* something in advance? Do you execute special breathing or yoga actions? Do you *"disappear"*? Do you listen to music? How do you motivate yourself one minute before you enter the contest?

✓ *Become aware of your rituals to enter the right psychic state of concentration.*

❒

➤ 5.5 How can you extend such a psychic condition, to profit as much as possible?

✓ *What really stops your flow? Pick up your answer from your past experiences,*

❐

➤ 6.1 Do you really know your strengths and weaknesses? Please isolate both and only pick three per each opposite segment.

✓ *Become aware of your S/W like a PRO.*

❐

➤ 6.2 Do you know which is the origin of your strengths? Which is the real cause (*physical – motivational – technical*) and how can you empower your personal strengths? Define a specific plan to do that.

✓ *You're now planning a program to develop our UPP: Unique Performance Proposition. So, you need to know the actual origin of your special uniqueness, first. Then you have to invest on that.*

❐

➤ 6.3 What is the real cause of each weakness that you know you have? How do you deal with that? Are you able to hide these weak points from your opponents?

✓ *Any human being has his/her virtues and defects. Even superstar athletes have weaknesses and defects, but they are able to hide them from their opponents, to deactivate situations that may allow these defects to emerge, and, as a preliminary task, they are perfectly aware of these defects/weaknesses and of the risk they run, in case their opponent hit them in their weak points. Be aware like a PRO.*

❐

➤ 6.4 What is your strategy to compensate for or to fill the gaps and cancel these weaknesses in the future?

✓ *A Contingency Plan (competition) and an Empowerment-Plan (Training Routine) is needed and you must apply them, after developing.*

❐

➤ 6.5 Do these weaknesses really jeopardize your performance? What really happens whenever they emerge and start expressing themselves? Which is your natural reaction?

✓ *Analyze your reactions, from time to time, when you allow your weak points to emerge during a performance.*

❐

➤ 6.6 Define an action plan to reinforce your personal strengths (and switch them into *"specials"*) and a contingency plan to properly react to your weak points.

✓ *Strengths are as much crucial as Weaknesses. You must quickly become aware of your strong points and you need to transform them into "Specials" to empower your UPP.*

❐

➤ 7.1 Which are the most frequent emotions that you believe affect (or may affect/reduce) your performance? Make a 5 items shortlist.

✓ *Start analyzing what may really affect your performance. Good or bad emotions: you need to take control of all that's running in your heart to succeed.*

❐

➤ 7.2 Why do these 5 emotions affect your performance? Which physical/psychic area do they influence and why?

✓ *SAME.*

❐

➤ 7.3 How do you believe you can take control of these emotions? Which are the symptoms that have emerged and which are proof that they are under control?

✓ *You need to catch the connection between these crucial emotions and their starting points (emersion).*

❐

➤ 7.4 How can you utilize and exploit these emotions?

✓ *A second stage is trying to understand how these emotions can be turned into energy, focus, and additional positive sources of competitiveness, and can support your performance.*

❐

➤ 7.5 Design a reaction plan: when these emotions come, you just have to follow clear and mandatory instructions. Considering the *"Trilemma"* model of reaction (*Fight-Fly-Freeze*), you chose to react (*fight*) then you have to *"act"* according to this plan.

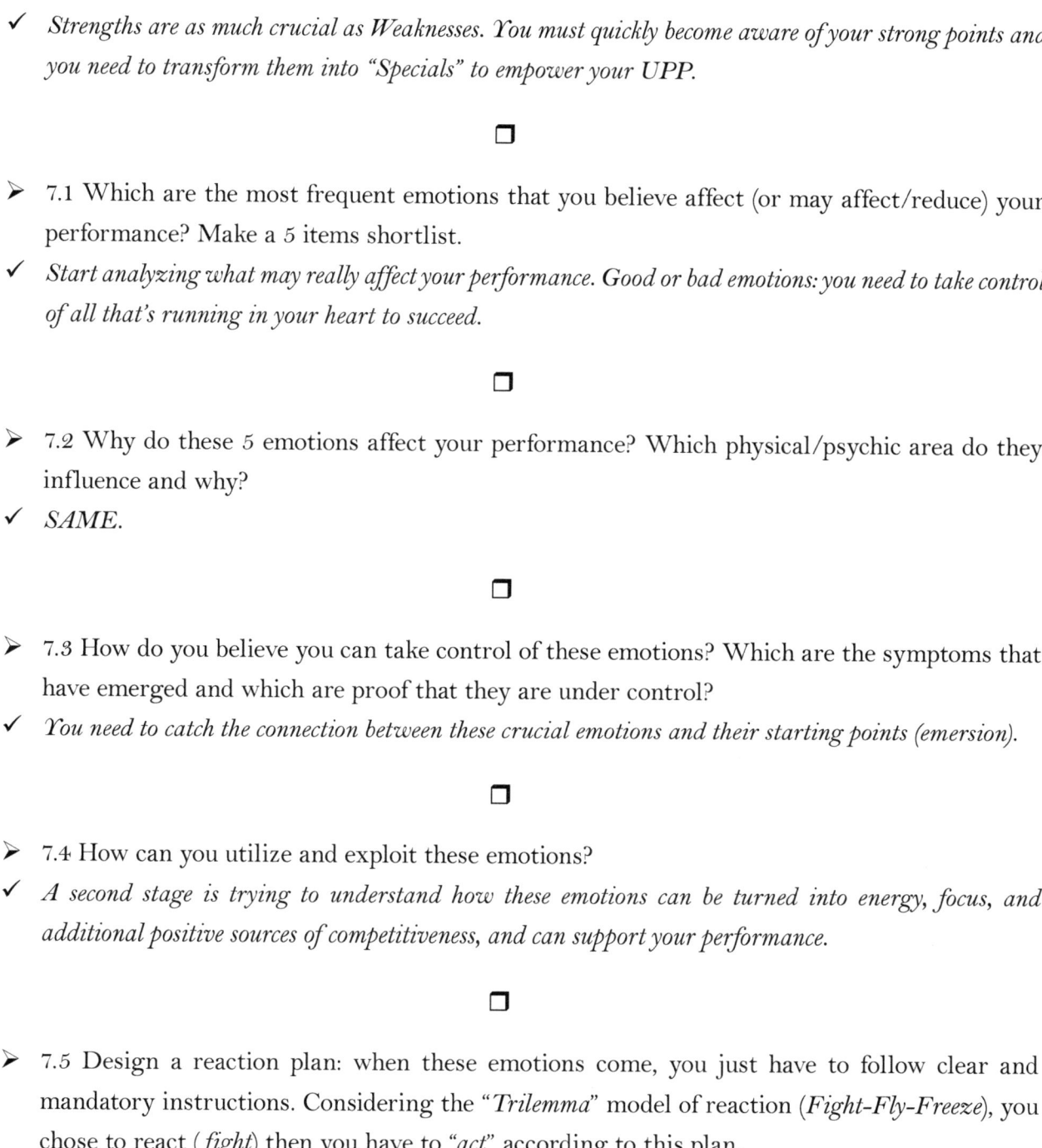

EMOTION	#1	SET OF ACTIONS A) FIRST ACTION B) SECOND ACTION C) THIRD ACTION
EMOTION	#2	SET OF ACTIONS A) FIRST ACTION B) SECOND ACTION C) THIRD ACTION

EMOTION	#N	SET OF ACTIONS A) FIRST ACTION B) SECOND ACTION C) THIRD ACTION

✓ *You are now switching from knowledge to action.*

❏

➤ 8.1 Are you familiar with alternative and *B-Planning*? Please explain your answer.

✓ *Become familiar with B-Planning like a PRO.*

❏

➤ 8.2 B-Planning is a matter of tactics and strategy, which means that something unexpected has happened and you are forced to invent another way to overcome and win. Which kind of events would force you to revisit your original plan?

✓ *Try to short-list predictable occurrences which may affect or jeopardize your original strategy.*

❏

➤ 8.3 Either you cancel these events or you find a way to elude the opponents' power, you're in need of a *B-Plan*: *Tactical Plan* (what to do and how) and *Strategic Plan* (why doing and how winning)

✓ *SAME.*

❏

➤ 8.4 Shortlist a scheme that includes the following and train yourself accordingly.

EVENT	#1	TACTICAL B-PLAN A) FIRST ACTION B) SECOND ACTION C) THIRD ACTION STRATEGIC B-PLAN D) WAY TO WIN THIRD ACTION
EVENT	#2	TACTICAL B-PLAN A) FIRST ACTION B) SECOND ACTION C) THIRD ACTION STRATEGIC B-PLAN D) WAY TO WIN THIRD ACTION

50 – Instructions & Recommendations

A Peak-Performer requires a huge amount of rationality and lucidity: you have to perform actions and gestures according to the appropriate plan which matches the current reality of the competition. This rationality cannot be executed if you are not provided with a strong sense of the situation: *What's happening? What should I do? Why should I act this way?* So become familiar with segmenting the situation, any time, any place.

Observe yourself while competing. See your emotions, feel those emotions, and analyze the decision-making process you apply in case of urgency, stress, and crucial choices. Look at this scenario from the outside, then catch the mistakes and come back inside: adjust your engine and fix the issues. *Hereandnowness*: do not allow your emotions to take control diverting you from your original plan. Observe yourself in your ordinary life. Observe yourself while you are entrapped in routine habits. You lie continuously to yourself and to others, you fall continuously into identification: father, mother, professional, athlete, friend, seller, buyer, man, woman, victim, and judge. You complain all the time and blame others: it's never your fault but theirs. You imagine things which do not exist and are not able to really understand and comprehend other's points, yet. You are subdued by your internal enemy and give him the power to govern yourself, every day of your life. Take action: strive against this useless routine. Take control of your life and then take control of your training program: you need to govern yourself before you can really govern events. You need to regain such control, otherwise, you will be acting by chance: sometimes you win, sometimes you lose, and sometimes you do not compete at all.

What you have to know is that, as an athlete who strongly wants to apply for being the champion, you do not need to suppress your emotions: you'd rather understand, change or exploit them as much as you can. In order to reduce their possible impact on your performance and to learn how to exploit their intrinsic energy, you need to know and explore primary emotions, first:

1. *Anger* → A strong feeling of displeasure and usually of antagonism. Anger is an acid which can do more harm to the vessel in which is stored, that anything on which it is poured.

2. *Discomfort* → Mental or physical uneasiness. You find yourself outside of your comfort zone, which is a great place to be, as you are pushing yourself through unfamiliar surroundings. You're doing something very different from your norm, your routine, from stuff you are familiar with and used. Discomfort, in fact, is the currency of success.

3. *Bitterness* → Distasteful or distressing to the mind.

4. *Disappointment* → Sadness or displeasure caused by the non-fulfillment of one's hopes or expectations.

5. *Resentment* → Bitter indignation at having been treated unfairly. You are very distant from "*Here and Now*": you are challenging the past. This attitude allows traumas and bad experiences to be present and coexist with the current ones.

6. *Guilt* → A feeling of worry or unhappiness that you have because you have done something wrong, such as causing harm to another person. You live your life in other people's expectations, opinions, and judgments.

7. *Shame* → A painful feeling of humiliation or distress caused by the consciousness of wrong or foolish behavior. You tend to internalize other people's beliefs.

8. *Anxiety* → Is an emotion characterized by feelings of tension, worried thoughts, and physical changes like increased blood pressure. You are stuck in the past or living in the near future. You care too much about everything, so you need to reconnect to the present: you need to achieve *Hereandnowness.*

9. *Worry* → The state of being anxious and troubled over actual or potential problems. Such a state puts huge pressure on the body and mind. Either you can change the situation or you can't: do not worry. Put your problem into perspective to give yourself mental clarity.

Each of these emotions, mixed or separated, may generate lots of stress on you, influencing your actions, reactions, and performance. Stress generates three kinds of consequences: (a) heart pumps faster – (b) breath becomes rapid – (c) blood pressure will raise. Instant self-suppressors are special hacks finalized to balance the emotional state when overbalanced by an upcoming/strong emotion. They operate through realism. Stress is addressed by planning, programming, making exercises, and training as realistic as possible to prepare the mind of the athlete for what is to be expected.

You need to apply a pattern that consists of three steps:

a) *Acknowledgement*: you need to know your emotions, their intrinsic cause, their possible danger, and the inner sense of each one.

b) *Acceptance*: you need to accept that not everything is under your control. The moment you accept responsibility for everything in your life is the moment you develop the power to change it.

c) *Take full responsibility*, define the emotional response, and take action.

Things under your control (you have to master and manage): *Your beliefs – Your attitude – Your thoughts – Your honesty – What you learn – How many risks you take – How kind you are to yourself and others – Whether or not you ask for help – How much effort you put in – How much time you spend worrying – Whether you care what others think about you – Whether you try again after a setback – How often you appreciate what you have – How much time you devote to training – How much confident you are – Whether you have a fixed or a growth mindset – Which kind of locus you developed.*

Things you can't control (you have to accept it): *Other people's thoughts – Other people's words – Other people's actions – Other people's feelings – Other people's behavior – External environment – External climate – External weather – Referee's attitudes – Rules and regulations – Suspensions – Your opponent's action – Your opponent's quality – Your opponent's strength – External reality.*

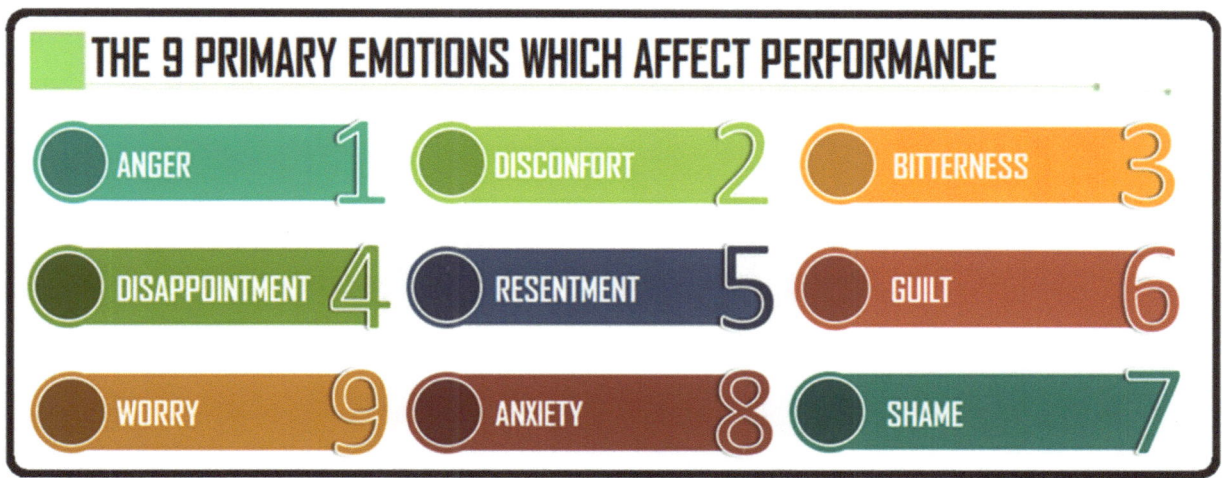

Average people and athletes are bogged down in details of every little problem related to their business, activity, and even daily routine: they are stuck and paralyzed. They are imprisoned by the impact of multiple solicitations coming from the external environment, which seem to create chaos: this chaos finally overwhelms everything. You do not need to take care of everything at the same time. Your pathway, your sports career, and even your life doesn't require you to have such a skill. You need to learn how to compartmentalize each problem and create a mental and emotional separation between the person and the problem. The first competence you have to develop to act effectively on reality is calmness, an inner state of peace that allows you to separate opinions from facts, threats, and risks from reality, and emotions from logic. What you ought to do is learn how to keep calm and apply your resources to one task at a time, when not-urgent.

## CHAPTER SEVEN

Self-Consciousness

51 – Definition

The power of Goals is much bigger than you can believe. If you apply yourself to the highest targets and accept to start the intensive process of training, which will lead you to achieve, many things will happen to you. You cannot become the World Champion of your sports discipline unless you go through peculiar aspects of your personality which strongly affect your performance. The whole of these elements will remain after your retirement from competitions because you should have consolidated them into your psychology and your arsenal. As a first attainment, you will have to develop a deep knowledge of yourself: the inner origin of your motivation as a sports professional and as a human being, your sense of responsibility, your fears and weaknesses, your uniqueness, your will, and your internal enemy. Your Goal forces you to clearly understand who are you now because you will progressively fill the gaps between this and the future version of yourself, that version which is capable to perform at maximum potential and to win the gold medal in the World Championship. To become that second and ideal version of you, you need to know the current one: its limits, its potentials, its psyche, its power, because you can only start on it, on the current version of you: that's your unique resource.

Self-Consciousness: Aware of oneself as an individual or of one's own being, actions, or thoughts.

> WITHOUT SELF-KNOWLEDGE, WITHOUT UNDERSTANDING THE WORKING AND FUNCTIONS OF HIS MACHINE, MAN CANNOT BE FREE, HE CANNOT GOVERN HIMSELF AND HE WILL ALWAYS REMAIN A SLAVE. SELF-CONSCIOUSNESS IS THE KEY FACTOR TO ACHIEVE THE POWER OF DOING.
>
> [GEORGE IVANOVITCH GURDJIEFF – ARMENIAN PHILOSOPHER, AUTHOR]

52 – Contextualization

Self-Consciousness is the huge result of a confrontation between *conscious activities* (training, efforts, sacrifices, persistence) and *subconscious activities* (automation, distinctive reactions, emotional skills). When a conscious mindset becomes capable to drive a subconscious mindset, you get self-consciousness and can achieve any result. That's why self-consciousness involves the mind, body, and spirit of an athlete.

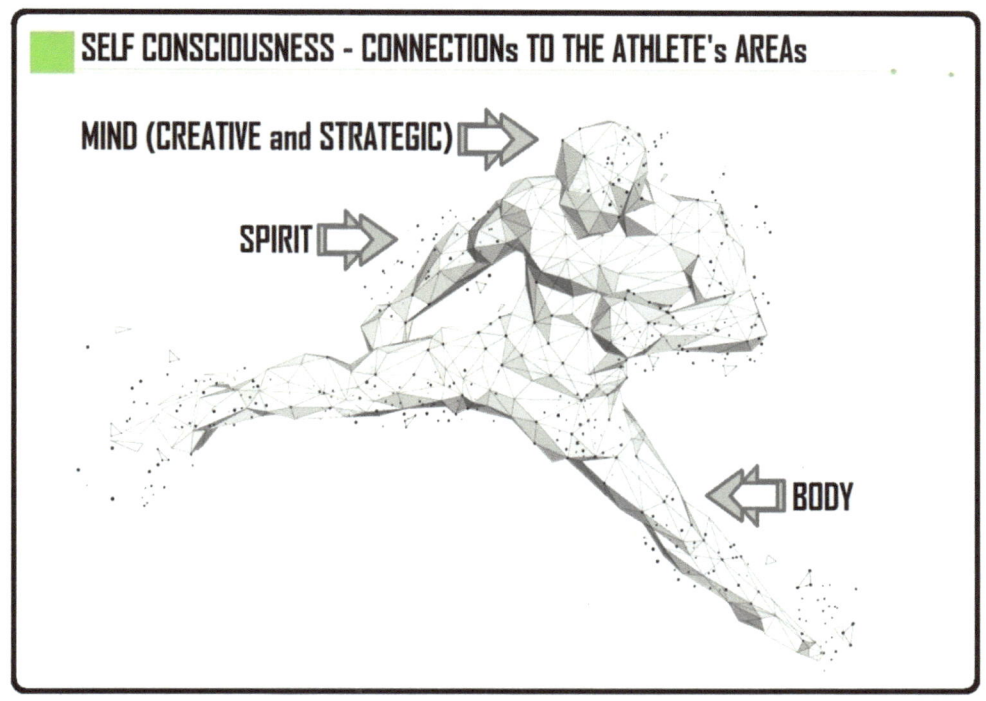

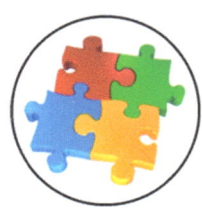

53 – Factors

Self-Consciousness features, which are significant for the development of the Champion's Mindset, are 10: (1) Self Confidence – (2) Criticism Management – (3) Strong Will – (4) Resistance to Flattery – (5) Uniqueness – (6) Framing the Failure – (7) Ambition – (8) Framing the Victory – (8) Inner Self Vulnerability – (10) Managing the Internal Enemy.

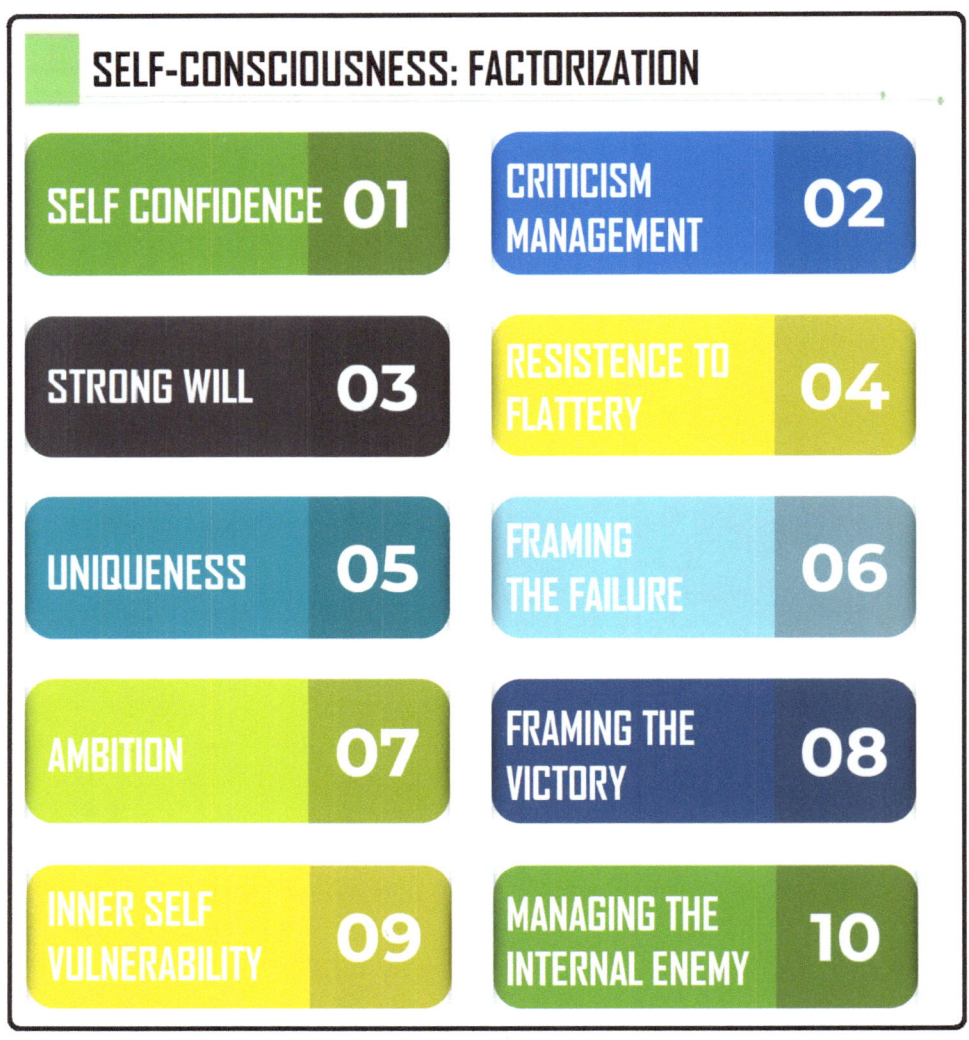

1) **Self-Confidence**: *Self-confidence is an attitude about your skills and abilities. It means you accept and trusts yourself and have a sense of control in your life.*

Believing in yourself in spite of others' criticism is crucial if you want to achieve. Criticism is a typical human behavior that cannot and must not be stopped (for social reasons), but quite often is also a strategy that is used to de-focus or demotivates the performer for two reasons: (1) emotional impact (which influences the inner state of the performer) – (2) psychic influence. If you are not provided with strong self-confidence you will find it very hard to invent special solutions and consolidate them into your style and strategy. You can effectively choose a strategy, a special approach, or an unconventional gesture and consolidate to your competitive style and practice only if you strongly believe in yourself. A Champion, in fact, is not an ordinary athlete. He has either overcome the others' criticism and audience/media judgments and the coach's prejudices on what is better and what is not, on what is possible and what is not, on what you deserve and what you do not. Nobody but you can make a decision on any aspect of your technicalities and of your sports career, but you need a personality and strong self-confidence to apply for such a chance. If you're not provided, you will fail as you are condemned to the state of an average athlete. Self Confidence, on the other hand, is also connected to another crucial skill which is named *"self-efficacy"*: the knowledge and confidence you are good enough (or excellent) in executing a specific task. You have to develop such Self-Confidence which is necessary to develop Self Efficacy which is useful to detect and empower *"specials"* and to learn and perfect complex and articulated gestures or strategies. In conclusion: no real Champion can ignore Self Confidence. Nothing is possible without such a skill.

> IF YOU DON'T HAVE SELF CONFIDENCE, YOU WILL ALWAYS FIND A WAY NOT TO WIN.
>
> [CARL LEWIS – AMERICAN WORLD CLASS ATHLETICS CHAMPION]

2. **Criticism Management**: *The act or an instance of making an unfavorable or severe judgment, or comment and the inner quality to ignore that and to keep on track.*

Criticism may be expressed in several ways: expectations from a special audience (and relevant delusions/disillusions), negative judgments from your coach, negative judgments from your opponents, from audience and fans, from press and media, and, finally, negative evaluations and judgments from yourself. Regardless of the others, the last ones deserve a short exploration. The judgments which are related to evident gaps and deviations from the performances' KPIs, which you have defined in advance, are acceptable, useful, and always true: you must take advantage of them. It helps you improve yourself and sounds like a test for your motivation. The subjective critics, e.g.: the ones which are based on non-evident aspects, sound like a discouraging judgment against you and are nothing but the voice of your inner enemy: you must handle them and prove him he is definitely wrong. Do not listen to the naysayers, do not believe in press predictions, do not believe others' sensations or predictable judgments: it's all a show. Your success needs your complete refractoriness to external judgment and strong adherence to reality.

> TO BEAR DEFEAT WITH DIGNITY. TO ACCEPT CRITICISM WITH POISE, TO RECEIVE HONOURS WITH HUMILITY: THESE ARE MARKS OF MATURITY, GRACIOUSNESS AND MENTAL STRENGTH.
>
> [WILLIAM ARTHUR WARD – AMERICAN BESTSELLING AUTHOR AND WRITER]

3. **Strong Will**: *A strong-willed person is determined. Your will is your desire or drive to do something, so a strong-willed person is someone with a powerful will.*

   After beliefs, emotions, and reactions, the will is the activator for actions. Is what is frequently known as a *"Call to Action"* (C2A). Actions are surely influenced by beliefs and by the availability of resources that can be activated, but if you're not enough provided with a strong will, nothing will ever happen. Will is the lightning that will light the fire, while motivation is the fuel to keep the fire on. Will is sacred. A weak will becomes weaker and weaker. A strong will becomes stronger, as long as you feed your career with the right motivation. Your will is a mix of internal desire, passion, and ambition to achieve. Its size neither depends on physical features nor depends on the talent and on other skills. It only depends on you and on your self-confidence and convictions to achieve, in the long term. On the other hand, the will of a mentally strong athlete not only allows you to start the training process and keep on the right track until you achieve but also provides you with the skill of dreaming big, of defining your big goal. If your will is scarce, your resources are scarce too, your chances to succeed are reduced, and your career quickly vanishes.

> THE KEY IS NOT THE WILL TO WIN: EVERYBODY HAS THAT. IT IS THE WILL TO PREPARE TO WIN THAT IS MUCH MORE IMPORTANT. THE MAN'S WILL IS ONE OF THE KEYS.
>
> [BOBBY KNIGHT – WORLD CLASS AMERICAN BASKETBALL COACH]

4. **Resistance to Flattery**: *Flattery (also called adulation or blandishment) is the act of giving excessive compliments, generally for the purpose of ingratiating oneself with the subject. Resistance to flattery is evidence of mental toughness.*

   Flattery hides threats, traps, and risks. You must accept that only hard work will give you back results build to last: if you catch a cheaper option, this means (1) that you're consciously or unconsciously looking for it (*Law of Resonance*) – (2) that you maybe deserve such a diversion – (3) that someone is offering you a false shortcut to success, to hit a target that is not what you're looking and working for, something which is not worthy. The outside world only gives you back what you actually deserve. Your sport will only give you back the success and the reputation which you have already paid with your efforts, your training, and your level of being. If you enter the trap of flattery, you're going to be given something in advance that you will be condemned to pay in the future and the latest you pay back, the highest the bill will be. The Champion follows the rules then works hard and then achieves. His final balance is always positive.

> FLATTERY IS A KIND OF BAD MONEY, TO WHICH OUR VANITY GIVES US CURRENCY.
>
> [FRANCOIS DE LA ROCHEFOUCAULD - FRENCH AUTHOR AND NOVELIST]

5. **Uniqueness:** *The state or condition wherein a competitive athlete is unlike any other else in comparison.* Uniqueness is not a technical skill, but a talent that belongs to the inner dimension of an athlete's (and of a generic professional) personality. It lives in the essence of any individual. Some special persons are provided with special skills which enable them to get the job done in unconventional ways. The awareness of such nonconformity added to strong self-confidence leads to the development of special gestures, special strategies, and a special approach to competition. The mix of all of these skills generates the uniqueness of an athlete. We are used to catching the unique gestures of an athlete when observing a competition, and we find it difficult to catch and appreciate the spiritual and personal uniqueness of any champion which lies behind. Any champion is unique and any champion is strongly self-confident because he/she has overcome others' prejudices until his/her success has come and has silenced anyone. Because uniqueness generates competitiveness and competitiveness generates success. And success makes you free.

> JUST RIDE THE ENERGY OF YOUR UNIQUE SPIRIT AND SIMPLY SUCCEED.
>
> [GABRIELLE ROTH – AMERICAN DANCER]

6. **Framing the Failure**: *The condition of not achieving the desired end: unsuccessful. Framing an unsuccess means interpreting the failure on a rational basis.*
When you switch to a higher level and apply yourself to a Peak-Performance career, you need to revisit the sense of failure. You have to define the failure, first. In short: the performance is the condensation and the projection of your current inner state added to your arsenal functionality and quality. If you do not succeed, this means that this mix is not enough to succeed yet or that, even if you have the potential, your performance has been limited by something (which is the same). In the first case, you have to work on that. In the second case, you have to isolate the actual causes of the failure. In any case, failure is a source of precious information: it's not a penalty, and it's never unfair or wrongful: sport is the most democratic and meritocratic possible dimension, the failure is always up to you. Big champions never fail: sometimes they win, and other times they learn something.

Many excellent careers owe their success to failures. Failure always generates disappointment and sometimes generates pain: pain is a special state which clarifies many hidden truths which need to be explored and accepted. Failures hide many precious lessons for whom want to succeed. The first step is that you need to develop the willingness to accept and the openness to catch and learn these lessons. This takes a huge humility. The second step is to adapt the sense of responsibility and apply these clarifications to what really happened. The third step consists of interpreting the match and of isolating the switch point which has determined the failure. Any failure, in conclusion, must be imputed to the right cause.

> FAILURE IS NOT GETTING KNOCKED OUT. IT'S NOT GETTING UP AGAIN.
>
> [MOHAMMED ALÌ – BOXE HEAVYWEIGHT WORLD CHAMPION]

7. **Ambition:** *An earnest desire for some type of achievement or distinction.*

Ambition is related to motivation, but is not the same thing. Motivation comes from inside, and lies deep in the heart of your inner being, while ambition is a kind of aspiration, in a sense, comes from rational features and considerations. Motivation can support ambition and vice-versa. Motivation is relevant to essence, while ambition is relevant to personality.

> HAVING THE AMBITION OF BECOMING AN OLYMPIC CHAMPION IS A WHOLE DIFFERENT AMBITION FROM WANTING TO BE THE GREATEST. THE SECOND INCLUDES THE FIRST.
>
> [DALEY THOMPSON – BRITISH WORLD CLASS DECATHLETE]

8. **Framing the Victory:** *A successful ending of a struggle or contest. Framing success means to keep on being humble, inside.*

Becoming a Champion is a process. It requires a sequence of competitions in a bundle of seasons, some of which are lost (failures), most of which are won (victories). You need to take profit from the failures and finalize the lessons learned to achieve crucial victories. It would seem easy to understand, but there are a few risks you may run, into achieving. The first one consists of the *"Loser's Syndrome"*, which is connected to the so-called *"Fear of Success"*. Except for very infrequent exceptions, all the champions have failed before switching to a higher level and before succeeding systematically. There is a stage, during an ordinary career, in which hard work has pushed the resources forward and the athlete is ready to win, but his/her psyche has not yet been informed of such good news. It's a matter of conviction and inner beliefs. Your body and your arsenal are ready to succeed, but your mind has no awareness and creates resistance. The *Loser's Syndrome* is based on the athlete's attitude to repeat past experiences (failures), ignoring any other aspects. Even if you are ready, this is not enough to win, because your mindset is not, and creates resistance. The *Loser's Syndrome* works against you until you start questioning *"what if"* and your imagination creates different scenarios of you succeeding in the competition. You are emotionally imprisoned by past pictures and past experiences and you'll keep being unable to win as far as you are not able to visualize your success: *"If you can see it, you can do it"*. You will become the champion when you feel ready to become, not before, and will switch from the loser's syndrome to the consciousness of the winner, with all the relevant responsibilities. The second risk you run is that you can impute too much importance to your victories, and you decide to quit learning and improving yourself, to stop training as hard as you got used so far. You start to believe you have become the champion and no one can teach or recommend you anything else anymore.

> THE MORE DIFFICULT THE VICTORY, THE GREATER THE HAPPINESS TO WIN.
>
> [EDSON ARANTES DO NASCIMENTO (AKA PELÈ) – WORLD CLASS SOCCER PLAYER]

9. **Inner Self Vulnerability:** *Openness to attack or hurt, either physically or in other ways. Susceptibility.* The inner self vulnerability is the essence of the individual which lies inside you. According to Behavioral Psychology, *Essence* is the real self of an individual, whilst *Personality* is the way this individual gets social acceptance from his/her community. Personality is stronger than essence, in a sense: it is capable to fit situations, feasible, and suitable. Personality is a matter of obeying the rules and following the instructions, essence wants you to be free. Essence must be protected by offenses and attacks coming from the outside, because when hit, it can generate very negative emotions which the individual is unable to stop: it is very difficult to stand up back, after a fall. Essence is the real source of intensity and of the inner power of any athlete, even if it is very difficult to access: it engages hidden and unknown energies and is able to exploit them effectively, at the occasion. For this same reason, the essence can easily determine the fall of a performance, when offended and hit hard. The inner self can easily ignore all that is meaningful but is very weak when the offense (or the special solicitude coming from the outside) hits the target. It just works as an electrical switch: when on, such an offense activates a strong, negative emotion (delusion, disillusion, fear) which is related to past trauma or to other inner individual features, or equally strong positive but dangerous emotions (rage, revenge, non-rational violence). A potentially good performance can quickly be jeopardized by the activation of such emotions, for they are ancestral, so strong that cannot be stopped or transformed. The *"Fight or Fly"* process is entered and you can only follow one of the two directions: no other rational change is possible. For these reasons, you must find the right way to go in deep and detect those few vulnerabilities which actually expose your inner self to huge risks. If you achieve in doing this exploration you are a step forwards. Then you have to find a way to control and protect these elements. You can start medicating and healing these aspects of your

essence or you can only learn how to manage the emotions which are activated when the internal target has been hit by your opponent or from other external causes. Such an achievement is a must-have for a Peak-Performer. The knowledge of these vulnerabilities is the first step to reducing the impact of attacks or even stopping the internal emotional reaction.

> YOUR ABILITY TO MOVE WITH EASE FROM INNER VULNERABILITY TO ISOLATION DETERMINES THE MAGNITUDE OF YOUR INNER SELF-RELIANCE.
>
> [AMY LARSON – AMERICAN ENTREPRENEUR AND PSYCHIATRIST]

10. **Managing the Internal Enemy**: *There is no greater pain that can be inflicted on you, than your own internal enemy. Your own thoughts will cause you more pain than anyone or anything.*

There is a dangerous individual everyone has to deal with, lifelong. Any person in this world cannot escape such a rule. This entity has got your same name, your same face, your voice, and your age: it is born with you. Has got your same friends, your same partner, and drives the same car: it behaves through your same actions. Unlike you, this person is full of fears and has always got concerned about your ideas and initiatives, on your non-ordinary behaviors. This person is always convinced that you are not able, not yet ready, or not capable. That neither you will succeed, nor you deserve to succeed. This person wants you average, mediocre, ordinary: a loser. This person doesn't want you to try, to strive for new challenges: the more you avoid, the better. This person wants your feet stuck on the ground: poor, dreamless, surrendered, condemned to an unhappy and unsatisfactory life. Wants you dead. This is your *Internal Enemy*. It lives within you, cohabits your same body with that special person whom you named "I" and tries to affect your rational brain. This person is not your friend. The problem is that most of the time, you even ignore that you are two. The second problem is that, whenever you realize this, you feel encouraged, because you believe this person will support you, and that you're not alone. In spite of these childish beliefs what you have to accept is that the entity is hostile. You have to realize that, then you have to develop a plan to catch it, push it against the ring ropes, and start hitting until you kill it definitely, once and for all.

> DEFEAT YOUR INTERNAL ENEMY. ALLOW YOUR INNER STRENGTH AND COURAGE TO EXPOSE FROM THE IMPRISONMENT MADE BY THE FEAR OF OTHERS' JUDGEMENTS.
>
> [MAITREE TAILOR – INDIAN LIFE COACH AND AUTHOR]

54 – Threats

Self-Consciousness is the final purpose of both a human being and a peak performer. He/she who is provided with *"self-consciousness"*, is equally given *"the power of doing"*, of changing and driving his/her life. Actions follow decisions, decisions follow criteria and criteria follow beliefs: if you want to change the final results of your actions, you'd better (and quickly) change your beliefs. If you are in lack of self-confidence, a strong will, ambition, and coherence, you are not an athlete, but only the pawn of a stronger athlete: you are part of the game and are only supporting others in achieving their conscious goals.

#	FACTOR	POSSIBLE THREAT
1	SELF CONFIDENCE	• Being fear-subdued • Overwhelmed by hurdles
2	CRITICISM MANAGEMENT	• Rage • Loss in self-confidence • Distorted performances
3	STRONG WILL	• External motivation • Depression • Alienation
4	RESISTENCE TO FLATTERY	• Easy seduction • Easy falling • Poor inner control/power
5	UNIQUENESS	• Routine addicted • Predictable • Average athlete
6	FRAMING THE FAILURE	• Never know the causes • No progress
7	AMBITION	• No actual motivation • No chances

8	FRAMING THE VICTORY	• Arrogant person • Distorted self-image
9	INNER SELF VULNERABILITY	• Always close to fail • Flickerness
10	MANAGING THE INTERNAL ENEMY	• Slave to fear • Victim of the Internal Enemy

1 If you're not provided with self-confidence, you'll always be looking for others' appreciation and confirmations and quite easy chances to succeed. You'll be hiding for the most part of your life. You will delude yourself into finding outside what you should be developing inside. Confidence in doing something comes from within, otherwise is obeying, in a sense, others' expectations. This kind of slavery means coexisting with fear and being overwhelmed by hurdles. Makes you stuck, in the long term.

2 Same for criticism: if you're in lack self-confidence you are longing for good judgments and appreciation and will try to protect yourself from bad and even constructive criticism. You'd probably avoid experiences, rather than approaching. Rage, additional loss of self-confidence and distorted performances will follow.

3 Strong will come from a strong desire to succeed and to make things happen your way. If your will is weak or even absent, this means that you're there, in the gym, because someone else is trying to motivate you, that you're striving to fulfill others' expectations. Alienation and depression will come to haunt you, in the long term.

4 No resistance to flattery drives you to easy falling and prevents you from developing and strengthening your control, inner power, and coherence. Without being centered you cannot transform yourself for the better.

5 If you do not recognize or accept your unique special skills you cannot switch to the higher level. You could become good, but an average athlete who is predictable and routinely addicted: same ordinary rules, same ordinary techniques, same ordinary results.

6 Failing in investigating your failures leads to demotivation, absence of real progresses, and expression of rage. This leads to frequent alibis and compliances, which keep you far from the ideal state of performance.

7 Ambition is connected to your desire: if your desire is strong, then your will is equally strong and will be supported by your ambition. Without ambition, there is no move, no contest, and no call to action. You are condemned to be a low-profile athlete.

8 A false vision of your victories can transform you into an arrogant person. You long for showing up your skills, competencies, and medals, ignoring that each level requires a switch. You'd rather have to celebrate, learn the lesson, and forget your victories.

9 You will never gain mental toughness until you protect your inner ego from offenses that may hurt you from within. You need to know yourself in deep, to explore the weaker part of yourself, in order to achieve.

10 You are not alone, down there in the heart of your mind: this needs to be clear, accepted, and understood. If you fail to accept such a truth, you'd better understand you're going to fail in performing at your max, your possible best. The best option is that you will perform well in mediocre competitions and mediocre in good competitions. The worst option is that you will be stuck because your internal enemy will easily convince the best and most courageous part of yourself that you're not enough skilled and that you'd better stay at home, rather than be publicly humiliated during an official competition. Then mediocrity waits for you: *no choice and no contest.*

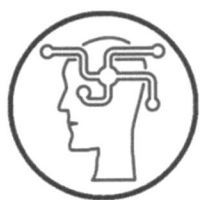

55 – Opportunities

Your self-confidence will lead to effectiveness and bravery. Will settle you for the highest results. Your emotional apparatus will become more and more balanced and you will have the power to affirm your uniqueness as an athlete and a human being. Finally, you will be able to cope with your worst opponent: *your internal enemy.*

#	FACTOR	STRATEGIC ADVANTAGE
1	SELF CONFIDENCE	• Stronger • Brave • Peremptory
2	CRITICISM MANAGEMENT	• Weighted • Balanced
3	STRONG WILL	• Motivation • Perseverance
4	RESISTENCE TO FLATTERY	• Tough athlete
5	UNIQUENESS	• Appreciation from the audience • Unpredictability
6	FRAMING THE FAILURE	• Seeing and learning the Gaps • Improving your Arsenal
7	AMBITION	• Motivation • Goal achievement • Energy extra-push • Pain suffering attitude
8	FRAMING THE VICTORY	• Balanced • Train like you never won, yet
9	INNER SELF VULNERABILITY	• A reliable person • A mean for your Sport
10	MANAGING THE INTERNAL ENEMY	• Mastering your ego • Inner calmness

1 Self-confidence will lead you straight to what you deserve. You will learn and strengthen self-effectiveness and will also improve your self-image as needed. Most of the residual factors which compose the sports mindset depend on such a crucial skill. Strength, sports bravery, call-2-action attitude, and peremptory action will be mastered due to your self-confidence.

2 You know what to listen to because you have become an essential person. So criticism management will enable you to look after the champion's advice, listening to only constructive criticism and judgment completely ignoring useless or fictitious descriptions of your failures/victories. What's useless is easily neglected by such an athlete.

3 Strong will and strong desire generate brilliant and incredible actions and ventures, stimulate a new form of bravery, and ensure motivation and perseverance. Strong will progressively lead you to be a resilient athlete, an individual who is capable to catch the chance in a threat and to overturn any difficult situations based on the inner and outer available resources. Which is one of the key skills of a winner.

4 Once you understand that flattery may only weaken you, your approach will change so much that you will never be given equivocal chances anymore. Your attitude will neutralize flattery. You have understood the danger coming from vanity, which prevents you from improving your true self-image and from speeding up your sports career.

5 Your uniqueness is crucial for building a strong UPP (*Unique Performance Proposition*), in spite of your physical and psychic limitations. After mastering your uniqueness, you can perform in high competitions without any stress or anxiety, because you know what to do for winning in the very advance. You only need to create the circumstances for your UPP to express itself.

6 The appropriate comprehension of the real causes which originated your failures will enable you and your coach to fill the gaps and improve your arsenal, as a consequence. You cannot escape this exercise if you want to act like a PRO.

7 Pain suffering attitude and extra-push of energy comes from your ambition. Strong will and desire, added to a huge ambition to excel and succeed, will enable you to face and overcome any kind of human possible sacrifices. *No-Pain/No-Gain* attitude can only be supported by your ambition. You need to recall the original motivation that brought you to start your practice and the sense of revenge that generated your dream.

8 You need to celebrate your victories, but you need to learn the lesson. After that, you need to forget your victories. You need to train as you have already won and to compete as you have never won anything yet.

9 The athlete who knows the inner and weaker part of him/herself is a step forward if compared to the other contenders, but is required to make action. If such an action is made, then you become a strong and reliable athlete, because your sport discipline can go through you without any barriers and unpredictable hurdles. Can express itself plainly.

10 Your bigger and most dangerous enemy is just yourself, your Ego. If you become the Master, you have completed more than half of your task. If you do not, you are wrapped around your fingers and will not ever be able to express yourself at your best potential. Peak performance can only be based on inner calmness and on silence which means your internal enemy is definitely off.

56 – Methodologies

The primary psychic factors related to Self-Consciousness are the following:

- Criticism Management —
- Uniqueness —
- Inner Self Vulnerability —
- Managing the Internal Enemy —

The methodologies for empowering these factors are based on emotional and psychic skills and competencies.

To better catch your uniqueness, you must preliminarily go through your inner characteristics. You ought to investigate your *"peculiar trait"*, which is what other people easily see in you and that, in most cases, you cannot see or you do not want to see. Such kind of feature talks about yourself: it surely includes one of the unique traits that you can exploit and should transform into a competitive skill. You have to catch your uniqueness, to detect which kind of technical (gesture) or tactical (action) may effectively fit such a feature and build a competitive solution on that. You then specialize this action and empower your UPP (*Unique Performance Proposition*). Your uniqueness is also determined by special attitudes and habits, something which you can perform easily and in a different way if compared to conventional ones. The methodology for exploiting uniqueness is based on the following steps: *define your physical peculiarities* → *define your peculiar trait(s)* → *study a way to effectively match physical features to your peculiar trait* → *include such a way into your set of actions* → *exercise, repeat and specialize the solution* → *secure and consolidate to your arsenal.*

Inner Self Vulnerabilities must be detected, first, and then isolated and cured. Such kind of activity must be executed apart from your ordinary training. You have to go through psychological methodologies which may also include self-autogenic training and/or relaxation and re-absorption. The cardinal principle is that, when you become able to catch and observe a problem, you really start to heal it in an almost automatic way. The light you bring upon the problem turns into medicine.

Criticism Management is quite often related to the voice of your Inner Enemy: it's your internal enemy the person who is giving resonance and voice to your audience, but you are not able to recognize the real origin, yet. To win your internal enemy and turn him into your partner and collaborator you must prove to him he is wrong and you are right. You can only do that through facts: you must take action and turn ventures into medals and success. Then you are able to turn him to silence.

PILLAR # 06 - SELF CONSCIOUSNESS

	TOPIC	GOAL	ACTION	EXERCISE	REPETITION
1	CRITICISM MANAGEMENT	Keep calm in the chaos Detect bad influences Reject bad influences	Distinguish fictitious from useful judgements Only listen to the second ones	Remember what you fight for Ignore anyone else	Lifelong
2	UNIQUENESS	Feel and discover your own uniqueness Turn into UPP (Unique Performance Proposition) Specialization	Take your peculiar trait Catch your special skills Turn to gestures and tactics	Select your unique talents Turn to specials Train – Automatize – Perfect your specials	Once per week
3	INNER SELF VULNERABILITY	Know your weaknesses Know how to react and manage circumstances	Explore your inner self Find your ISV Connect to offences	Create dangerous scenarios Wait for emotions arrival Automatize reactions	Once per week
4	MANAGING THE INTERNAL ENEMY	Reduce the game against Your Internal Enemy Exploit your energies Coping with YIE			

57 – Practical Techniques

Criticism Management is crucial when you're getting close to the top: your mental toughness is strongly tested. You start ignoring others' judgments and select people whose judgments are crucial or significant to you. Decide only to fulfill them, if strictly necessary, but always keep in mind that you only report to yourself. As for managing criticism, you should apply the following easy rules: (1) listen honestly for a critic's intention – (2) decide if feedback is constructive or destructive – (3) thank those who offer constructive criticism – (4) avoid exploding in the face of constructive criticism – (5) minimize encounters with harmful people – (6) make plans to act on constructive criticism.

Experts believe that willpower is like a muscle: you need a Strong Will, definitely. To a certain extent, you can build it up over time. On the other hand, you can also overuse it by constantly denying yourself one thing after another. This *"willpower depletion"* may weaken your ability to resist temptations. Although your willpower may be fatigued in the short term, it can be strengthened over time. Willpower tends to be greater if you are working toward your own goals. If you're making the sacrifice for someone else, it's more of a drain on your willpower. There is some advice that may empower your will and willpower when needed: (1) don't take on too much at once: *one thing at a time* – (2) plan ahead and always visualize your current self (CS) and your future self (FS): you are striving for the second to emerge – (3) avoid temptations and diversions as much as you can – (4) reward yourself, when you deserve it – (5) don't have a fixed mindset: ask and get support from others, when needed – (6) stay connected to your dreams, constantly – (7) make reasonable goals and achieve.

Resistance to Flattery is a skill that is included in your self-control, emotions, and ethics included. You could start with the following steps: (1) be honest with yourself – (2) recognize a potential temptation – (3) visualize yourself resisting temptation – (4) consider the long-term consequences – (5) distract yourself – (6) don't give yourself a choice.

Any true champion has exploited his/her Uniqueness, in a sense. You need to know your unique talents and use them with respect to the sport's technical rules and regulations. You have to adapt your talents to specific gestures: this kind of personalization will enable you to rely on special solutions to overturn disadvantaged situations. Once you have tested such a special solution you need to strongly secure it to your arsenal, with lots of repetitions.

Failure and victory are two sides of the same coin: F/L/F: *Feast* → *Learn* → *Forget*. You neither have to punish and blame yourself nor blame others and complain for something wrong that has happened. Nothing wrong happened: you simply failed. (1) Find calmness – (2) analyze – (3) impute the appropriate causes – (4) isolate each cause and find the connection with your weaknesses – (5) work on your weaknesses and start filling the gaps – (6) correct your self-image – (7) learn the lesson – (8) go back to training. Framing the Failure will quicken your career.

Ambition is connected to both vision and goal setting: you must have these 3 features strong and consistent. Let your ambition grow up consistently according to your sports goals. A psychological self-analysis is required to understand where you really want to go and what you really want to achieve. The answer to these two questions defines the size of your ambition.

As we already know failure and victory are two sides of the same coin: F/L/F: *Feast* → *Learn* → *Forget*. Framing the Victory, in a sense, requires prudence: you could easily fall into a trap of becoming arrogant and affecting your self-image. You need to: (1) become calm again – (2) look for possible mistakes (you did, in spite of your victory) – (3) celebrate your victory – (4) learn the lesson – (5) forget. Your self-confidence, self-effectiveness, and self-image will be empowered as a consequence, but you need to be quickly back on track. You must prepare yourself for the next tournament.

Go in deep and explore the enemy, the Inner Self Vulnerabilities. Find out your inner self's points of weaknesses. Then you have 3 options: a) you prepare to live with – b) you develop a strategy to protect your ISVs from offenses – c) you start healing your ISVs: strong action is needed. Keep in your mind that your ISVs are the actual causes of the emotional gaps in your emotional balance: they cause wrong emotions which lead to wrong actions (paralysis included) and reactions.

The real enemy is not your opponent: you can train, you can work hard, you can strive the hardest to be better than him/her and finally, you can succeed. Your opponent is visible and tangible: you can get a big bundle of information related to his/her personality, attitudes, approach, and strategies. The real enemy lives inside you, but, in most cases, you are unaware of this strange cohabitation. Your worst enemy is your Internal Enemy. This dangerous individual must be hunted down, put on the ropes, and eliminated forever. You need a safe and effective strategy to contrast him, otherwise, you could imagine you won it, while he just hid for a bit.

You need to know how your Internal Enemy works so that you can contrast him effectively. (1) *Your Internal Enemy floods you with impulses.* No indulgence will ever destroy your life, but that's what's so insidious about your Enemy because he is reducing your potential. Your life becomes focused on self-gratification, rather than on fulfilling your inner potential. You try to turn inward. At first, all you will probably find is a vast emptiness; a void you've always tried to fill with the outside world. But if you're patient, you'll find an unexpected source of abundance arising from within the void. Over time, by filling yourself up from the inside, your whole relationship with the outside world will change: you'll be able to bring something to the world, rather than trying to extract something from it. Such a principle is called *Inside-Out Approach*. (2) *Your Internal Enemy convinces you to disengage from the world.* You create energy when you engage with the world, and you destroy energy when you withdraw from the world. The reality is that we all have access to an infinite source of energy. Life's energy comes from the meeting, not disengaging from, the demands of life. Contrast your Internal Enemy by taking action and empowering your engagement with the world in spite of escaping it. (3) *Your Internal Enemy gets you to give up in the face of setbacks.* What he actually does is convert the disappointment into *all-pervading darkness* that smothers every part of your life, a deep hole that feels impossible to climb out of. You must create hope out of despair. You must train yourself to be resilient. That's the ultimate reason why the world knocks you down: you need to train yourself to get back up again. (4) *Your Internal Enemy stops you from recovering when you are wronged.* Instead of recovering, you "*reinjure yourself*" by replaying what happened over and over again. If you stay in this "*victim*" state too long, you stop taking the emotional and creative risks that are essential to living a full life. In the long run, you lose relationships, opportunities, and chances for revenge and success. There's only one solution: you must *learn to die an emotional death* and accept all the hurt feelings in your heart. (5) *Finally, your Internal Enemy wants to be right and wants you to agree with him.* Be confident, take strong action, and prove him to be wrong. This will progressively weaken him until you will manage to silence your Internal Enemy.

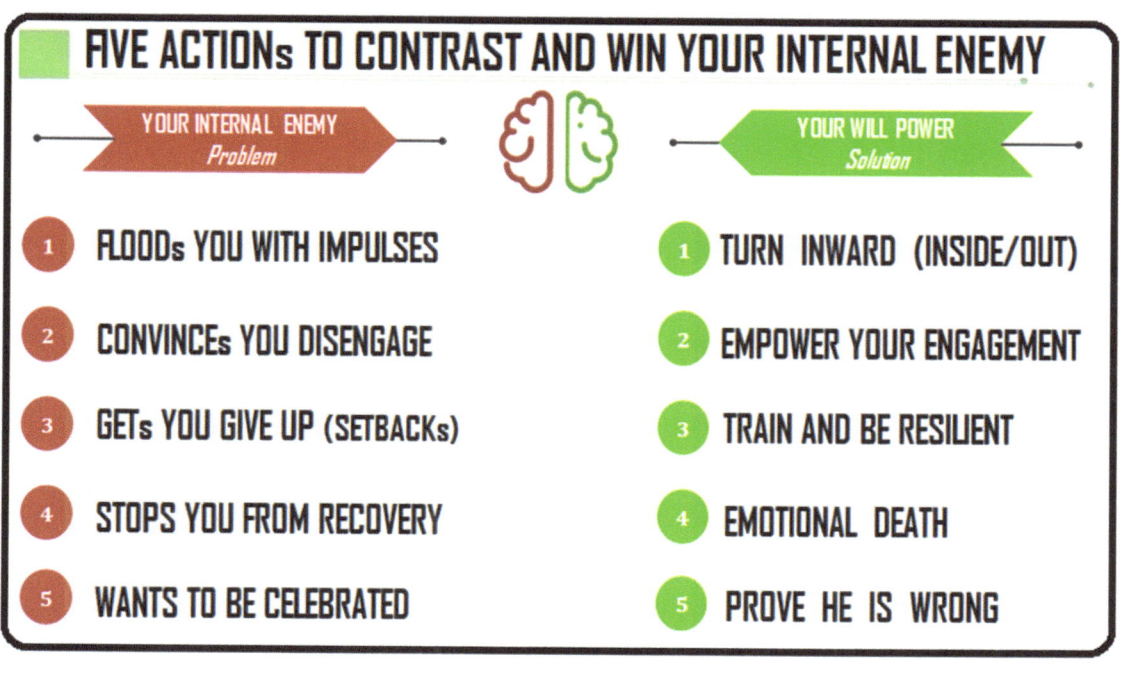

58 – Powerful Questions

Use these questions to force yourself (as an athlete) or your coachees to switch to a higher mental perspective and unlock additional energy to keep being in the right direction. All the questions require specific and honest answers which may also take a few minutes or more, to be developed.

➤ 1.1 How do you define and decline *"Self-Confidence"*? Do you believe you're already provided with this skill? Why?

✓ *It's crucial that you become aware of your current state. You have the task of confessing whether you feel/are self-confident or not. Much of the work depends on how honest your confession is.*

❑

➤ 1.2 Which activity/situation/event do you feel not comfortable with, scared, weak, or non-confident? Shortlist and explain the reasons why.

✓ *SAME. You need to recall these situations because the whole that you neglect and ignore will return back oversized.*

❑

➤ 1.3 Each fear always hides a specific desire: to do something, to have something, to happen or not to happen something, to escape something else. Go through this and try to isolate these strange desires hiding inside you.

✓ *The one who has no desires is free from any fear, Buddhism declares. Fears emerge because related to some hidden desires. According to a sports perspective you need to detect which are these hidden desires, because you have to cope with them, in spite of escaping. Otherwise, they will become your boss and will keep your feet on the ground.*

❑

➤ 1.4 Make an action plan to catch and cancel the origin of these fears, including the chance to prove to your inner enemy that *"he/she is wrong"*.

FEARs	DESIRE RELATED	REACTION	HOW TO COPE WITH
FEAR-#1			
FEAR-#2			
FEAR-#3			

✓ *Start planning a kind of psychological healing to strengthen your hidden self.*

❑

➤ 1.5 Explain the limiting beliefs which lie behind your lack of self-confidence.

✓ *Start making your hypothesis and have a confrontation with your coach, if possible. What you cannot overcome inside will emerge outside and will affect both emotional balance and physical performance.*

❑

➤ 2.1 In your opinion who is in charge of judging something? Why?

✓ *Judgement may be considered appropriate/inappropriate, fair or unfair, true or false: it's only a matter of subjective perspective. But, at the same time, judgment is crucial and necessary (the Referee's judgment). So you have to cope with it.*

❑

➤ 2.2 How do you react to appreciation and why? And to contemns? Why?

✓ *Your resistance to judgment is tested.*

❑

➤ 2.3 Why others' judgment is so important to you?

✓ *SAME.*

❑

➤ 2.4 Criticism is important for you for two reasons: (1) it includes a message for you (whether true or false) – (2) is a chance, an exercise to practice emotional control: how do you handle this?

✓ *SAME.*

❑

➤ 3.1 How strong is your will? Present a few events and gives details to confirm your belief.

✓ *Will is facilitated when you're "in the flow" of excellence. You'd better detect your Will-Power when challenging adversities.*

□

➤ 3.2 If your will is so strong, would you be willing to introduce a totally unproductive habit and practice it for at least 3 weeks? Why are you so sure? Make some examples.

✓ *The introduction of an unproductive habit and the repetition (short-term) is a challenge to your will, in a sense.*

□

➤ 3.3 Now just brainstorm and select one new productive habit and introduce it into your daily routine for 21 days and act accordingly.

✓ *From the mental experiment to action. Find this habit, consolidate it into your daily routine, and secure it in your arsenal.*

□

➤ 3.4 If you do not respect your commitment: *why do you think you deserve to become the champion?* Maybe you believe in luck, don't you?

✓ *You already know: believing in luckiness means believing in misfortune as well. This means that you have a strong external LOC which will become stronger and stronger in the future. No control over external events. Means you are a pawn, even though you are not aware of that.*

□

➤ 4.1 You believe a champion *works on the rock*, don't you? So what do you think about *easy chances?* How do you pay for that, in the future?

✓ *Your inner beliefs are tested. The sense, size, and quality of your final purpose are tested. Your Code of Ethics is tested too.*

□

➤ 4.2 If goals are to be accomplished with hard work, how do you think flattery is being returned back? Do you like to create debts in your life? Why?

✓ *Your attitude to be a creditor/debtor is tested.*

□

➤ 4.3 Hard work, and only hard work, will return you back results: how do you handle this? Does it resonate with your convictions?

✓ *SAME.*

□

➤ 5.1 Is there anything so special belonging to you, which may be considered *"unique"*? Can you take advantage of it? What kind of additional gestures/strategy/training should you add, to make your uniqueness transformed into a *"special action"*?

✓ *You need to discover your gift and your special talent and give it a real chance.*

❐

➤ 5.2 Isolate your strengths and list the ones which are connected to your uniqueness. Then transform these into *"Specials"* (e.g.: special actions that you are able to execute easily and effectively to hit a target when needed). How can you profit from them?

✓ *The process of capitalizing on your special talent.*

❐

➤ 5.3 Develop a strategic plan which enables you to apply your specials and express your uniqueness.

SPECIAL	SITUATION	CREATING A SITUATION	EXECUTION	GOAL
SPECIAL-#1	*Favourite Situation*	*How to create this Situation*	*Technical Instructions*	*What for?*
SPECIAL-#2				
SPECIAL-#3				

✓ *Physical and Mental Conditioning for making your Specials actually emerge during the competition.*

❐

➤ 5.4 Design, train, and reinforce your UPP (*Unique Performance Proposition*), so that you can easily and frequently use and apply it during a competition.

✓ *SAME. Structuring your UPP as a "ready-2-use" tool.*

❐

➤ 6.1 Failure is important because it always teaches you something significant: why? Explain in detail.

✓ *Your current approach to failure is tested.*

❐

➤ 6.2 Describe some failures and what these failures have thought you.

✓ *SAME.*

❑

➤ 6.3 You lost: what kind of defeat was that? Technical? Tactical? Strategic? Emotional? Find the correct answer and try to find the real cause of your defeat.

✓ *You are guided in exploring the sense and the process of your failures. You have to catch the mistake.*

❑

➤ 6.4 Failure is a test and a master: you have to profit from the defeat, always. Write a pattern to do that, including the following:

PRG.	Tournament	Kind of Defeat	Cause/Origin	Mistake	What to avoid	Lesson to learn
#1						
#2						

✓ *SAME, according to a special pattern.*

❑

➤ 7.1 Is your ambition strong enough that enables you to leave everything, to accomplish your goal? What (or whom) are you connected so strongly that prevents you from acting accordingly? Why? What does this element mean for you? Why so significant?

✓ *Your ambition, commitment, and devotion are tested. You are required to make crucial comparisons and benchmarks.*

❑

➤ 7.2 What this fear is telling about you yourself?

✓ *The answers that you gave actually define possible limitations to your full devotion. Remember that your final goal requires you to be fully committed, to a full-time job toward your golden dream.*

❑

➤ 7.3 What amount of effort your ambition is capable to bear and why? Where do you find these energies?

✓ *Same. The size of your ambition is tested, in spite of what you think about it and yourself.*

❑

➤ 8.1 Are you scared to win? Why? What is this fear telling about you?

✓ *Your attitude to success is tested. Your possible "Fear of Success" is tested and explored.*

❒

➤ 8.2 Who is *"The winner"* and why?

✓ *Your sense of success is tested.*

❒

➤ 8.3 What really happen to you, when you win? What do you think you can learn after you win a tournament?

✓ *Your inner "Self-Improvement" attitude is tested, even with regard to successful events.*

❒

➤ 8.4 Is there only one way to win or did you already experience different declinations of a victory? Please explain.

✓ *SAME.*

❒

➤ 8.5 How would you like to win your ultimate world championship? Explain tactics, technicalities, and gestures, then figure out the scenario and start training accordingly and prepare yourself to do that in the official tournament.

✓ *Your imagery and visualization capabilities are tested. Your (current) level of readiness is tested as well.*

❒

➤ 9.1 What really drives you to tears? Which kind of pictures/events/situations make your heart tremble? What really causes your commotion?

✓ *Start exploring the weaker and feminine parts of your inner self.*

❒

➤ 9.2 Explain the reason why and try to find the origin of each of these causes.

✓ *SAME. You start exploring details.*

❒

➤ 9.3 How these elements: (1) present in a performance (shape/emotions/gestures) – (2) can affect your performance?

✓ *SAME. You start going down deep in your inner self.*

❒

➤ 9.4 How do you believe you can deal with these inner vulnerabilities of your internal dimension? How can you take control of that?

✓ *Starting this brainstorming may enhance your task.*

❐

➤ 9.5 Design a plan to handle that and make sure they do not interfere with your performance anymore.

INNER SELF VULNERABILITIES	WHEN (EMERSION)	RISKS	HOW TO COPE WITH
ISV-#1			
ISV-#2			
ISV-#3			

✓ *Developing a "Reaction-Plan" may enable you to manage the issue, in the long run.*

❐

➤ 10.1 What do you think is your strongest enemy and why?

✓ *Your self-awareness is tested.*

❐

➤ 10.2 Who is belonging the voice of that person who continuously talks to you?

✓ *SAME, from a different perspective.*

❐

➤ 10.3 What does your internal enemy prevent you from figuring out? (about your capabilities, your qualities, and your goals).

✓ *The Internal Enemy power starts by preventing you from visualizing successful events and only stops when making you stuck.*

❐

➤ 10.4 Which activities does your internal enemy prevent you from doing? Which decisions? Which chances?

✓ *The details of the previous concept.*

❐

➤ 10.5 How can you better deal with him? Can you manage to handle a parenthetical confrontation with him or are you only his favorite victim? Explain.

✓ *Start a manly confrontation with your internal enemy.*

❑

➤ 10.6 How often do you suffer his power?

✓ *Start a systematic exploration of your internal enemy's interference in your ordinary life. Start being aware of such a hostile person inside.*

❑

➤ 10.7 Develop a kind of reasonable talk to oppose him, then make your promise and commit yourself to prove he is totally wrong.

✓ *Develop rational arguments and reasoning to oppose him, when needed.*

❑

➤ 10.8 List the most important things your enemy does not want you to do or to be involved in, take each of these elements and develop a pattern that includes the following stages and act accordingly:

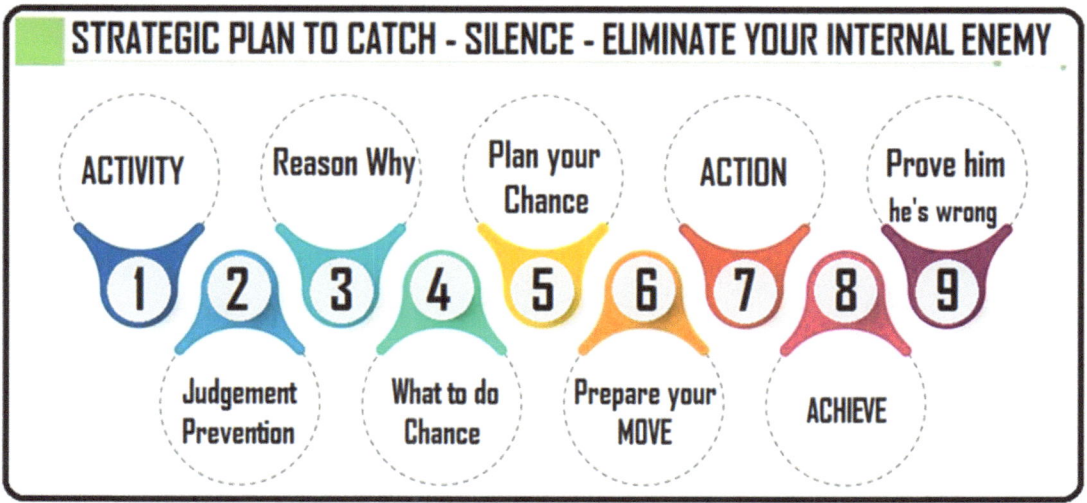

✓ *Start developing a program to contrast your Internal Enemy*

❑

➤ 10.9 Develop a personal strategy to put him on the ring rope, to beat him, and to kill him definitely.

✓ *Your personal internal enemy must be eliminated. When you're able to do that, you will start to express yourself as a free human being and as a free athlete.*

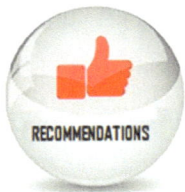

59 – Instructions & Recommendations

Apart from the cycle of action, which describes the way the decision is made, if you do not take action, you cannot transform your reality. Your condition is the same unless you take action. Action, on the other hand, is initiated by a decision, but is driven by will. Strong will is everything. Strong will is connected to strong desire: an inner and unstoppable pulsion to achieve something. Find your motivation and let it be your boss. Listen carefully to your voice tone and let your will take action. Test it, develop, and strengthen your willpower unless you succeed: everything depends on it, in any area of your life. When you prove to yourself that your will is strong and your actions can transform reality, you will equally strengthen your self-confidence: *I see → I make a decision → I initiate an action → I engage my will driving this action → I succeed → I feel adequate → I feel self-confident → I rely on my resources → "I can do that"*. So take action, aggressively, achieve your results and become tougher and tougher. Then come back to your expectations and realign your ambition and your aspiration to your higher level of self-confidence: the two elements cannot be asynchronous.

Start realizing you feed a hostile individual who wants to prevent you from doing. Observe, listen to his voice, and learn his strategy. Once you feel strong enough, engage your energies and start the fight: you have to face and beat him on his battlefield. You know the rules (5: *see above*), you know his strengths, and you know how much the impact of his action is, over your life and career. Engage the fight and make him silent, once and forever. Your decision-making process will become quicker and quicker. Your willpower will become stronger and you will take action more frequently. You won't be stopped and stuck anymore.

If you want to become a champion you need to develop a resistance to external judgment and criticism which needs to be generated inside, as the consequence of a mental switch to the upper level. PROs and champions actually evolve to a higher level of consciousness where outside approval is no longer necessary. There is still a kind of gratification and sense of emotional compensation coming from the external approval, but the champion is no longer motivated to take action to achieve this acceptance. The champion is motivated by *self-expression*, which means affirming and confirming their creativity through their sports performance. It's a kind of *emotional and psychic evolution*: from proving themselves to be that champion (*first stage*) they quickly evolve to the state of expressing themselves (*upper level*). Such a mental attitude is hugely significant to understand the champion's mindset. The contender, the high-level athlete who wants to become the champion is motivated by the urge to prove him/herself, to demonstrate to himself (and to others) that he/she can succeed and be the best. The champion, e.g.: the contender who has overcome all the hurdles, barriers, and adversities and has already become the champion, is no longer motivated by such a mix (internal/external). The act of proving oneself is based in spirit and rooted in the fear of not being good enough (*lack of self-effectiveness*), while the act of expressing oneself is based in spirit and rooted in the love and passion to share and celebrate that any person is unique and is provided with a special talent. Expressing oneself is a natural process that has no attachment to anything and anyone. Leadership is first *being*, then *doing*. Everything the leader does reflects what he or she is. Therefore, leadership is about expressing yourself, not proving. That's the reason why you need to learn how to switch from the basic level (*proving*) to the next (*expressing*): you cannot be the champion until you are convinced you to need to prove something to someone.

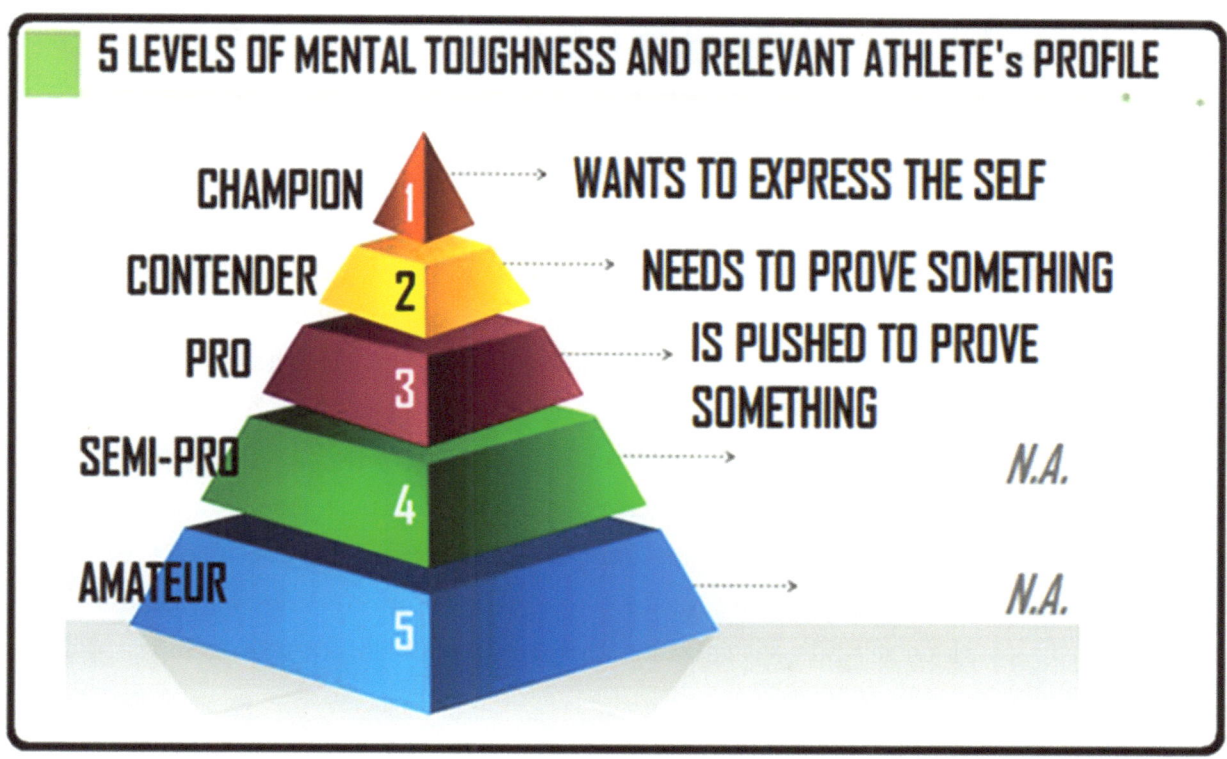

In fact, both champions and top/peak performers belonging to any field of sport and business are pushed from the inside to improve their performance, ever and ever. They are committed to never-ending personal, sports, and professional growth. For such a reason they are so-called "*Growth Mindset Provided Persons*" (GMPP). They are willing to fail on their way to success. The typical self-talk of the champion is something similar to the following: "*I cannot fail, I do not fail. I can only learn, I can only grow, I can only win*". The core principle behind such a skill is the "*learn and grow*" attitude. Such skill requires a propensity to risk, criticism resistance, and, finally, strong self-confidence, which through you can lock your internal enemy and take action repeatedly. *Learn and Grow mantra* is one of the so-called "*world-class beliefs*" of top performers. Champions cannot escape such a mental hack to succeed.

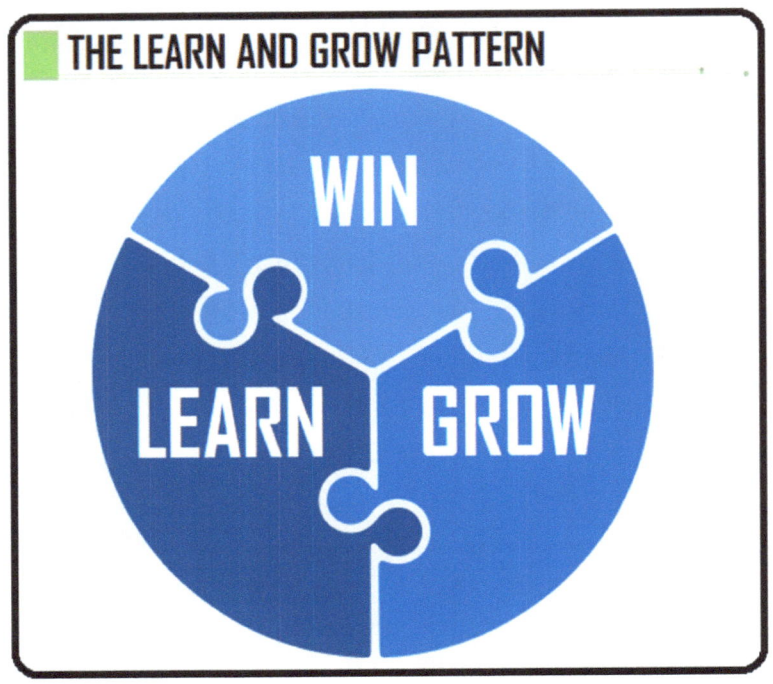

As for Self-Image, we must accept the current psychological theory according to which everyone on the planet is inferior and superior to everyone, in some way. Everyone is unique, just like you and me. People are provided with multiple kinds of intelligence depending on their personality, style, experiences, cultural roots, language, inner beliefs, and individual talents: artistic, mathematical, emotional, rational, and physical. Champions strongly believe the question is not *"Are you smart enough?"*, but *"How much are you smart? How can you get smarter?"*. As a consequence, we realize that the self-image is the real foundation of their success. Self-Image really affects the way a champion approaches business, life, and sports training and competitions. Besides it determines the size and scope of the vision they create for their entire life. You ought to detect who you currently are (true self-image) and start creating your self-image for the future. You need to work on self-talk, visualization, imagery, and, obviously, your technical skills.

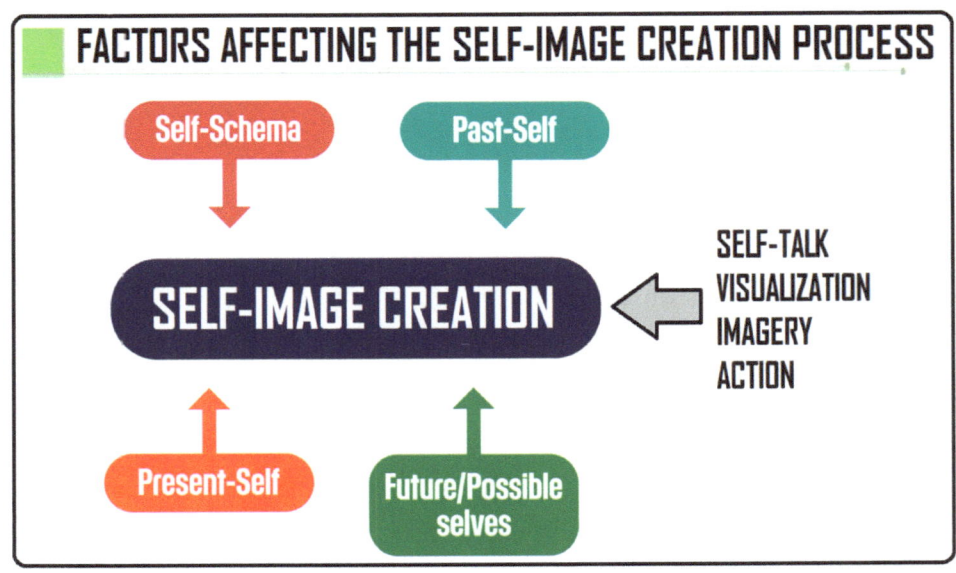

## CHAPTER EIGHT

Adaptation

60 – Definition

Adaptation is fulfilling the imperative rule which had been given by mother nature, a principle that is strongly endorsed by the instinct of survival. Self-defense, self-protection, and adaptation are the primary consequences of such an imperative: no living being can escape such a rule. In short: only the individual who is capable to adapt his/her resources to the external environment, threats, risks, and hostilities, is destined to survive. Adaptation is not an option, is the only way to survive and improve your state in a competitive environment that is unregulated, hostile, and full of possible risks. The sports arena, considered from a large perspective, is such a case: a highly competitive and dangerous environment in which you need to overcome your opponents to achieve. The whole of athletes who belong to a specific sports discipline can rely on their resources (arsenal), but they need to learn how to handle all external environments, including, and not limited to, their opponents. The athlete must adapt himself, his/her mindset, and his/her physical resources to several elements, some of which can be considered dynamic variables and the residual are constraints:

a) Rules and regulations;

b) Referees' judgment, style, and approach;

c) Sports discipline physiology and biomechanical gestures;

d) Experts, Press, and Media criticism;

e) Hostilities coming from opponents/coaches and institutional entities;

f) Physiologic constraints (individual's resources and limitations);

g) Possible health issues;

h) Sports Injuries;

i) Possible psychic issues or syndromes;

j) Internal Enemy;

k) Possible past traumas;

l) Possible family issues;

m) Personal responsibilities;

n) Time availability (to devote to training);

o) Age;

p) Food and diet;

q) External environment (contest location);

r) Enemy contact (competition's occurrences);

s) Disadvantage situations (competition development);

t) Light, weather, and climate conditions;

u) Diversion and suspension;

v) Demotivation coming from failures;

w) Unpredictable hurdles;

x) Unpredictable chances (rules – environment – opponents).

All of that said, it appears evident how much difficult an effective adaptation to all these segments really is. And this is the plain reason only a few individuals have the nerve and the appropriate capabilities to do so. And these people are the Champions.

Adaptation: Any beneficial alteration in an organism resulting from natural selection by which the organism survives and multiplies in its environment.

> THE MEASURE OF INTELLIGENCE IS THE ABILITY TO CHANGE.
>
> [ALBERT EINSTEIN – NOBEL AWARDED PHYSICIAN]

61 – Contextualization

Adaptation basically affects and influences your mind, because if you manage to adapt yourself to a stressful change, your mind will get benefits from such a transition. Your mind, at the same time, actually influences the adaptation process, because the solution you need to find will be recommended by your (current) mind. To enhance your adaptation skill, therefore, you need to enrich your mindset.

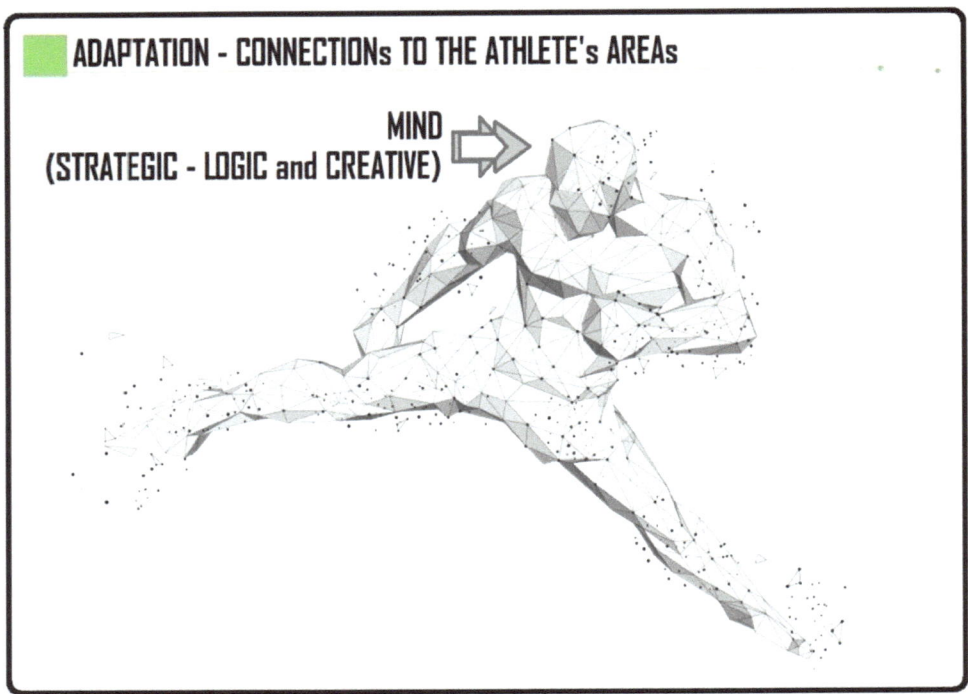

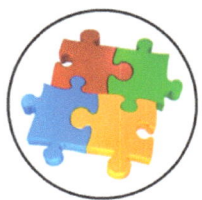

62 – Factors

Adaptation features, which are significant for the development of the Champion's Mindset, are 5: (1) Learn from Failures – (2) Suspension – (3) Injury – (4) Hurdles – (5) Resilience.

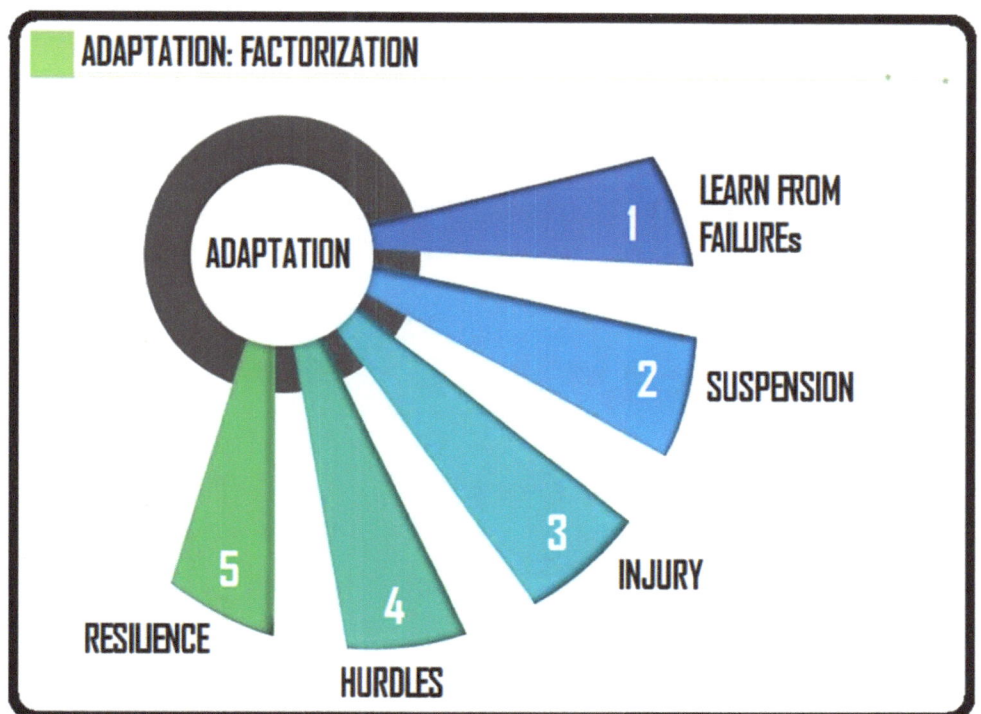

1. **Learn from Failures**: *Learning from failure describes processes and behaviors through which athletes, individuals, groups, and organizations gain accurate and useful insights from failures and modify future behaviors, processes, or systems accordingly.*

Failure cannot be escaped. Failures can determine depression, lack of motivation, and self-confidence decrease, and can structure the *"past-related patterns"* which are responsible for *Loser's Syndrome*. Can frustrate the ambition of an athlete. This is what is called a *"Fixed Mindset"*, which is an attitude (and an inner belief) according to which talent is not developable. There is another approach, completely different and opposite: the *"Growth Mindset"*, the mental attitude to learning, which is used by champions and high-caliber performers. According to the Growth Mindset attitude, failure is so much important and even necessary as victory actually is, because only when failing and falling down the ground you actually have the chance to know exactly who you are, which are your current limitations, how much huge your motivation is, how much higher your commitment may get and, finally, which are the real gaps which still prevent you from winning, from becoming *"the Champion"*. A fixed mindset is typically refractory and resistant to failures: it actually prefers avoiding a challenge, rather than approaching. For this reason, the athlete who has got a fixed mindset learns slowly, avoids risky experiences and threats, and is hugely affected by failures, falls, and injuries, when they occur. The dynamic or growth mindset is open to changes, risks, threats, and oversized efforts and is attracted by long-term goals. It definitely approaches, rather than avoiding. As we already know, we ought to learn from failures; there are a lot of things unsaid within a match or competition that has been lost: mental approach, strategy, preparation, technical lacks and gaps, physical shape, wrong self-image and many other aspects which are related to mindset and performance. What you have to know about failure is that is not a penalty, so you don't have to punish yourself or feel ashamed, and you don't have to be afraid of that. You'd better explore. Understand and declare to yourself *"never more for such a reason"*, then you walk your way and look forwards, to another tournament.

> I'VE MISSED MORE THAN **9000** SHOTS IN MY CAREER. I'VE LOST ALMOST **300** GAMES. **26** TIMES, I'VE BEEN TRUSTED TO TAKE THE GAME-WINNING SHOT AND MISSED. I'VE FAILED OVER AND OVER AND OVER AGAIN IN MY LIFE. AND THAT IS WHY I SUCCEEDED.
>
> *[MICHAEL JORDAN – AMERICAN WORLD CLASS BASKETBALL PLAYER]*

2. **Suspension**: *The act of stopping something from happening.*
Suspension is the temporary interruption or termination of an activity. This block can be voluntary and is normally called a *"stop"*, but it can also be involuntary; in this second case, it becomes *"the criticality"*, since it prevents the exercise of a function (or all, at the same time) preliminary to the activity, hindering the achievement of the business sport. In the battlefield, intuitively, the suspension of the activity is represented, in most cases, by an injury of such an extent as to prevent training (and competition) for 6-8 months (at least), thus compromising the entire season. The second reason, in terms of frequency and percentage, is the recurrence of unsportsmanlike behavior so serious as to determine the exclusion from national or international competitions (for example the positive result in the anti-doping analysis or overt bad faith during the match). In all cases, the suspension of months/years can lead to the collapse of the career of a professional sportsman: the athlete could suffer a psychophysical trauma such as preventing him from returning to compete at a sufficiently high percentage of his original potential, or the act unsportsmanlike could be so relevant (for its reputation) that will forever expel him from the competitive circuits. Essentially there are causes of liability directly ascribable to the subject (fault and bad faith) or to causes which, although not directly ascribable to the subject (in good faith), still determine devastating effects. The athlete's temperament and inner motivation can give him a second chance.

> SUSPENSION IS NOTHING BUT A TEST. JUST TAKE YOUR TIME, PREPARE YOUR MENTALITY TO BE TOUGHER THAN EVER AND DON'T QUIT. WHETHER YOU'RE A WARRIOR, YOUR TIME WILL COME.
>
> [GLITTER JEAN SUDOMYO – SERBIAN WORLD CLASS SPORT COACH]

3. **Injury:** *A particular form or instance of harm.*

   Injuries occur very frequently, during a high-caliber sports career. They may either influence a sports season or completely jeopardize the aim of success of an athlete. If a serious injury occurs, you could be condemned to a limited version of yourself as an athlete, for you will always be unwilling to repeat those gestures and those situations which caused that issue, in the future. This is the mental pattern that is named *"Circumstances Avoidance"* and which easily turns to *"Chances Avoidance"*. Not only your opponent is easily informed of such a new attitude (*Compulsive Reaction pattern*), but you will progressively reduce your chances by voluntarily (or unconsciously) erasing those peculiar situations and/or technical gestures that you consider dangerous. It's very hard and equally difficult to overcome such a problem, even after you have fixed the issue and your body is physiologically intact. Is a mental barrier that nobody can ensure you will overcome. This is the reason why, if you want to succeed, you have to learn how to limit the possibility of being injured seriously. Strongly warming up your muscles' districts in advance, detecting the risk and learning how to manage it effectively, learning how to apply a true costs/benefits balance, checking a true physical shape, and making the right decision attending/neglecting a specific tournament (if you don't feel well) are only a few hacks which you need your mental arsenal to be provided, to prevent injuries occur as much as possible.

> HEALING IS A MATTER OF TIME, BUT IT IS SOMETIMES A MATTER OF OPPORTUNITY.
>
> [HIPPOCRATES OF KOS – GREEK PHYSICIAN, MEDICAL PRACTITIONER]

4. **Hurdles:** *An obstacle that you are expected to overcome.*

   Even when we are enough prepared and have developed an excellent Action Plan, we cannot aspire to any result if we are alone: everything is achieved in the relationship with another subject, within *the System*, which is the set of elements that compose the competitive arena: the player, his/her opponent(s)/contender(s), a rules-set, a referee, an appropriate location. The playing field and the opponent, in its internal and external declination, are determining factors without which it is not possible to achieve any purpose in life (which is further to self-survival). We have to be aware of our opponents, this is an intuitive fact. And we have to respect the rules, and this is less intuitive. The *External Adversary* can inspire us (the opponent), but he/she does the opposite job: he represses us, rejects us, hinders us during the activity and especially during the confrontation; he/she postpones our goal, frustrates our efforts and complicates our business. He/she enters into a partnership with the *Internal Adversary* and creates an almost indissoluble bond. These two subjects actually live in symbiosis: they speak psychically and understand each other perfectly; one reveals our weaknesses to the other, just before the moment in which the attack is launched, our uncertainties, our fears, and the other one acts accordingly with perfect timing: a nod is enough and we find him/her in front of us. They live and thrive in symbiosis: for this reason, both must be defeated. If I defeat my Internal Adversary then I have some chance of winning his/her counterpart, otherwise, my victory will be unfair, undeserved, or impromptu. The Playing Field complicates the existence of the subject, often co-opts the Internal Adversary to itself, and facilitates the External Adversary, as evidence. Yet it also plays a role of inspiration for the subject: it presents him/her with an orthodox scenario and educates him/her to respect rules that could lead him/her to success, if respected. It shows him/her away, without revealing the pitfalls. Finally, there is the Internal Adversary: the *Alter Ego*. He is the only, authentic opponent of every human being who wants to measure and improve him/herself. Rejects represses, frustrates, distracts, and dissuades the individual. His greatest satisfaction consists of procuring a paralysis that keeps his roommate in the confined space of aphasia, sloth, indolence, self-pity, and fear: I would say *mediocrity*. He hardly manages to go that far, but his ultimate job is to demotivate us and to achieve this result through picking from the past (to highlight and celebrate traumas and burning failures), to remind us about our incompetence, our weaknesses, our blackmails. He is very adept at making us forget current successes, skills, and resources; he resizes all that or simply proceeds by generalizations, distortions, and trivializations. His way of communicating is very simple: he speaks to us in the first person (indicative tense), he is direct, and he formulates peremptory sentences of three, a maximum of five words, yet he is strong: he exercises a gigantic power over our psyche. The power of the Internal Adversary is inversely proportional to ours: he is powerful as long as we grant him his power. He must be hunted down, displaced, and annihilated. Obtaining this result takes time and commitment: it must be put to the "*a-contrary*" test. You have to prove to him that he is wrong about everything. The only tool that allows us this kind of inner upheaval is doubt: you need to suspend the disbelief (the lack of self-confidence) and show him that he was wrong. In most cases our Internal Adversary proceeds by prejudices, drawing them from a past that he has contaminated: it is necessary to gather these false opinions and put them in the corner of the ring, isolate them from the facts, and test the results of contrary action. There is no "*Cold Turkey*" process to get rid of the Internal Adversary: you have to proceed through small compromises. It takes time, you need to act in the opposite direction until you achieve small results: from that moment on, the limiting belief is seriously questioned and you can progressively succeed in reclassifying it as *pure opinion*, almost always unfounded. *If it's not raining, it's not training*, they use to say (*Navy Seals*, specifically, during outdoors training sessions). Average people and athletes want things easy, they want to keep themselves in their comfort zone. Comfort zone, as we already know, prevents you from testing your real potential, because everything great requires risks to be taken, and problems to be fixed: you cannot become a top performer until you decide to face adversities and jump into your discomfort zone. On the other hand, champions believe that if you remove the adversities, you remove the victory, definitely. They tend to view adversities as challenges through which learning and growing occur. If you set yourself to becoming a champion, one day, you need to understand that stress, pain, risks, and struggle are the key factors to becoming a mentally tough individual. You have to test yourself in your discomfort zone, as much realistic as you can.

> NEVER LET YOUR HEAD HANG DOWN. NEVER GIVE UP AND SIT DOWN AND GRIEVE.
> FIND ANOTHER WAY, BUT DON'T QUIT.
>
> [SATCHEL PAIGE – AMERICAN WORLD CLASS PROFESSIONAL BASEBALL PLAYER]

5. **Resilience:** *The capability of a strained body to recover its size and shape after deformation caused especially by compressive stress.*

Only high-caliber athletes and Peak-Performers are provided with this skill. It comes from a special mix of mental attitudes and skills, from one side, and of physical and physiological ones as well, from the other side. Your brain, when making the crucial decision of striving harder to overturn a bad situation, must rely on an intact body, an attitude to sacrifice, on the availability of new and hidden energies which will be engaged and addressed toward a new and specific direction. That's why resilience is surely driven by your mindset, but needs the support of your body, in the long run. There are lots of circumstances and events that both actually influence or reduce the potential of an athlete (while performing during a competition), and even prevent his/her future career (risk of quitting). Serious medical issues, serious psychic issues, personal and financial problems may cause huge stress and impact, anxiety and even panic, unpredictable changes occurring during the training program, an unexpected situation of disadvantage during a crucial competition (Olympic Games or World Championship), unfair accuses/criticism by media (doping), legal issues, death of a close relative, mental issues and insanity: all of these occurrences are more frequent than expected. Any athlete had been required to face and overcome at least one of these events or circumstances during the sports career, before becoming a champion. In fact, we cannot select or avoid lots of such events, we can rather decide how to react to issues, crises, and hostilities. As a human being, any athlete can make a free decision in crucial times, depending on inner aspects. Such a choice is discriminant and marks the real difference between an ordinary athlete, who is condemned to be an average sportsman, and a champion. Any sports record, any day of glory, and any champion's goal hide an interesting story, and this story includes difficulties, hurdles, failures, lots of falls, and get-ups. Resilience is an inner quality of being. It is connected to the ancestral instinct of survival and can be considered a peculiar declination of the spirit of adaptation of all living beings, animals included. If you are resilient, you welcome the difficulty, the change, and the upheavals and you question yourself on how to overturn this bad situation, then you try to take control and employ the available resources to achieve the original goal or a new target, if the first has vanished. If you are resilient, you know how to transform a crisis into a chance. If you are resilient, you are resistant in a world that is changing, dynamic, and hostile. If you are not, you can only hope to win everything you can until bad times come, which may not be enough to reach your targets. Resilience is not an ability, but a skill. Can be developed, improved, and strengthened. It is no limit. It's an opportunity.

> OUR GREATEST GLORY IS NOT IN NEVER FALLING, BUT IN RISING EVERY TIME WE FALL.
>
> [CONFUCIUS — CHINESE PHILOSOPHER, FOUNDER OF CONFUCIANISM]

63 – Threats

If you do not learn how to adapt to external changes and hostilities, you will be overcome by your competitors, who actually know how to better adapt to you and your arsenal. If your mindset will keep being fixed and does not learn how to adapt to different scenarios, you will be quitting very fast. No adaptation, no results. Your brain will continue to apply old patterns and will easily convince you that you're not enough skilled. Your internal enemy has won.

#	FACTOR	POSSIBLE THREAT
1	LEARN FROM FAILURES	• Complaining attitude • No real improvements
2	SUSPENSION	• Complain attitude • Quitting
3	INJURY	• Demotivation • Depression • Quitting • Fear subdued
4	HURDLES	• Distorted self-image
5	RESILIENCE	• Quitting • Settle to second place

1 What you fail to learn from bad events will automatically strengthen your fixed mindset. Your current beliefs related to your inadequacy will be strengthened and will join a set of compliances that become second nature. But nothing ever happens by chance and whenever you fall, you can get a lesson learned. It only depends on your attitude. Anyone fails, before succeeding. Your fixed mindset prevents you from doing and questioning: you only want to archive the failure and pretend that it never happened. You're losing a chance and you're empowering your External-LOC: *I have a really small power in my personal world and I cannot address the events.* Low-profile athletes typically blame others for their failures.

2 If you're not passionate and motivated enough you will find stuck when a suspension occurs, for any reason. If you are not provided with a strong self-improvement attitude and patience you may be driven

to stop and even quit your practice. You need to accept a suspension and try exploiting it as a chance to improve your arsenal through unconventional ways.

3 Injury must be accepted as much as suspension. They both come for specific reasons even though have been generated by different causes, but the very first hurdle which needs to be overcome is acceptance. Only a great champion can approach such an event calmly and in a centered way. The arrival of a small or serious injury can create a loss in motivation, when preventing you from partaking in a crucial competition, and can imprison you in a fear cage, limiting your arsenal as a consequence.

4 Hurdles are on the way. Hurdles are your personal motivator, your best coach: they show you what to do and how did. In hurdles and barriers lies the original sense of the sports challenge. If you avoid hurdles, you're settling for being a mediocre, low-profile athlete. You have decided to stand for small goals. Hurdles are the best exercises to challenge yourself and prove yourself you can work it out. Hurdles avoidance turns you to be a loser.

5 If you avoid, rather than approaching, you are escaping hurdles, and obstacles, you are stopped by barriers and upheavals. But mental toughness, just like resilience, is generated, determined, developed, and strengthened through adversities. You have to face hostilities and come through: there is no other way.

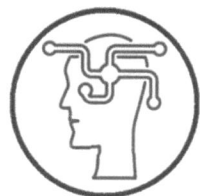

64 – Opportunities

Adaptation is one of the main keys, is a mental trigger that fixes lots of impactful and upheaval situations. Mindset takes charge, then the body operates and correct behaviors would follow. Adapt your arsenal to dynamic circumstances if you want to succeed.

#	FACTOR	STRATEGIC ADVANTAGE
1	LEARN FROM FAILURES	• Enhancement • Mental toughness
2	SUSPENSION	• New skills • Rescheduling attitude
3	INJURY	• Good recovery • Stronger • More careful
4	HURDLES	• Challenges • Self-confidence increase • Motivation
5	RESILIENCE	• Life-learning athlete • Overcoming humiliation

1 Once you have understood failures are precious, you can regain the opportune calmness after the rage and you can start learning the lesson. Then you integrate such a lesson and you can even forget. Learning from failures enhances your resilience and gives you back the motivation you have lost.

2 The most appropriate approach to suspension recommends diverting from your primary activity to enhance your physical shape and to learn new useful skills. Then you turn back to reschedule your sports competition agenda and come back to your primary training program. Acceptance facilitates the coming back to the flow.

3 The comprehension of the real causes which lie behind an injury can facilitate acceptance. Once your recovery is completed, you will be more prudent, but stronger: it only depends on you.

4 When your hurdles have been overcome, this means you're ready for the next level: a new set of hurdles is ready and you are required to be stronger, more precise, more strategic, and tougher. It's used to say: *when the going gets tough, the tough get going.* This means that you need to look for hurdles during your sports career because only a strong attitude to challenge will increase your self-confidence and your self-effectiveness and will make you tougher.

5 Resilience will transform you into a *life-learning athlete* and will give you the right perspective on any failure. Will keep you on track until the end and will finally enable you to interpret events and overcome humiliations, if any. Resilience ensures a constant enhancement of your skills.

65 – Methodologies

The best and very difficult way to quicken your sports career consists of exploring what you did, as soon as you can. So, Learning from Failures is one of the keys. Analyze and find out the real causes which have activated the failures and connect these causes to technical, emotional, or tactical elements. Once this connection is clear, start working on such gaps.

Once a Suspension occurs, for any reason, you first start to accept, then you reschedule every task and switch quickly to alternative activities which may keep you training and protecting both your physical shape and your mental balance.

The injury comes, as we know, and even though we didn't expect it, we need to accept its arrival and make a compromise with our current goals: they need to be postponed, at least. Here is a set of recommendations you ought to follow in case you get injured: (1) accept the injury – (2) allow healing – (3) restore full range of motion and function in the injured area – (4) regain normal gait – (5) regain muscle strength – (6) regain endurance – (6) regain skills – (7) regain confidence – (8) come back to ordinary training routines – (9) come back to competitions.

There is no champion or top performer in any contest who has not overcome Hurdles. Hurdles, barriers, hostilities, and adversities are the battlefield of mental toughness. They all pushed you forward and prepare you both for your incredible success and for the opposite: failures, stress, and depression. You can only become resilient if you have faced and overcome lots of hurdles. So welcome your hurdles: plan your action, take action, and overcome. Then settle yourself for huger hurdles and start back the cycle.

Resilience is crucial, a must-have of the Champion. Resilience can only be developed (and empowered) by going through adversities. You need to go through lots of crucial adversities until you learn to love hurdles, barriers, and problems. You need to become a *problem-solver*. You fall down and stand up many times and keep on being on the right track. You only have to follow your destiny: it will surely present some kind of opposition between you and your success. Be patient, keep on believing in yourself, just keep on track, and never quit. A champion is not a rock, a champion is a problem-solver.

PILLAR # 07 - ADAPTATION

	TOPIC	GOAL	ACTION	EXERCISE	REPETITION
1	LEARN FROM FAILURES	Detecting real faults and huge mistakes – Improve and do not demotivate - Framing the failures and find the appropriate causes	Dissect the failure Catch the mistakes and errors Find the causes – Connect with gaps	Create specific scenarios Test the skills to fill the gaps Repeat lots of that	Once per week
2	HURDLES	Adversities strengthen mindset Skills enhancement – Mindset improvement	Pick hurdles and all your mental barriers	Create specific scenarios Apply to preliminary circumstances - Repeat lots of that	Once per week
3	RESILIENCE	Fall and stand up Transformational skills Keep being on the right track	Assess all possibilities Select one Go through the necessary steps Achieve your result	Long Life job	

66 – Practical Techniques

Adaptation comes from the attitude of learning from failures and is the projection of your inner technical and strategic quality, in a sense. It includes resilience and strong will, as well. Learning from Failures, in short, means learning the lesson, in the framing failures attitude. Suspension management is connected to self-improvement skills: you need to accept it and start enriching your arsenal with additional skills and competencies. (1) Calmness – (2) re-definition of your goals – (3) re-schedule of crucial upcoming events – (4) go back to training.

The injury must be healed and the body of the injured athlete must be recovered from both a physical and psychological and emotional perspective. You should immediately stop the injury, then you should prevent injury escalation, and find the motivation back. Again: the usual steps which you should go after are the following: (1) become calm again (rage is erased) – (2) accept (the injury and the relevant suspension) – (3) compromise (with your body, your emotions and your goals) – (4) healing process (no physical training) – (5) progressive coming back to training – (6) progressive mental arousal – (7) coming back to contests.

Hurdles must be considered the best friend to improve your skills. Hurdles require you to be intelligent, fast, dynamic, and open. Require your extra efforts to achieve. They really want you better than your current state. Hurdles are the antagonist and are there, outside you, only because (and until) you have not yet fixed them. Hurdles are the main tools to quicken your pathway to success. The huger the hurdles, the quickest you succeed.

Yes-attitude facilitates the process of transformation: transformation (or adaptation), caused by a change in environmental conditions, does not necessarily generate pain, but *"resistance to transformation"* surely does. Resilience is the most effective way to accept such a transformation, overturn a disadvantaged situation and catch new chances. Developing resilience consists of behaviors, thoughts, and actions that can be learned by anyone. There are 4 main skills/capabilities, which enhance/facilitate resilience: (1) the capacity to make realistic plans and carry them out – (2) an affirmative view of self and confidence in your strengths and capabilities – (3) communication skills and problem-solving – (4) the ability to cope with strong feelings and emotions. There is, finally a set of 10 recommendations you should follow and implement to your habits, if you want to secure a strong resilience to your mindset: (1) *make connections*: with close family members, friends & others. Accepting help and support is hugely important so your close friends and relatives can listen to you and strengthen your resilience – (2) *avoid seeing crises as insurmountable problems*: you cannot change that a highly stressful event happened to you, but you can change how you interpret and respond to these events – (3) *accept that change is a part of life*: focus on the events you can make different – (4) *move towards goals*: develop and achieve only realistic targets, one at a time – (5) *take decisive action*: don't detach from the problem and wish it would just go away – (6) *look for opportunities for self-discovery*: learn about yourself; may feel a greater sense of strength even while feeling vulnerable, gain an increased sense of self-worth and appreciation for life – (7) *nurture a positive view of yourself*: develop confidence in the ability to problem-solving – (8) *keep things in perspective*: keep things in a broader context. Compare your current self with your future self and make the second emerge – (9) *maintain a hopeful outlook*: optimistic outlook, visualize what you want rather than worrying – (10) *take care of yourself.*

67 – Powerful Questions

Use these questions to force yourself (as an athlete) or your coachees to switch to a higher mental perspective and unlock additional energy to keep being in the right direction. All the questions require specific and honest answers which may also take a few minutes or more, to be developed.

➢ 1.1 Based on your personal experience are there "*fair failures*" as opposed to "*unfair failures*"? Which are the ones and which are the second? Which is the element that clearly distinguishes fair from unfair?

✓ *Your awareness and knowledge of "the rules of the game" is tested.*

❑

➢ 1.2 Did you ever lose one competition due to an unfair judgment or to an unfair action made by your opponent? Why do you define "*unfair*"? What did really happen? How did you react to your defeat?

✓ *SAME. You're required to go down deep into the topic.*

❑

➢ 1.3 Who is only responsible for a *fair victory*? Who is only responsible for a defeat? Same persons? Why?

✓ *You're required to catch the paradox of your previous judgment (if any).*

❑

➢ 1.4 Even a defeat is an experience: how can such an internal burning fire be useful for you? Why?

✓ *Your attitude to lessons-learning is tested.*

❑

➢ 2.1 How do you react to an unexpected suspension of your activity or to a postponement of a competition you were waiting for? Why? Your opponents are suffering the same, so what?

✓ *Same tools, same potentials, same resources: so why a suspension is so impactful? Maybe your rage hides an alibi?*

☐

➤ 2.2 What kind of additional skill could you develop during such a suspension? *Physical/psychic:* something which you have neglected so far. How could you take advantage of this period of time?

✓ *Switching problems to opportunities.*

☐

➤ 2.3 Could you possibly create scenarios simulation to check and train and enhance your resources and arsenal accordingly? How would you set for this project?

✓ *From theory to practice. Exploit your chance instead of waiting.*

☐

➤ 2.4 Suspension only challenges your patience, doesn't it? So, develop a strategy to transform your anxiety into energy and train harder.

✓ *SAME.*

☐

➤ 3.1 Try to isolate and find out the real cause which determined the injury. *Physical ↔ Psychic:* understand the real origin.

✓ *Go back to your injury and explore the real causes which have generated that. Try to rebuild back the complete event and find the connections between emotional, psychic, and physiological features.*

☐

➤ 3.2 Develop a plan to accept the injury.

✓ *The first stage to heal your injury is acceptance.*

☐

➤ 3.3 Develop a plan to transform such an injury into an opportunity to: (1) understand something – (2) enhance some skills – (3) learn something new.

✓ *Your self-improvement attitude and resilience are tested.*

☐

➤ 3.4 Set up for the physical and psychic recovery: don't quit. The gold medal has only been postponed, but it is still waiting for you to catch it.

✓ *SAME.*

❐

➤ 4.1 How do you currently define and handle hurdles and problems, in general?

✓ *Your attitude to challenge adversities is tested.*

❐

➤ 4.2 What are the most frequent hurdles which you must face during your training sessions, personal life, and tournaments?

✓ *Start exploring the hurdles systematically.*

❐

➤ 4.3 Make a pattern that includes the following:

AREA	PROBLEM	CAUSE	EVIDENCE	IMPACT (1/10)
LIFE				
TRAINING				
TOURNAMENT				

✓ *SAME, according to a special pattern.*

❐

➤ 4.4 Each problem includes internal hardiness: just find out what and where this origin lies and explore its size. Be aware of the inner cause of the problem.

✓ *SAME.*

❐

➤ 5.1 How do you happen to win? When do you *"feel comfortable"* and easy, in winning? What does it really happen?

✓ *Start exploring which kind of feelings you have, when you are riding the flow.*

❐

➤ 5.2 What does happen in your mind when you fall into a disadvantageous situation (score) or when your opponent misplaces your original plan? Explore and explain the following: *self-talk, physical reaction, physical evidence,* and *final result.*

DISADVANTAGE SITUATION	SELF TALK	PHYSICAL REACTION	PHYSICAL EVIDENCE	FINAL RESULT
SITUATION-#1	YOUR INTERNAL ENEMY SPEECH	WHAT HAPPENS TO YOU	WHAT YOU REALLY DO	WHAT HAPPENS FINALLY
SITUATION-#2	SAME	SAME	SAME	SAME

✓ *Check according to a special pattern.*

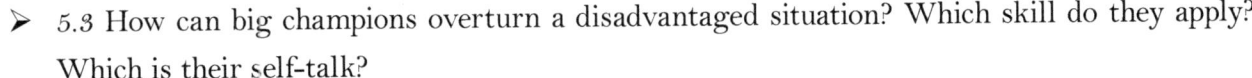

➤ 5.3 How can big champions overturn a disadvantaged situation? Which skill do they apply? Which is their self-talk?

✓ *Your knowledge of the rules of the game is tested.*

➤ 5.4 Are there tournaments or situations which you consider as *"hopelessly prejudiced"* and lost? Who has decided they are lost? Who is speaking?

✓ *Recall the exact internal conversation you have inside when you get close to surrender. This "self-talk" surely affects your performance and quickens your failure.*

➤ 5.5 Plan, schedule, and apply a workout finalized to overturn a difficult situation which includes the following, then feed this pattern with any issues:

PROBLEM PREJUDICE	APPLICATION (STARTING POINT)	EXERCISE TRAINING	MONITOR YOUR PROGRESS
SITUATION-#1			
SITUATION-#2			

✓ *Start empowering your mental toughness and your resilience according to a precise action plan.*

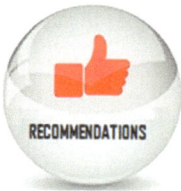

68 – Instructions & Recommendations

Hurdles are the best representation of opportunities, in competitive sports. A hurdle is nothing but *a chance of learning*, structure, or test a skill. You need to become passionate about hurdles, problems, and barriers: they represent a sample of what you will find on the battlefield. There is a problem and there is you. You have two options: a) escaping the problem – (b) preparing yourself to fix the problem. Option (b) would increase your mindset: success is on the other side of the risk. You need to take the risk of failing and engage yourself to fix the problem. Once you solve the problem you will be awarded because an additional skill has been developed or tested: you proved to yourself you can do that. Option (a) is the loser's choice and will keep you still. You will always find a reason *"not to do"* something. Victory is on the other side of your comfort zone: if you keep moving easily, you'll never test your full potential and you'll never become a champion. You need to take a risk and go over the boundaries of your known world. Easy problems will bring you easy results. You need to feel uncomfortable, in danger, or even inadequate, to learn how to succeed in sports as well as in business and life.

Many athletes have been close to death, for many reasons, before succeeding. Some others have been going through humiliation and pain, before declaring to themselves that *"enough is enough!"* A residual part has overcome all their mental barriers before applying to become a winner: height, weight, age, culture, nationality, religion, and location. No one has had an easy life, an easy career, or an easy pathway. Injuries, financial issues, cultural gaps, lack of chances, family issues: you have to be stronger than that, to succeed. Resilience is the skill that supports you in switching from a *near-miss* to a new chance of success. You have to accept it, find a compromise with yourself, correct your self-image, and re-engage your resources because you must finalize a new and different goal, provided with a new timeline. You have to temporarily revisit your expectations, but you need to understand that you are still alive, and if you keep being balanced, healthy, and mentally strong, you can achieve your goals. Because they are still within your reach. You have to convince yourself about that: life added to a strong will, is the basic tool to re-engage your everything. It's up to you. It's always been.

CHAPTER NINE

Courage

69 – Definition

Courage means doing the right thing at the right moment, in spite of risks, fears, and threats which might prevent you from doing. A professional athlete, in fact, is a brave individual: he/she is not making decisions anymore: the situation requires a specific solution and that solution is executed. There is neither decision nor choice: the PRO must obey. If you are still in a state of fear (low propension to risk added to inner self-vulnerability and low self-confidence), the action might not be executed correctly. This means that the action is not effective. For such a reason you need to learn how to perform well and you have to master that gesture. Technical and emotional skills empower self-confidence and self-confidence generates courage.

Courage: Courage is a mental or moral strength to venture, perceive and withstand danger, fear, or difficulty.

> HE WHO IS NOT COURAGEOUS ENOUGH TO TAKE RISKS WILL ACCOMPLISH NOTHING IN LIFE.
>
> [MOHAMMED ALÌ – BOXE HEAVYWEIGHT WORLD CHAMPION]

70 – Contextualization

Courage actually affects your mind. Heart and spirit may activate the proper and prompt action (or reaction), but the mind actually drives the action. A conscious mindset can effectively lead to the courage to do the right thing and fix a crucial and dangerous problem.

Courage, in fact, is not a matter of physical talent or technical skills. Courage is rather a matter of psyche. The individual's mind resists the powerful and almost unstoppable pattern of the *"Instinct-Trilemma"* (*Fight-Fly-Freeze*) and finally makes the emotions silent, then makes a quick decision and takes action. We are used to seeing and evaluating the actions of an individual, because they are quite evident, and appreciate the effects of these actions, but courage is an inside-out process that takes place in the mind.

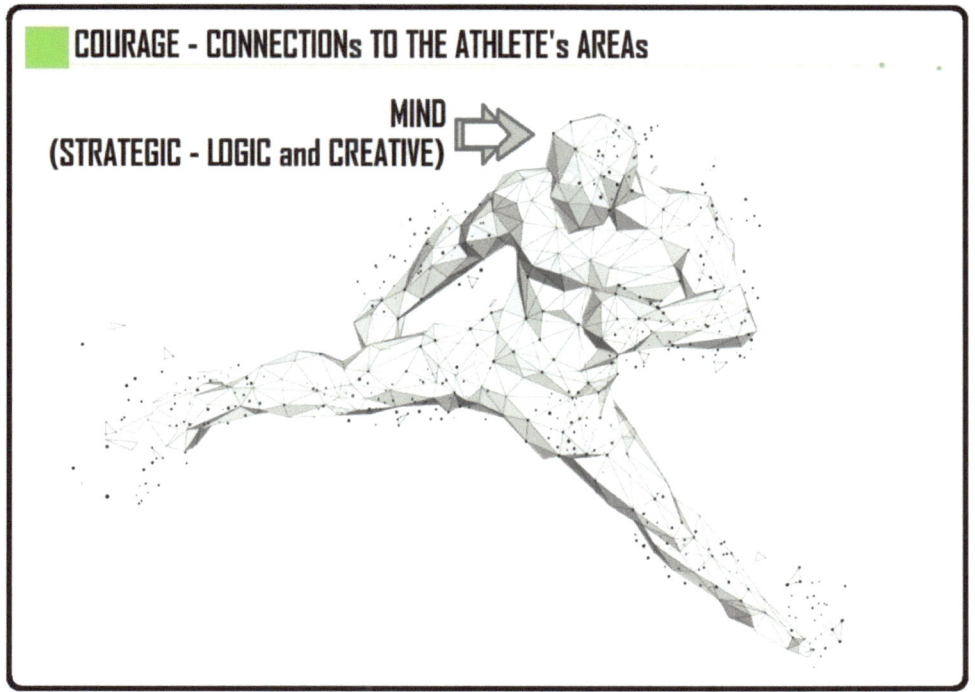

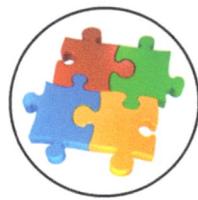

71 – Factors

Courage features, which are significant for the development of the Champion's Mindset, are 6: (1) Propension to Risk – (2) Risk Management – (3) Non Conformity – (4) Internal LOC – (5) Fearlessness – (6) Responsibility.

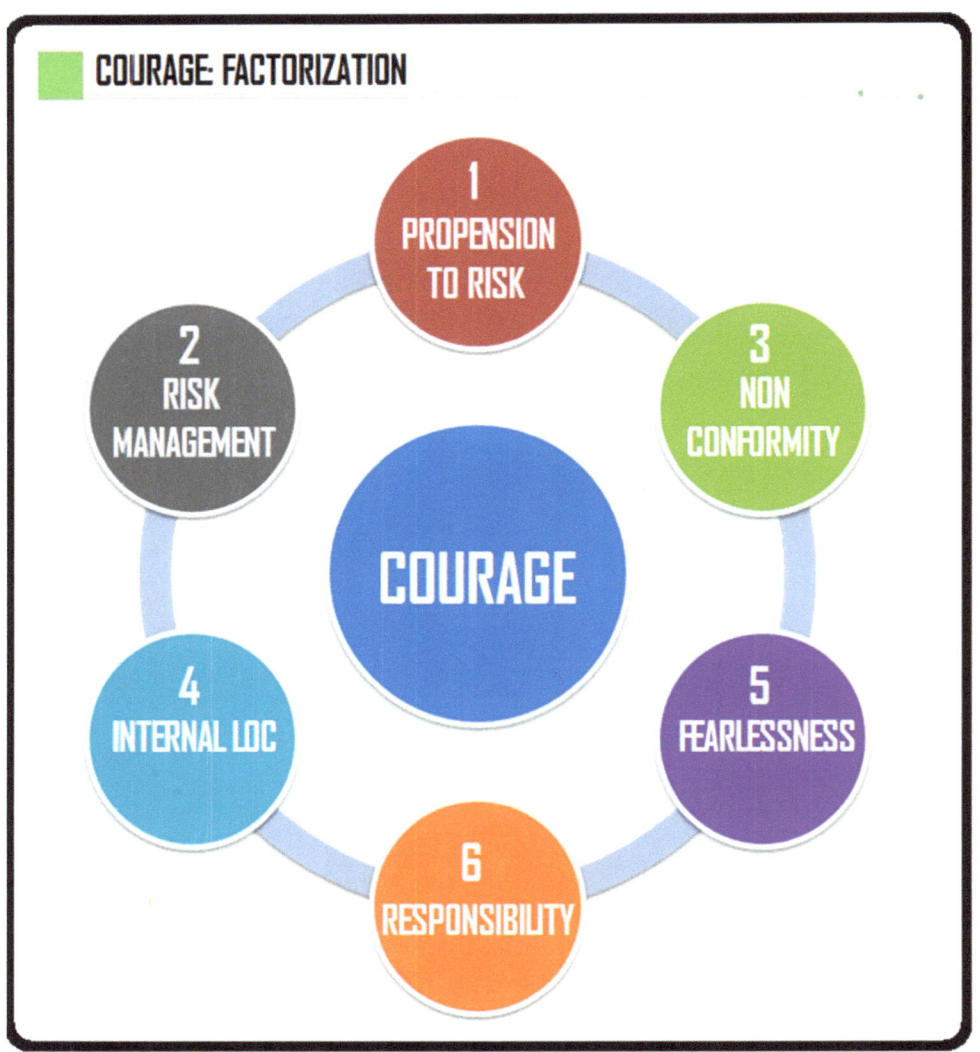

1. **Propension to Risk:** *Risk is the possibility of something bad happening.*
   Any huge target requires a huge risk to be taken. Any huge accomplishment requires you to risk something before you accomplish it. No big target is easy to achieve: I am neither talking about

sacrifices and efforts nor about technicalities and physical skills. All of that is *"quantity"* and quantity, in fact, is only a matter of time and commitment, which is the basis of being (and feeling) a sportsman/woman: no doubt that it is within the reach of every athlete. I am rather talking about *"quality"*, something very difficult to develop, even if not impossible, but equally crucial. If you really want to achieve, you must accept that you have to run a risk and you will run risks as easily as you have got an inner attitude to do that, the so-called *"Risk-Appetite"*. The stronger and more natural this attitude, the quickest the results arrive. The first risk you must become familiar with to run is *the risk to fail*. This is not as easy as it seems, because all human beings are provided with a special attitude which is called *"propension to certainty"* (or resistance to uncertainty): if you are not able to modify such a propension, you will never become a champion within. You must become familiar with exposure to failure. There are athletes who have this propension to risk as an innate skill, while others feel limited or stuck if approaching uncertainty. Nevertheless, this risk must be run, otherwise, there is no contest. The other risk you must take is the risk of consuming all the energies, in your performance: *the risk of being emptied*. A champion knows how to balance energies, but when the situation requires an extra push, he/she also knows where to engage the energies and exploit them without fear. He/she does not ever save energies for the way back: is not his/her concern. The only thought is focused to reach the target and the champion will grant all his/her resources for this purpose without additional concerns. If you really learn how to exploit everything you are provided with, you have no alibi: the champions avoid excuses, for they already know everything is up to them. The third risk you have to run is a *technical risk*: any sports discipline has special moves and gestures which lead the performer to a higher score (or to a situation of significant advantage), but which equally require a higher risk: *failure exposure*. Many times, something unexpected occurs that needs your quick and strong reaction and also affects your original strategy. You are consequently forced to adopt risky strategies to balance the situation. When risky events happen, you need to get ready to fulfil your propension to risk and to quickly apply what the situation actually recommends. You take a high risk to achieve a high result: you need to handle this balance, otherwise, the risk may overcome the benefit. Lots of additional risks you need to become familiar with to handle, if you want to become a high-caliber athlete. You need to develop a particular skill that somehow involves your inner analytics: catch the best solution, size the risk, balance the risk with the benefit expected, then apply the solution. You are running a risk, in fact, but you are increasing your propensity to risk.

Courage and bravery are kinds of *self-referential skills*, in a sense. You can develop bravery by being brave: no other possibility is an option. Becoming a brave athlete (and a brave individual) starts with taking action after you take a risk of such an action, in case of evident threats or adversities. Champions have got straight to the point: they know facing their biggest doubts, fears, pains, and worries are the ultimate challenges to achieving their goals and therefore they actually exercise a huge amount of bravery and courage throughout their lives and sports careers. In fact, they realize that they need to take action if they want to change reality, so the bravery they develop during the battle for their dreams is nothing but a direct consequence. As a recommendation to develop or empower your courage, you ought to follow these steps: (1) shortlist seven things/activities you have always been afraid of and assign a score: 7 is the highest, 1 is the lowest – (2) pick one of them, average score (3-4 points) – (3) start investigating everything related to this activity, to the risks, the threats and also the connection to your emotional balance – (4) convince yourself to take the risk – (5) start taking action: *do this thing*. The so-called *"Circle of Courage"* is a model of individual development based on the principles of *belonging, mastery, independence*, and *generosity*. The Mentally tough athlete, the athlete who set him/herself to become the champion, ought to develop bravery and courage for a few specific features included in the 2nd and 3rd quadrants:

2nd quadrant (*Mastery*): (1) achievement – (2) success – (3) motivation;

3rd quadrant (*Independence*): (1) leadership – (2) inner control – (3) confidence – (4) autonomy.

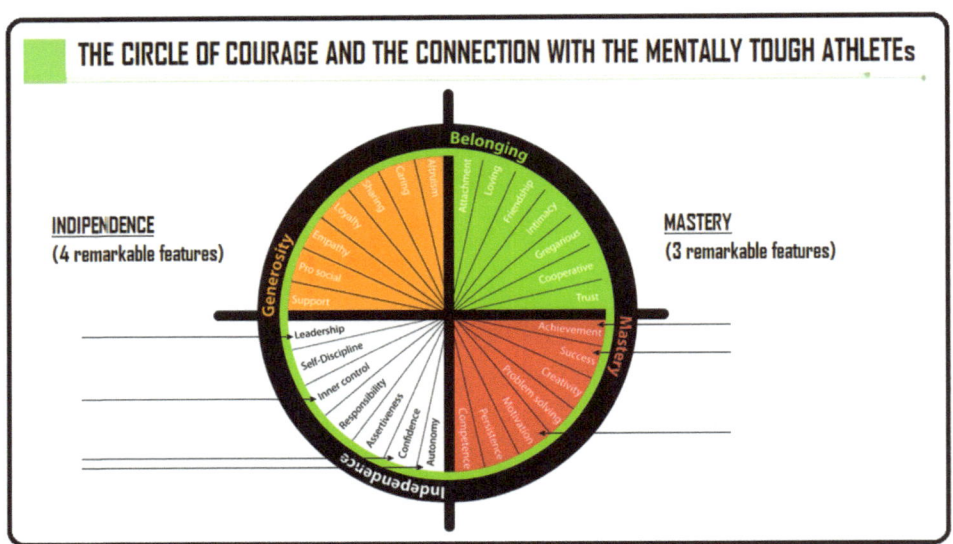

THE CIRCLE OF COURAGE AND THE CONNECTION WITH THE MENTALLY TOUGH ATHLETEs

INDIPENDENCE
(4 remarkable features)

MASTERY
(3 remarkable features)

IF YOU ARE NOT WILLING TO RISK THE UNUSUAL, YOU WILL HAVE TO SETTLE FOR THE ORDINARY.

[JIM ROHN – AMERICAN BESTSELLING AUTHOR, MOTIVATIONAL SPEAKER]

2. **Risk Management**: *The forecasting and evaluation of specific risks together with the identification of procedures to avoid or minimize their impact.*

Together with *Time, Risk* is one of those critical issues that, if handled carelessly, can lead to the collapse of a project. What we consider useful here to underline is the subject's perception of risk and the impact this aspect generates as a consequence. Risk is connected to success, it is immanent in the path of achieving any challenging result. It is the very concept of *"challenge"* that evokes it: if there is a challenge, then it means, by definition, that the amount of psychic and physical commitment required is decidedly superior to any routine task or activity; this also means that the pathway includes additional dangerous and risky aspects which cannot be assessed, because they are unknown. The inconsistency of our modest forecasts associated with the fluidity of the future, which *"semper incertum est"* (fate is always uncertain) and certainly does not protect us from threats, whether internal or external, determines the emersion of risk. Risk is the currency with which success is paid: *"Assess and take your risk and then take action"* the managerial motto suggests, without fear of being proven wrong. Playing the game while taking a certain risk means getting out of your comfort zone. In our comfort zone, everything is familiar to us. We find ourselves immersed in a perfect combination of physical and psychological comforts, small difficulties that are perfectly manageable without affecting our nervous tension, obstacles that are not very significant and never really prejudicial, and the occurrence of sudden episodes, manageable by changing the program of the day.

The Comfort Zone is the substance of the routine that keeps us, like a cog, in the standard process of average and mediocrity (political scientists call this same standardized phenomenon *"mediocracy"*). The assumption of risk, intuitively, coincides with the abandonment of the Comfort Zone that switches to the Discomfort Zone, an area open to operations that could hide threats and obstacles which are unknown (intensity/form), but certainly offers enormous opportunities, equally unknown. Anyone who wants to move from the universe of the average to that of success and excellence is forced to cross the path of discomfort and, consequently, to take the responsibility of managing risks. For many Top/Peak-Performers of all fields, the risk is a necessary element in their journey, it is the fuel of their motivation, the fuel that keeps them awake, in a trance state, to devise the best solutions and reach the goal. The motto of the members of the English SAS is *"Who dares, wins"*, switched to the sports dimension it sounds like *"Who plans, wins"*. Beyond brocades, mottos, and proverbs, what often keeps us from daring is not the lack of courage, but the invasive presence of fear. Courage, in fact, is not opposed to fear: Courageousness is an individual who acts *"despite"* fear suggests the opposite; *courage coexists with fear.* The problem arises when fear, which is essential, because required by the instinct of self-preservation, goes beyond its role of alerting the subject thus paralyzing and preventing him/her from deciding, acting, or reacting. The brave subject takes the risk and acts despite fear. The appearance of fear testifies to the transition from a comfort zone to a discomfort zone. Since it is an instinctive mechanism, fear must certainly not be removed, also because it improves concentration, accelerates actions and decisions, and strengthens the will to try again, in case of failure; it has rather be managed. When fear is triggered by exceptional stimuli (a full-blown threat, for example), a defense mechanism is activated which, in sports jargon, is called *"Reaction Trilemma"*: Fight, Fly, or Freeze, (or fight, fly or become paralyzed). The worst instinctive reaction that can happen is the third because it offers the whole target to the opponent and the impact, at that point, is extremely powerful. Other psychodynamic characteristics related to the sports personality determine the exercise of one of the other options (*fight-fly*). This is what happens on an instinctive, prehistoric, and reptilian level: very effective reactions, but far from logic and rationality. If you want to contrast fear you need to learn how to mediate between instinct responses (*Instinct-Trilemma*) and rational decisions: while doing that you are *"taking a risk"*. Fear is controlled by self-confidence, which is inversely proportional to the degree of self-efficacy (subjective) and self-esteem (equally subjective). It is also manageable through a sense of self-irony that displaces one's internal enemy (which supports and corroborates the feeling of fear). Fear is also manageable through the continuous, systematic, and passionate study of failures; this kind of analysis, if conducted in a sincere way, develops the intuition to *guess the dangers*, anticipating them. The very awareness of *"expecting"* a threat, in a path of discomfort (risk), transforms the *unexpected* event from a threat into a simple obstacle. Finally, fear can be controlled by the attitude of constantly keeping it at bay, offering it the food that it desires; if the object of fear is death, let us constantly offer it this thought: let us keep the mind focused precisely on death; this attitude, typical of the Samurai of the Japanese Middle Ages, exorcises the fear of death in the long run. Managing risk, in essence, means *learning to live with it*, in most cases (PLW: *Prepare to Live With*). It is a part of the job of those who want to excel. You just have to accept this truth: the ways to manage risk come as a direct consequence of applying to become number one.

> RISK, THEN, IS NOT JUST PART OF LIFE. IT IS LIFE. THE PLACE BETWEEN YOUR COMFORT ZONE AND YOUR DREAM IS WHERE LIFE TAKES PLACE. IT'S THE HIGH-ANXIETY ZONE, BUT IT'S ALSO WHERE YOU DISCOVER WHO YOU ARE.
>
> [NICK VUJICIC – AMERICAN SPORT COACH AND MOTIVATIONAL SPEAKER]

3. Non-Conformity: *Failure to match or act like other people or things or a conscious refusal to accept generally accepted beliefs.*

We have already spoken a lot about both uniqueness and how peculiar skills of an athlete should be *"specialized"* and pushed to excellence, so that can be finalized in *"specials"* and to strengthen the UPP: *Unique Performance Proposition*. If appropriately endorsed, uniqueness leads to higher competitiveness and becomes the main resource of a champion. What we have to better focus on, now, is that the uniqueness of an athlete also benefits from the contribution of his/her non-conformity. Extraordinary people are frequently provided with equally extraordinary skills and attitudes. Extraordinary features are *"beyond ordinary"*, which means that there are people who have got unconventional skills and qualities which we can also name *"incompliant"* because they do not comply with standards. They are *"non-conformist"* persons and non-conformist athletes. That makes sense if we consider that the hugest champions seem to be provided with supernatural skills and qualities. What we have to understand, for our specific purpose, is that such an inner non-conformism, when present, must be fed and protected until your personality is strong enough to express itself with as much freedom as possible. The competitiveness of an unconventional athlete is something operational and tangible: needs time, space and open-mindedness to be expressed in the tangible world (the competition, the contest). If we realize we have special skills, we have the personal obligation and commitment to protect them from accusations and judgments from others and to give them the best way to express and affirm themselves. We ought to understand how such a skill might be employed for the final purpose (the victory) and then make them a strength, rather than being ashamed of it (because non-compliant with standards and conventional approaches). For such reasons non-conformity sounds like a huge skill for the Champion: you need huge self-confidence to become who you really are, to behave as you really desire, in a world of conventions.

> GREAT THINGS ARE NOT ACCOMPLISHED BY THOSE WHO YIELD TO TRENDS AND FADS AND POPULAR OPINION.
>
> [JACK KEROUAC — AMERICAN BESTSELLING AUTHOR]

4. **Internal-LOC**: *Locus of control is the degree to which people believe that they, as opposed to external forces (beyond their influence), have control over the outcome of events in their lives.*

Being aware means answering certain seemingly trivial but very powerful questions: *Who am I? Where I am? Where do I want to go? Why do I want to go right there? What choices does my vision involve? What sacrifices am I willing to make to become myself?* Exhaustively answering these questions requires considerable internal work and energy expenditure, but you cannot escape that. The answers include the motivation to action: we cannot ignore such a task. The LOC (*Locus of Control*) expresses the tendency to make the outside world responsible for the events and the impact they have on our personal life. Those who tend to complain and shift responsibilities to the outside have an external LOC; vice versa, those who believe they have been the *"cause of the problem"* or in any case have actively taken part in the determination of an event (*contributing cause*), have a strong internal LOC. Self-efficacy consists in the subjective perception of high competence in a specific area of activity (*"I know how to do that thing well"*), while Resilience does not need to be described. Well, it is neither enough to define the goal, nor to devise an action plan, if you do not first work strictly on your inner matrix. A man who wants to assert himself is aware of himself (self-image as sincere and truthful as possible), has a very solid internal LOC, calmly admits he has areas of self-efficacy, and, above all, is a resistant subject. The combination of these four elements determines the onset of motivation which, little by little, is ridden by the conscience. It manages to activate the resources that are congruent, in quantity and quality, with the effort required to achieve the result. The *Inner Matrix* evolves by challenging our original hypotheses and those limiting beliefs that had kept us stuck. The goal: the same goal that we had intuited and were unable to represent before, today appears specific, detailed, and within the reach of our abilities. The goal, that same goal, is within our reach simply because it was conceived. That goal is the source of the action. Take Action. Your goal will follow.

I AM NOT WHAT HAPPENED TO ME. I AM WHAT I DECIDED TO BECOME.

[CARL GUSTAV JUNG – SWISS PSYCHOLOGIST AND PSYCHIATRIST]

5. **Fearlessness**: *The quality of having no fear. Strength of mind to carry on in spite of the danger.*

The term *"fear"* originates from a distortion of the Latin word *"pavor-paveris"*: fear. This term, in turn, derives from the verb *"fear"* substantiated: *"timeo-es-ui-utum-ēre"*. The root of the verb *"timeo"*, in essence, can be traced back to the origin of the Latin verb *"timēre"*. Linguists and codicils believe that the root of the verb fear originates from ancient Sanskrit: *"tam-rà"*, in the literal meaning of *"obscurity"*, properly alludes to a state of obscuration, disturbance, dulling of the mind. Fear, therefore, has been considered for millennia as the condition in which the mind (therefore: *the rational center*) is darkened by an external agent or an internal agent. It is generally understood as the feeling of strong worry, insecurity, and anguish, which is felt in the presence or at the thought of real or imaginary dangers. Professor Umberto Galimberti describes fear in his Dictionary of Psychology with the following words: *"Primary emotion of defense, caused by a dangerous situation that can be real, anticipated by prediction, evoked by memory or produced by fantasy. Fear is often accompanied by an organic reaction, for which the autonomic nervous system is responsible, which prepares the organism for the emergency situation, arranging it, even if in a non-specific way, to prepare the defenses that usually translate into attitudes of fight and flight."*

Fear is, in fact, a brilliant stratagem that nature has organically inoculated in the living being, which has allowed a strategic evolution of the species, but which has its roots in uncertain and very often misleading. You are afraid of a real threat (which is reasonable and correct), but you are also afraid of an imaginary or eventual threat, which leads to serious problems and uncontrollable pathologies. If it is clear that fear is a contingent tactic that collaborates with the survival instinct, by which the principle of self-preservation is governed, then it will be equally clear that the source of fear (of all fears) is the *fear of death*. It takes different forms and different declinations from man to man, based on experience, the degree of internal/external LOC (*Principle of Responsibility*), deep and latent beliefs, and age. Fear of loneliness, sense of inadequacy, vanity, immanentism (inability to project oneself in the future), inaction, egocentrism, ineffectiveness, mendacity, presumption, victimhood, self-pity, nihilism, identification: all these disabilities, incapacitating and limiting, are psychically related to the fear of death according to a regressive internal dynamic based on the sedimentation of emotional slime that stratifies, year after year, decade after decade, and finally returns to the subject an unbalanced response (the disorder) that can degrade into a real pathology. When focused on an imaginary object or on the possibility that a truly unlikely event occurs, fear turns out to be a terribly harmful element, harmful to the balanced structuring of the personality, hostile and averse to the achievement of results, intended in a perspective of *"evolution of the generic individual"*. Fear must be found, faced, broken down, explored (origin, effects), compromised (negotiated), silenced, or definitively annihilated. When it does not determine real immobility, fear contaminates the rational center of the individual, makes it dysfunctional, determines a psychic/emotional discrepancy, and, consequently, impacts the path of action, in the cycle of success. It basically contaminates the decision-making process (when taking action), but even more often it inhibits the decision itself (inaction). It envelops the primary emotions, pollutes and poisons them by stealing the energy of passion and any other quality useful for evolution or simple manifestation, and transforms an opinion (*limiting opinion*) into conviction (*limiting belief*). From that moment on, the interpretation of reality, which forms the basis of the "*individual representation of reality*" that each individual constructs through his/her own individual perceptual system will be unequivocally based on the "*limiting beliefs*" generated and fed by fear, regardless of the form that this has assumed, settling into the personality of the subject. Until we eradicate these convictions, consequences of specific fears, we are condemned to the failure to which those same convictions aspire, because either everything changes or everything repeats itself forever. It is evident that fear is the intangible representation of our "*Internal Enemy*", which also runs a very tangible power over us, taming our behaviors.

> ONCE YOU BECOME FEARLESS, LIFE BECOMES LIMITLESS.
>
> [ELIO D'ANNA – ITALIAN PHILOSOPHER, LIFE COACH]

6. **Responsibility:** *The state or fact of having a duty to deal with something or of having control over someone.*

Responsibility is certainly a critical element for various reasons. First of all because very often the subject officially burdened with certain responsibilities, fails to fulfill the expectations of those who assigned them, entering into a condition of stress, high psycho-physical tension, and psychological pressure. In the second instance, there is often a dystonia between the attribution of responsibility and the power to make decisions and transform them into actions, to fulfill that specific responsibility. Responsibility is a fundamental element for managerial management as it is for the achievement of any sports result. Responsibility "*includes everything*". Moreover, in common words, some individuals are accused of being "*irresponsible*" in the precise sense of being unaware of the consequences of their actions, or of consciously ignoring them, which should make us reflect. A responsible person simply "*responds*" to the results of his/her actions or is he/she also required to evaluate the consequences of these actions in advance, and therefore to correct them at the decisional stage? In the first case, he is simply a *man of his word*, in the second case he is a *strategist*. Are these elements sufficient, even when combined with each other, to define a responsible person? Is there something missing? The term "*responsibility*" is hardly used, we almost always speak of "*reactivity*", or "*responsiveness*": the quality/ability to offer a quick, timely response, but above all congruent with the scenario and what is happening during the competition. Yet, intuitively, the moment of confrontation with the opponent is a partial moment that does not represent the complexity (and quantity) of the work and commitment of the athlete. As decisive as it is, the competition represents only the apex of effort and concentration, the moment of evidence. We could say that training is *work*, while the match is just a *stage*. There are two kinds of responsibility: *Real Responsibility* (which is a very rare and equally powerful element) and *Mendacious* or *Fictitious Responsibility* (which is completely inconsistent). The first comes from within, it is a quality of being and takes the power needed to be sustained just from the inside. Generally, it is refractory to titles or proxies (it does not need it), it is resistant to criticism, it expresses itself in an evident and tangible way and it is recognized and appreciated by the subjects who benefit from it. The second, otherwise, arises from the outside, it is a *defect of being*, it is fragile and vulnerable because it is based on negotiation (*do ut des*), it is temporary (it is linked to a contractual term), it is considered a weight (or an aggravation) and ends up being detested, blamed and hindered. Finally, responsibility testifies to the quality of the goal we have set ourselves to achieve. "*I want to be the world champion*", he will have confessed to himself any champion of any sport one day, when he was still very far from his goal. That *personal statement* has the force of a contract. He/she took responsibility and that responsibility gave him/her back the resources, a path, and the opportunity to become the best version of him/herself, one day. This assumption gave the strength to fight, attention, concentration, two legs and two arms to be reared patiently, with constancy, a head to protect and a mindset to be strengthened, year after year. If otherwise, the responsibility comes from the outside (*Outside-In Process*), then we must be wary: there will be catastrophes. (1) It may be that the set goal is not (or is no longer) "*ecological*" or coherent and in harmony with other goals achieved (family, personal interests, economic interests); (2) it may be that the goal is not (or is no longer) "*corresponding*", in the sense that the athlete is no longer really motivated to achieve it; (3) it may be that he is not actually able to direct or handle pressure with sufficient emotional distance, being overwhelmed by events; (4) it could be that the athlete has difficulties in making rational decisions, because they involve too many resources close to him (sense of guilt); (5) finally, it could be that he is not sufficiently competent to carry out the role. In all these cases it fatally happens that the level of psychophysical stress exceeds the *Performance Balance Point* so far (the so-called IPS: *Ideal Performance State*). Ultimately, the responsibility of an athlete should be intended as a long-life "*journey into being*" in search of one's motivation and the definition of everything we wish to sacrifice to achieve a goal, an enhancement of such a goal, remembering that everything, always, springs from an "*inner yes*", that everything is born in the invisibility of our essence and then solidifies in reality. *Visibilia ex invisibilibus*, Latin used to say: the visible comes from invisible.

RESPONSIBILITY IS ACCEPTING THAT YOU ARE THE CAUSE AND THE SOLUTION OF THE MATTER.

[GEORGE IVANOVITCH GURDJIEFF – ARMENIAN PHILOSOPHER, AUTHOR]

72 – Threats

If you cannot handle uncertainty, then you have to know that you can learn how to cope with it. If you don't want to, you'd better become familiar with failure. Even though it is not evident to our eyes, no real goal is achievable without running a risk. A sized and pondered risk, but a risk is run, definitely. If you don't learn how to detect, size, and manage risks, you are condemned to the first level of competition: *victory is always uncertain to happen* because is affected by possible occurrences which you did not predict in advance. You are condemned to improvisation, to a feeling of being unprepared. If you don't learn how to cope with fear, you are condemned to permanent psychic imprisonment. About the threats in case of violation:

#	FACTOR	POSSIBLE THREAT
1	PROPENSITY TO RISK	• Losing chances • Talent locked
2	RISK MANAGEMENT	• The unexpected turns to failures • Incorrect reactions
3	NON-CONFORMITY	• Routine • Non-risk-taking athlete
4	INTERNAL LOC	• Complaining • Fear of external environment • Difficulties turn to inabilities
5	FEARLESSNESS	• Behaviours imprisoned • Creativity is locked • Paralysis
6	RESPONSIBILITY	• Constant complaining • Suffering others' plans • Rage and bad emotions

1 You prefer avoiding rather than approaching: your fixed mindset will prevent you from succeeding because only in the heart of the action, the chance comes out clearly. You will lose chances and your talent will be kept locked and unknown.

2 Unpreparedness is what happens to whom doesn't feel well in facing uncertainties and, when forced, cannot manage to handle and overturn the situation. You will react incorrectly because you will fall into the *"Instinct-Trilemma"* (Fight/Fly/Freeze) without any plan in your hands. Unpredictable occurrences will lead you straight to failure because you do not know *"what to do"*, or how to react.

3 Conventional routines drive conventional athletes. Conventional athletes are not champions, but can only aspire to be good/average athletes. Your arsenal will remain poor and locked, limited by your weak attitude to risk-taking.

4 Risk-avoidance, unwillingness to learn from failures, unfamiliarity to deal with uncertainties, and compliance to conventional rules will slowly bring you towards a loser attitude: systematic complaining, alibis, fear of eternal environment, and, finally, the progressive transformation of your current difficulties into inabilities. All of these preventing features depend on your inner belief that the world controls you in spite of vice-versa.

5 Fear and being scared of fear itself lead you to psychic imprisonment. You enter a vicious circle from which you cannot escape easily. In fact, fear is crucially important because forces your attitude to focus on risks, pressure, and threats. You do not have to put your fear *"in front of you"*, but *"behind you"*, so that you will feel motivated to run, to take action, and to execute tasks. If you do not face and overcome your fear, your creativity will remain locked and your best potential behaviors will remain unknown because imprisoned by invisible chains. So take action, rather than postpone.

6 The world wants you as its slave. The world needs most of the people feeling psychologically imprisoned and limited to support the choices and the projects of a few ones, who take responsibility for their business. The first segment is the workforce which is needed to achieve the projects of the second segment of people. You need to decide which segment you want to belong to. If you take full responsibility, you will be given all the resources needed to achieve your goal: physical, mental, and financial. Otherwise, you will always be complaining, suffering others' plans, and full of rage and bad emotions.

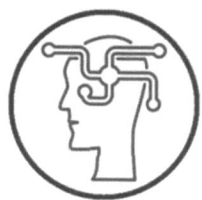

73 – Opportunities

When fearless, you become brave and courageous. You can actually affirm yourself as an intact human being. You are capable of acting according to your will and ethics to fulfill your desires, in spite of reacting to offenses that somehow are related to fear. When fearless, you can catch your uniqueness and turn it into a competitive weapon to succeed. When fearless, you are free: ready to succeed in any contest you like.

#	FACTOR	STRATEGIC ADVANTAGE
1	PROPENSITY TO RISK	• Catching more chances • Talent is unlocked
2	RISK MANAGEMENT	• No huge surprises • Appropriate reactions
3	NON-CONFORMITY	• Free expressions of your uniqueness
4	INTERNAL LOC	• Control your world/sports-career • Creates chances to victory
5	FEARLESSNESS	• Living your inner essence • Being one • Integrity
6	RESPONSIBILITY	• Internal LOC very high • Increasing your arsenal according to your will

1 A strong propensity to risk will enable you to catch more chances, not only during competition but even in ordinary life. Your sports career will be enriched accordingly. Your talent will progressively be unlocked and you will start thinking bigger. Even your self-image and your self-confidence will be awarded and empowered.

2 Managing the risk in the appropriate way will enable you to control the tournament from a strategic and tactical perspective. You will react accordingly to surprises because you should have already planned them in advance. You will switch to the second level of the competition: *Compete after winning.*

3 Self-confidence, added to a strong self-image, will facilitate catching and exploiting your inner special talents. Your uniqueness will become one of your weapons in winning the competitions. You will enter the winners' cycle.

4 When you understand that everything depends on you, that everything which you may control must be under your unique control, you have entered that special pathway to become a champion. You will not complain anymore about anything and you will create circumstances to apply your uniqueness and chances for victory.

5 Fearlessness will free you and will allow you to behave as *"one"*. Will progressively lead you to spiritual and social integrity

6 *It's none of your business: it's my business!* This might be the statement of the responsible athlete, in a sense. Everything depends on you, every goal is up to you. Great responsibility, but you're equally given all that you need to execute such a responsibility. Your huge goal will give you resources: the huger the goal is, the better the resources will be. Your Internal-LOC will be increased accordingly and you will become good at increasing your arsenal depending on your will and your efforts. You define the limit because *you are the limit*, and you bear this in your mind very clearly.

74 – Methodologies

The primary psychic factors related to Adaptation are the following:

- Risk Management —
- Internal LOC —
- Fearlessness —
- Responsibility —

The methodologies for empowering these factors are actually based on psychic skills and competencies.

Precisely explore and study any crucial action and shortlist everything which may happen as a consequence, if you made that action. Try separating possible risks from threats and from current risks. Then learn how to quickly assess the risk by applying a cost/benefits mental model, then make your decision. For any action, for any circumstance, for any level of competition. Try this during a gym training session before applying to an official match. Try, experiment, assess the result and understand. Do this lots of time, then you get ready to use risk assessment during an official competition.

Risk Management will enable you progressively decrease your fear. Why? Because you are experiencing what fear is, because you're actually confronting the risk of an action that creates fear. Because you're progressively embracing your fear and you will become able to put fears behind you and run towards success, in spite of keeping them in front of you and being stuck. Face your fears in any possible training session: run against your fears, so that you can destroy them, finally.

Responsibility and Internal LOC are strictly connected and recall your self-confidence, your self-effectiveness, your ambition, and your sense of control. Create lots of circumstances rationally, and consciously, and turn these circumstances into achievements. Experience continuously your power to affect, adapt and create reality and you'll be increasing both your Internal-LOC and your sense of responsibility.

PILLAR # 07 - ADAPTATION

	TOPIC	GOAL	ACTION	EXERCISE	REPETITION
1	RISK MANAGEMENT	Apply bravery to competition Exploit each opportunity Reduce the risks	Think of an action Breakdown the risk connected Assess the risks Find a solution	Create situations Make your choice and finalize See the risk running (in action)	Once per week Long Life work
2	INTERNAL LOC	Full control of external events Strong mix of Mindset Tools Philosophic attitude to victory	Create conditions Enter the contest Do the job and finalize	Find the internal causes of effects (outside-in process) Make the right connections	Long Life job
	FEARLESSNESS	Express your inner self	Explore your inner self Haunt your fears See the cause of your fears	Create fearful scenarios Go through those scenarios Face your fears and win	Long Life job
3	RESPONSIBILITY	Internal LOC increase All things related to you The owner of your own destiny	Select your project Take full ownership Finalize time-bounded targets	Pick the effects Find the connections Explain reasons and causes of these connections	Long Life job

75 – Practical Techniques

The "*Yes-Attitude*" will enhance this skill: take action, have fun doing lots, and do not be scared of failing. This is a good definition of Propensity to Risk.

Risk Management is strictly related to the propensity to risk and is crucial to catch multiple chances during a competition. You need to: (1) realize the presence of a risk – (2) decline the risk (quality/size) – (3) define the impact of any risk (low/medium/high) – 4) prepare a contingency plan for any risk – (5) manage the risk: *erase – reduce – prepare to live with* – (6) go to action and perform at your best.

You need to be provided with strong self-confidence to affirm your precious Non-Conformity because you might be contaminated by possible effects of criticism coming from your opponents, coaches, companions, and even from your audience. You must be compliant with the code of ethics and the rules of the sport, but you should not ever give up your uniqueness. So take action, affirm yourself, and ignore criticism and blame coming from outside. Make your results talk on your behalf.

Internal LOC is strictly related to both your code of ethics and your inner philosophy and sense of responsibility. Consciousness is the key, added to your sense of responsibility. These two generate beliefs that activate resources; decision follows, then action and achievements. You need to understand what is really under your control. Try realizing that, most parts of the events you have been involved in: (1) either had been influenced by you (when conscious), (2) or you were completely subjected (unconscious).

Self-confidence, added to a strong self-image and to self-control, can facilitate the emersion of a crucial state, for the Champion and the Peak-Performer: *fearlessness*. If you want to get such a crucial state you need to develop those skills first, and you will equally get a kind of courage that enables you to do the right thing at the right moment with the appropriate amount of energy. Fearlessness is achieved by taking decisive actions and proving to yourself that: (1) you can do that, you can achieve, in spite of your original fear – (2) nothing crucial happens if you fail – (3) you can take profit from both a victory and from a failure: lots of lessons to learn, to prepare yourself challenging your fears again. Before taking action, you ought to find the real causes of your fears, which are directly related to the exploration of your inner self vulnerabilities.

When you get a strong sense of Responsibility you feel any business you are involved in is totally yours: you respond to yourself about resources, motivation, organization, and results. Your sense of responsibility can only be developed as long as you work on your internal-LOC empowerment. In addition to that, you can apply these crucial recommendations: (1) stop lying to yourself and to others – (2) do not identify any more – (3) do not express negative emotions – (4) stop making excuses for yourself – (5) stop complaining – (6) learn how to manage your resources – (7) overcome procrastination – (8) be consistent and stick to your schedule – (9) start realizing nothing ever happens by chance – (10) start realizing your life is the projection of your conscious activities and of your level of being. In short: if you want to counteract your external LOC, you must resist routine habits.

76 – Powerful Questions

Use these questions to force yourself (as an athlete) or your coachees to switch to a higher mental perspective and unlock additional energy to keep being in the right direction. All the questions require specific and honest answers which may also take a few minutes or more, to be developed.

> 1.1 Do You think you feel comfortable in presence of risk? Why? Are you able to manage the risk? Are you capable of declining all the risks connected to an event? I mean: *possible, current,* and *actual* risk?

✓ *Your attitude to risk-propensity and to uncertainty is tested. Your ability in running a risk is tested as well.*

❏

> 1.2 What is the difference between *possible, current,* and *actual* risk? Explain.

✓ *SAME.*

❏

> 1.3 Define expected and unexpected events: do risks only come from unexpected events? Why?

✓ *SAME.*

❏

> 1.4 What is your natural reaction against *actual risk* (threat)? How do you handle that?

✓ *Your level of resilience, of adversity-challenging, of managing the risk is tested.*

❏

> 1.5 Do you think a tournament might be won without running any risk?

✓ *Your opinion is required, but your answer is equally testifying the size of your commitment.*

❏

> 1.6 Do you think you have to win *"managing the risk"*? How do you assess the risk?

✓ *Risk assessment is not a talent, but a competence that needs to be developed.*

☐

➤ 1.7 Any risk is hiding a big opportunity: talk about that, and explain your point on this subject.

✓ *SAME. The two points are connected: any competition includes risks (to be run), which can be turned into chances.*

☐

➤ 2.1 Risk may influence your behavior when performing: how do you react in such a case? Which kind of chances may be hidden in a huge risk?

✓ *SAME.*

☐

➤ 2.2 *Fight/Fly/Freeze* added to *Routine/Disturb/Emergency*-Model: explain the connection, based on your experience.

✓ *Help yourself using the following pattern:*

	(WORK)	FIGHT	FLY	FREEZE
ROUTINE				
DISTURB				
EMERGENCY				

☐

➤ 2.3 Risk escalation: maybe facing the upcoming risk could reduce the final impact: how much are you confident with this? Why? Explain through an experience in an official tournament.

✓ *Your familiarity with Risk-Running is tested.*

☐

➤ 3.1 Rules: what do you think about rules?

✓ *You need to be aware of your actual level of discipline. This figure depends on your definition of "Rule".*

☐

➤ 3.2 A champion is familiar with *breaking the rules*: what is your opinion about this topic?

✓ *Your opinion is asked. Your answer includes your openness or limiting belief about this topic.*

☐

➤ 3.3 You think you have *some kind of uniqueness*: how much do you feel confident in expressing your eccentricity, your *unique electricity*? Do you know how to express it in an unpretentious way?

✓ *Honest and better knowledge of yourself is needed.*

❒

➤ 3.4 How much are you sensitive to others' judgments? How come? Why do you need to fulfil others' expectations? What do you believe this judgment may add to your training and to your performance?

✓ *Your sensitivity to others' expectations can destroy your performance. You need to be aware of such a risk.*

❒

➤ 4.1 In your opinion: why does an event happen? Why does this event happen the way it happens?

✓ *Your sincere opinion on this topic is strongly needed. Your future depends on your opinion and position on this matter.*

❒

➤ 4.2 How much influence do you think you can have on the external environment? Why? How do you think you can increase this percentage?

✓ *The strength of your Internal-LOC is tested.*

❒

➤ 4.3 What is the limiting belief preventing you from taking charge of everything which happens to you, in your small world?

✓ *SAME, from another perspective.*

❒

➤ 4.4 When you fail: whose is the responsibility? Whose is the fault? Why?

✓ *SAME, from another perspective.*

❒

➤ 4.5 There are two possibilities: (1) being a *pawn* – (2) being the *chess checker*. Which segment do you belong to? Which segment you would like to belong to? How do you prepare yourself to have such an influence on the outside world?

✓ *SAME, but you need to go in deep and formulate your powerful conjectures to overcome.*

❒

➢ 5.1 What is "*fear*" in your opinion?

✓ *Your definition, which is probably based on your past experiences and on your current and unresolved issues, is required.*

❒

➢ 5.2 How does fear influence your behavior and your performance?

✓ *Your psychic balance, the quality of your self-image, and your sincerity are tested.*

❒

➢ 5.3 What are your fears? Which desires are these fears connected to?

✓ *Start exploring your fears.*

❒

➢ 5.4 Find a way to connect to your internal and hidden side: you ought to catch your real fears and explore them. Remember: when you are capable of seeing your fears, you have started the process of self-healing.

✓ *As soon as you "see" your fears, you've already started the process of healing. So start at the soonest.*

❒

➢ 6.1 Are you a responsible person? Why do you define yourself this way?

✓ *Your definition is required.*

❒

➢ 6.2 What is the connection between reliability and responsibility?

✓ *SAME.*

❒

➢ 6.3 Being responsible means that you are the sole owner of your business: are you such a person?

✓ *Is that ever really possible? Are you such a kind of person? Explain the reason why, bring yourself the evidence.*

❒

➢ 6.4 Are you such an athlete?

✓ *SAME, from a sports perspective.*

❒

➢ 6.5 What do you think you need to prove to yourself that everything is influenced by your sense and behavior related to responsibility? How think you can increase such a conviction?

✓ *Start developing powerful conjectures on that.*

❏

➢ 6.6 In fact responsibility means that becoming a world champion only depends on you and on your level of being. Do you think that this sentence is true? Why?

✓ *Your inner Code of Ethics is explored and tested.*

77 – Instructions & Recommendations

The PRO attitude makes you do the right thing in the appropriate situation: the technical and tactical circumstance asks the contender for a special solution and the solution comes in the form of execution. The champion's mindset overcomes such an essential pragmatism. The champion applies the best solution which fits both circumstances, time, and requirements, and finalizes the action to a mix of elegance, effectiveness, and technical beauty. The champion is provided with a complete repertoire and can rely on a strong arsenal. The battlefield is the way to express his/her UPP (*Unique Performance Proposition*). Doing the right thing at the right time according to excellent technical standards. You need to overcome fear, to perform in such a way. Fear of failing, first of all, of not being lucid enough in that crucial moment, of getting wrong. The champion knows that everything may never happen, but he/she has focused *on controllability* and acts accordingly. There is no compromise: the champion chooses the best solution and executes his/her possible best. When in the flow, the champion *cannot even choose*: the gesture and the action express themselves on the battlefield. The actions obey to circumstances and cross the champion to express their best.

Do not ever think that the crucial victory may come by chance. Nothing great may ever come unless great efforts have been engaged. Your crucial victory will be something you have built precisely, the set of circumstances which match your strong action.

As we already know, *Fear* is one of those crucial items which may definitely influence the emotional balance of an athlete and, as a consequence, may strongly affect, reduce or even invalidate the performance, in any field. Fear is a natural, powerful, and primitive human emotion. It involves a universal biochemical response as well as a high individual emotional response. Fear forces an individual to cope with the *Instinct Trilemma* if you're not trained to offer a different and rational response: *Fight – Fly – Freeze*. Fear is crucial and powerful, but fear is even necessary and irrepressible. Nevertheless, fear might be managed, reduced, and mastered. That's what you have to do.

Fear is controlled with confidence – The first way to contrast fear is to mature a strong perception of being prepared to face it and such an inner perception can only be developed with preparation. Training, preparation, and direct experience of fear are 3 primary tools to cope with fear. People feel naturally scared by the unknown, is a natural emotional response, is human, and, finally, is a direct consequence of the instinct of self-preservation: *avoiding the unknown*. Coping with fear, therefore, is a matter of becoming lucid and rationalizing the cause of fear: such activity requires strong training and preparation. Skills and training are practiced constantly to the point where it becomes second nature (it puts an *automatic response* in the brain's computer) to the point where it becomes even boring, so that, when an athlete is facing a threat, he/she already knows how exactly defusing that situation. Such a strategy includes the following: (a) definition of the cause of the fear and of the fear itself – (b) the creation of realistic scenarios/simulations which even include a real threat – (c) taking action in the situation and fixing it – (d) when effectively fixed, do lots and lots of time.

Fear is controlled with humor – Laughing in the face of fear has been proven to be one of the most effective ways to reduce stress, panic, and all the emotional impulses which emerge in case of fear. Some Champions and Peak-Performers set themselves a challenge to laugh every day on selections courses to lessen the strain and pressure. In fact *"Humor is about playing with ideas and concepts"*. So, whenever we see something as funny, we're looking at it from a different perspective. Humor is another way to utilize imagery and mental visualization. In short: when we apply humor to a crucial and critical situation, equally not urgent, we are unconsciously exploiting our skills of imagery and visualization, we are exploring the risky situation, in a sense. Such an attitude lets another perspective clearly emerge and affirm itself on the original one. You can easily resize the risk and regain control and self-confidence, time by time.

Fear is controlled by keeping it at the forefront of your mind – This mental hack was intensely utilized by the ancient warriors of ancient Japan. Both *ancient Samurai* (but also *Thai warriors* in Thailand) got used to keeping fear at the forefront of their minds. They were trained to have death (and all the fears which from death descend) as their primary thought in their mind: continuously, systematically, intensively. The core principle was that the real warrior, to be courageous, brave, effective, even honest, and spiritually intact, had to think about death any time of the day. A samurai should always be prepared to die: whether his own or someone's else. If he engaged in combat fully determined to die, he would have overcome his opponents and would have been alive; if he wished to survive in the battle, he would have surely met death. The amazing thing about fear is that when you run to it, it runs away. Another way to express such a concept is that postponing, due to fear, makes you a coward while taking action defeats fear. So you have to assess the risk and you need to take action: you have to embrace your fear.

Fear is controlled by studying failure – Spend time studying failure: analyze, learn the lesson, and forget. All too often we focus on the successes of others, overlooking their failures. But if we did both, including analyzing failed plans, we would dispel fear as we then apply that information. Studying victories and applying their lessons exactly whilst expecting similar outcomes is just as illogical as repeating mistakes and expecting different results. Sway that fear by analyzing your plans from all angles, different perspectives, and rational criteria. Navy Seals use to say that the word *"FEAR"* spells itself out: *False Evidence Appearing Real.*

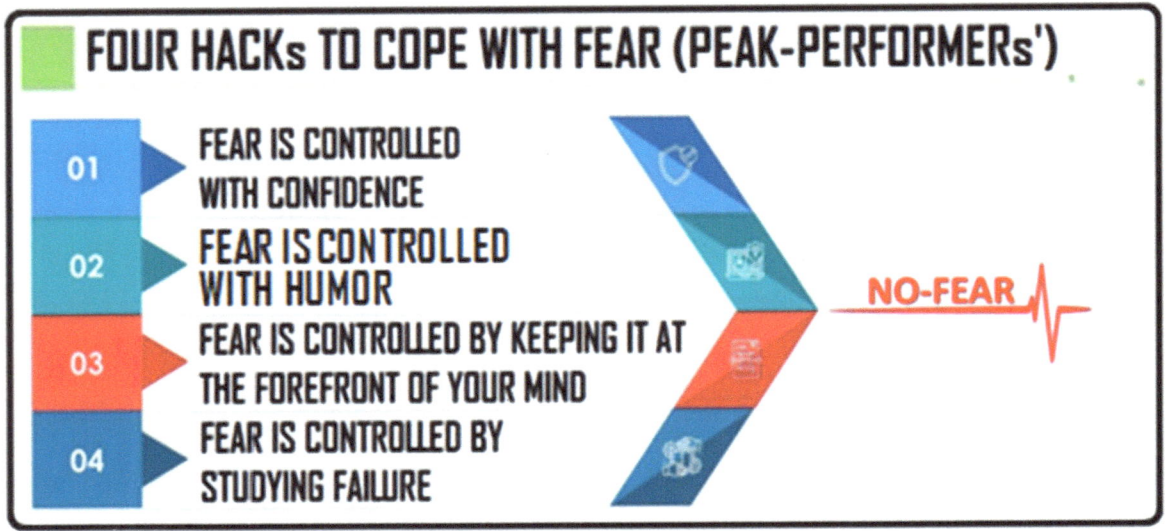

You need to learn how to play your game mentally. Such a practice is very effective and is very frequently utilized by champions, peak performers, and soldiers. They learn how to cope with difficult or crucial situations in their mind: the systematic and continuous repetition of visualization generates "*imagery*", which is a kind of psychometric skill very useful to face crucial situations without stress. You learn to play your game thousands of times, to fine-tune your movements and gestures, to fail and correct your moves and strategies and stand back. You learn how to win, before winning: a kind of theoretical training to prepare you to handle victories and success. The core concept which lies behind such a practice is that "*if you can imagine it, you can achieve it*" (and vice-versa). You know that visualization will be of benefit to you when you realize you want to control the way you act in a particular situation. Using visualization, athletes have been able to face their fears, of heights or open water (for example). You need to follow the 5-steps process to strengthen your imagery skills:

1) *Relax the body.* Spend five minutes taking deep breaths and sitting quietly, undisturbed.

2) *Picture yourself in a stressful situation*, the situation you want to change, but you performing calmly and in control.

3) *Visualize the scenario* with as much detail as possible, appealing to all five of your senses. Imagine the weather, the people around you, the sights, and the smells. Imagine your opponent, the referee, or the audience. Try to hear the noises of the match, the shot of the start. Try hearing your name spoken by the megaphone.

4) *Be realistic.* If you are imagining running a marathon, for instance, imagine being hungry, hot, and tired as you would be on the day. Nonetheless, imagine yourself overcoming those obstacles. See the obstacles and see yourself overcoming them: see your efforts, see your face, see your inner smile.

5) Focus on how you feel after your success. How does the success make you feel? Attach yourself to that feeling. Create an *emotional anchor.*

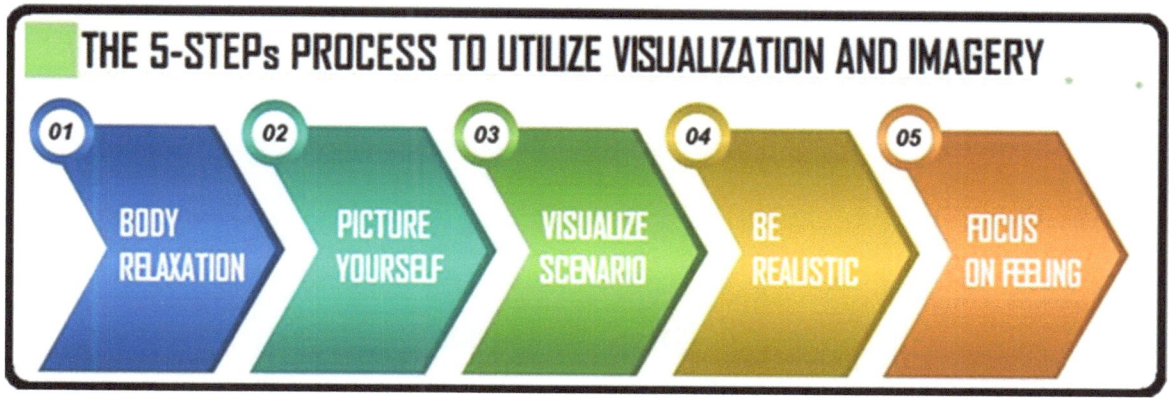

Amateurs, low-quality athletes, and individuals tend to create invisible barriers which surround them. They find themselves imprisoned in a mental jail. There are no iron bars preventing them from escaping, only limiting beliefs. The primary conviction which holds these individuals back from moving and from setting for a career jump is the responsibility: they are convinced that they are (and will ever be) victims of the powerful people, of the government, of the outside world, including rules, poverty, unluckiness, hurdles, illness. The champions have a completely opposite perspective: they deeply feel and rationally know the world is abundant and start operating supported by their spirit-self. They really think they are responsible. The three stages of the evolutionary process are the following: *I am a victim → I am not responsible for what happens to me → I take responsibility → I am completely responsible.* You need to become a responsible person and athlete, so you will progressively tend to be unafraid, aggressive, an ultra-competitive warrior who approaches life and competitions like a battle. As soon as you take responsibility for your life and career, your internal LOC will start increasing, as a consequence.

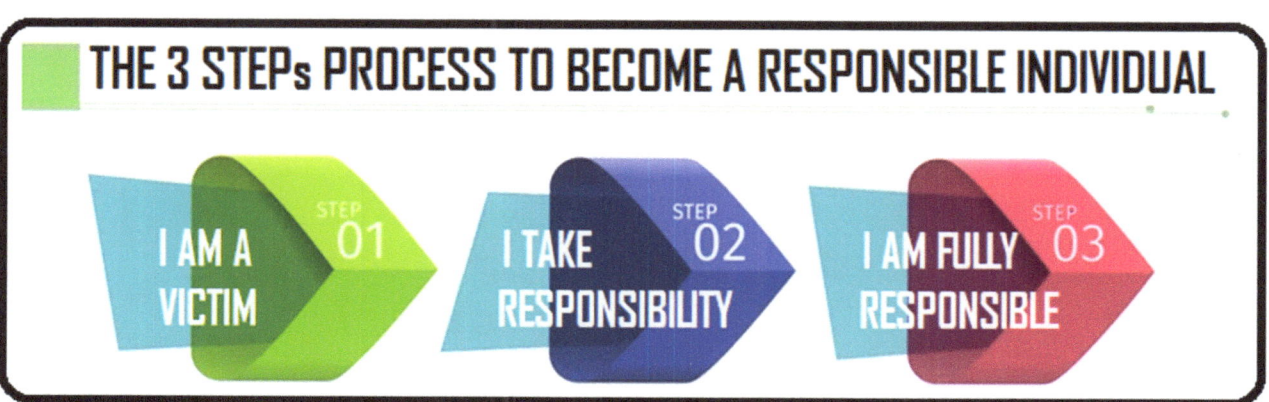

CHAPTER TEN

PEAK PERFORMER's PROFILES

78 – The Five MINDSET's TOOLs

The *8 Pillars Model* can be made simpler. I am talking about a match with another quicker model which is called *"5 Tools Mindset"*, according to which the Sport Mindset can be factorized into 5 integrated tools which include the whole that we have gone through until now and that, in the best case scenario, work together at the unison. Each of these 5 tools must be considered *"complete"* and gives it contribute to the final goal (*the Mindset*) in harmony with the other tools. There is a clear connection between the two models and among the relevant Pillars/Tools:

1. Courage + Physical Training mental features ↔ *STRONG DESIRE*
2. Self-Consciousness ↔ *CONSCIOUS AWARENESS*
3. Tactical/Strategic mental features ↔ *SUBCONSCIOUS MIND*
4. Adaptation + Tactical/Strategic mental features ↔ *FOCUS*
5. Clarity of Destination + Self Consciousness ↔ *SELF-IMAGE*

The *5 Tools Mindset*, as far as the *8 Pillars Model*, affirms that only when these 5 tools are present (and are enough developed) and work together in the unison, coexisting in the same individual, the *Peak-Performance* emerges (The *Contender*). This easy model enables us to present a short list of the profiles of the performers, changing significantly the characteristics and the features depending on the total absence or the mis-functionality of one of the tools (or more). You are required to understand *who you are* (which is the profile that better fits yours) before applying to *who you want to become*. This model can easily facilitate your understanding of which profile you currently belong to and, as a second step, you must start applying the relevant recommendations included in the profile.

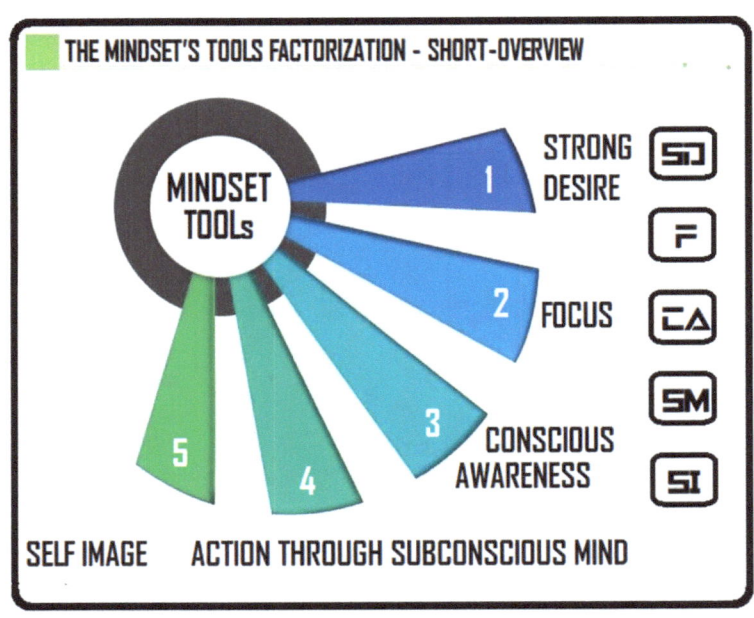

79 – The Performer's Profile

As a recap we already know the performance of a generic athlete, no matter if practicing an individual/collective or situational/endurance sport discipline, depends on four areas:

1) Coordinative capabilities
2) Conditional capabilities
3) Technical and Strategic competences
4) Psychic competences

We have previously divided the *Psychic Skills* into 8 Pillars, which include the whole of the primary and secondary psychic, mental, and emotional skills (55, to be precise). We have declined each of these Pillars into the relevant factors and we have gone through any of these, enriching the topic with details, advices, and recommendations. These Pillars define the structure of the Sports Mindset and we have also simplified this model into a *5 Tools Mindset Model*, which presents only 5 Factors (or *Tools*). What you have to recall to your mind is that the IPS (*Ideal Performance State*) of a Champion comes from the first 3 physical areas (1: Coordinative capabilities – 2: Conditional capabilities – 3: Technical and Strategic competencies) added to the Sports Mindset. The perfect Sports Mindset is represented, in fact, by the 5 Tools Mindset model. Just figure out a piece of hard and precious rock made up of 5 fundamental elements present at a state of remarkably high quality, five dynamic elements that coexist and collaborate effectively and consistently.

This is what you need to achieve if you want to switch to the higher level, if you want your psycho-physical engine to start doing incredible things entering the flow of the peak performance. You must first develop each of the components (the 8 Pillars – the 5 Tools) and then make them cooperate and work together at their best potential. You need to work hard to achieve this special *rock piece* if you want to succeed, because quality always beats quantity.

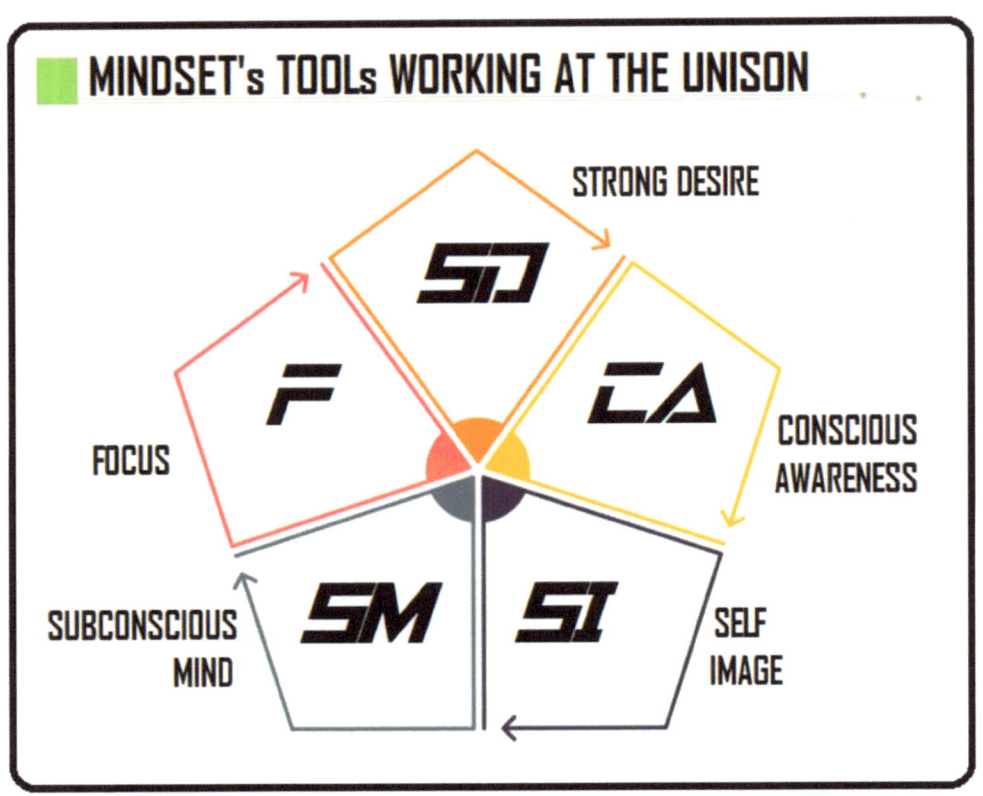

80 – The Rookie

The Rookie is the kind of athlete who *has not done enough*, yet. For this reason, most part of the Rookie's training program is based on conditioning, technical gestures, and on actions. To the Rookie everything is new and for this reason, the coach, the companions, and the instructions are crucial. *The subconscious Mind* is totally absent or does not work properly, because the automated, instinctual, and subconscious routines which deal with tactics, strategy, and the state of inner self-perceived consciousness, are all skills which need a very robust athletic and technical background, on which basis they can be developed. In fact, the Rookie is a good athlete, full of motivation and great potential, but very far from performing at a higher level. He/she is actually what the evidence reveals to be: *no hidden virtue, no hidden skill, and no strategic spirit at all*. It's all action, push, and extra-push of energy, which ought to be appropriately driven and addressed toward a strategic goal.

Characteristics: The Rookie Profile Performer:

- His/her conscious thoughts process everything.
- Is driven by a strong desire and a strong motivation.
- Most of the residual mental tools work properly.
- Needs evidence: observation of actions, learning by doing, emulation, receiving frequent coaching sessions.

Temperament: Aggressive, direct, determined, willing to learn, easy-taking actions, willing to have multiple experiences.

Strengths: Motivation, determination, sacrifice, devotion.

Weaknesses: Weak strategic tools and competencies, low self-image, a soldier rather than a warrior, depending on the team and on the coach.

Missing Mindset Tool: *SUBCONSCIOUS MIND*

Call To Action: Development of the Subconscious Mind (→ Tactical/Strategic mental features):

- Needs to learn and apply Tactical gestures and actions.
- Needs to develop a stronger Vision and to refer to the big-picture, constantly.
- Needs to become familiar with Strategic Planning, with B-Planning, and to apply and execute Strategies.
- Needs to enhance all the competencies related to self-consciousness.

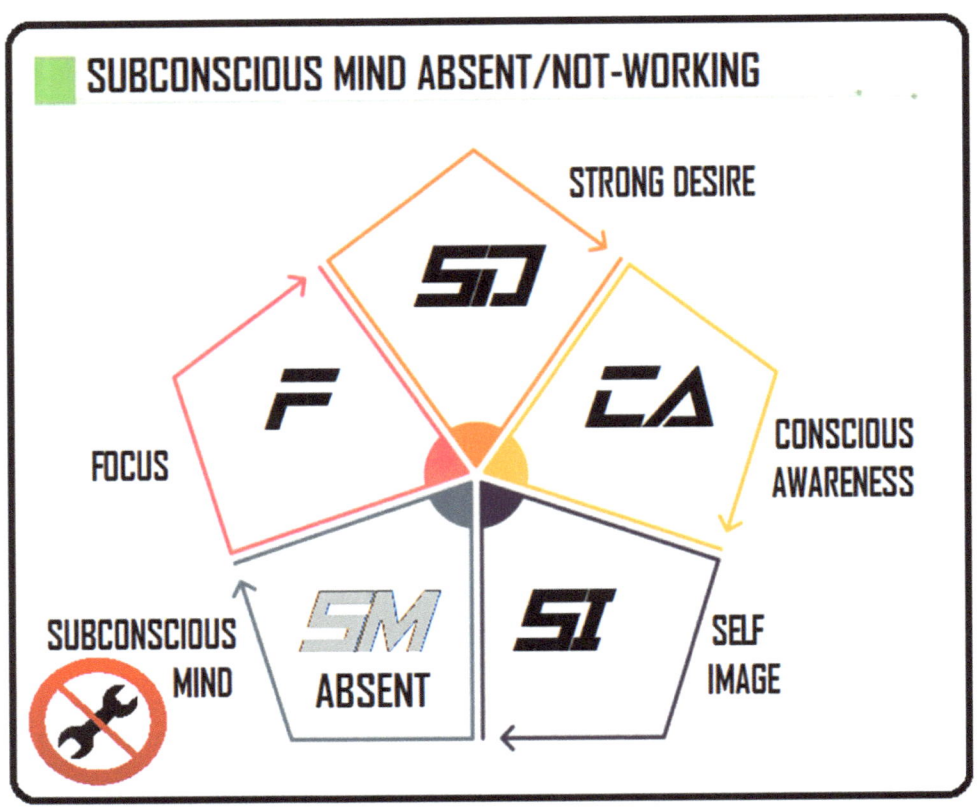

81 – The Spectator

The Spectator is the kind of athlete who is strongly passionate and even determined to struggle and to train harder and harder, but is strongly scared of confrontation with others: coach, companions, opponents, competitions, and even collective training sessions. The Spectator is basically afraid to venture up, to experience new missions, to go to action. He/she is not provided with good endurance and with adequate physical shape, even though the other tools are managed and even mastered at a good/high level.

Characteristics: The Spectator Profile Performer:

- His/her conscious thoughts and fears prevent actions/ventures.
- Is driven by psychic and rational desires.
- He/she keeps very high control of emotions and pulsions.
- Most of the residual mental tools work properly.
- Needs lots of confirmations before entering the contest.

Temperament: Calm, submissive, fearful, polite, avoids contact, avoids any involvement, low-profile attitude.

Strengths: Emotions control, self-improvement attitude, critical-thinking attitude.

Weaknesses: No self-confidence, fear, scared to take action, low propensity to risk, physically exhausted, lots of psychic barriers.

Missing Mindset Tool: *STRONG DESIRE*

Call To Action: Development of the Subconscious Mind (→ Courage + Physical Training mental features):

- Start taking action to get more comfortable.
- Let the courage emerge, to venture up.
- Increase the training sessions (*frequency* + *intensity*) and force any kind of physical confrontation.
- Develop a self-effectiveness attitude (*do once good, then do lots*).
- Challenge and combine fears + what creates obstacles.
- Develop perseverance and persistence.

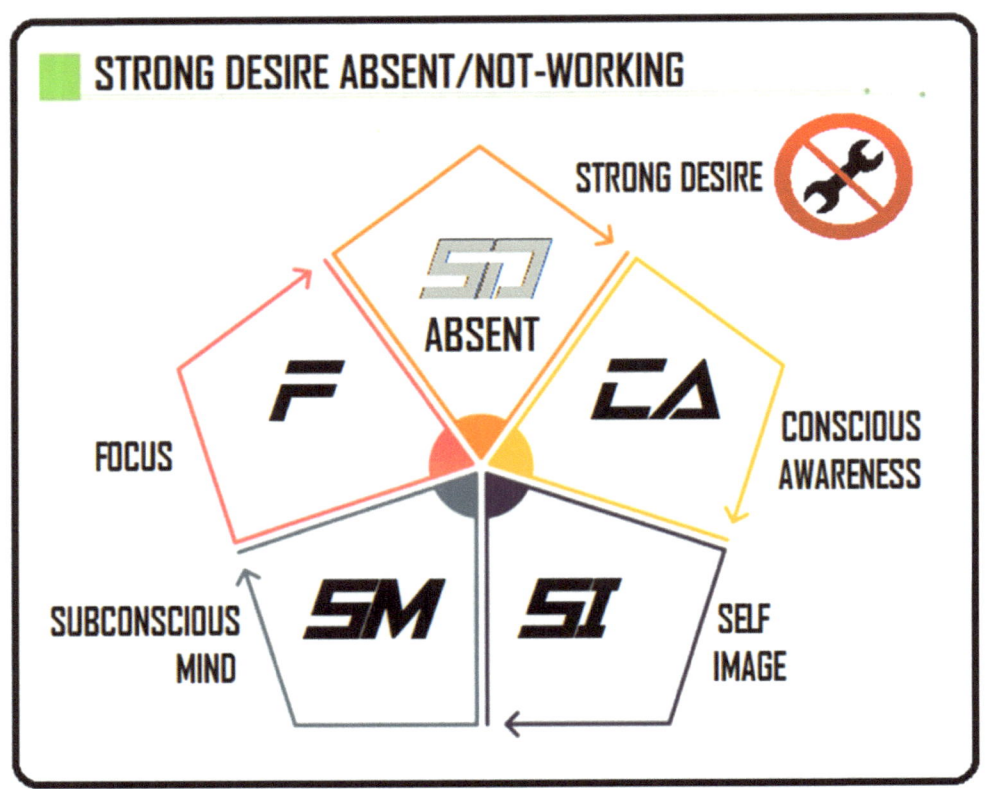

82 – The Participant

The Participant is the kind of athlete who has started to take action so far and the results which have been easily achieved had strengthened his/her self-confidence and self-effectiveness. Participant partakes in any event, any collective session, and masterclass and usually enjoys and succeeds.

Characteristics: The Participant Profile Performer:

- Partakes in any sports events (training sessions, competitions, masterclasses).
- Always strengthen his/her self-confidence in achieving new targets.
- Most of the residual mental tools work properly.
- He/she is focused on what seems needed to be done (his/her own belief).
- Wants to succeed.
- Does not think of him/herself as a winner (yet).
- Considers him/herself as a good *"Team Player"*, but nothing more.

Temperament: Calm, polite, humble and correct, discreet, an orderly soldier.

Strengths: Humility, contributions to the team, spirit of sacrifice, low profile, no useless showing up.

Weaknesses: Profile lower than expected and deserved, inner resources unawareness, talent locked, always needs to be coached, comforted, and encouraged.

Missing Mindset Tool: *SELF IMAGE*

Call To Action: Development of the Self Image (→ Clarity of Destination + Self Consciousness):

- Having fun and succeed, (*feast → learn → forget*).
- Inner exploration and start understanding what he/she really deserves.
- Start understanding he/she has the other tools and only needs to feel inside ready for the next level.
- Try acting *"as-if"*, during the competition, win the competition, and empower his/her self-image.

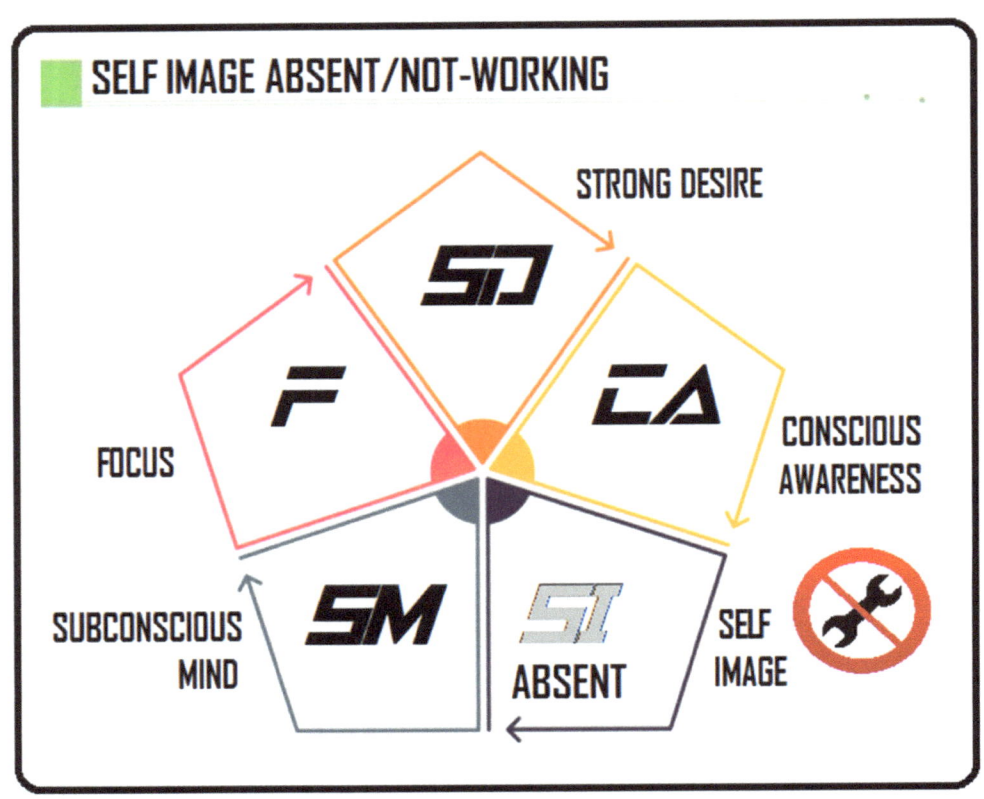

83 – The Prima Donna

The Prima Donna athlete is a non-balanced kind of athlete. In most cases, he/she is a *natural*, which means that is provided with lots of natural skills and competencies, but does not strive to improve his/her arsenal, because is overwhelmed by a false and intolerably higher self-image than deserved and expected.

Characteristics: The Prima Donna Profile Performer:

- Vanity prevails over all the rest.
- He/she is an exhibitionist and always attends every possible event.
- Not more focused on improvement.
- Not willing to do extra work, when needed.
- Arrogant and unwilling to get advice and recommendations.
- Relies too much on natural abilities.
- Does not have a real desire to make sacrifices.

Temperament: Arrogant, exhibitionist, strong-temperament, self-confident, always happy and optimistic.

Strengths: Natural, good/excellent skills and competencies, know the rules of the games, attract people, innate leadership attitude.

Weaknesses: Totally wrong self-image, arrogant, unwilling to struggle, to learn and to self-improvement, to question and challenge him/herself.

Missing Mindset Tool: *SELF-IMAGE*

Call To Action: Development of Self Image ($\rightarrow$ Clarity of Destination + Self Consciousness):

- Go back to basics to empower humility and redefine the Self-Image.
- Try managing better his/her internal enemy and deaseing the ego.
- Quitting identification process: needs to contrast routine's traps (identification – complains – lies – imagination – consideration – showing off).
- Needs to be scaled back by coaches and by failures (and learn the lesson).

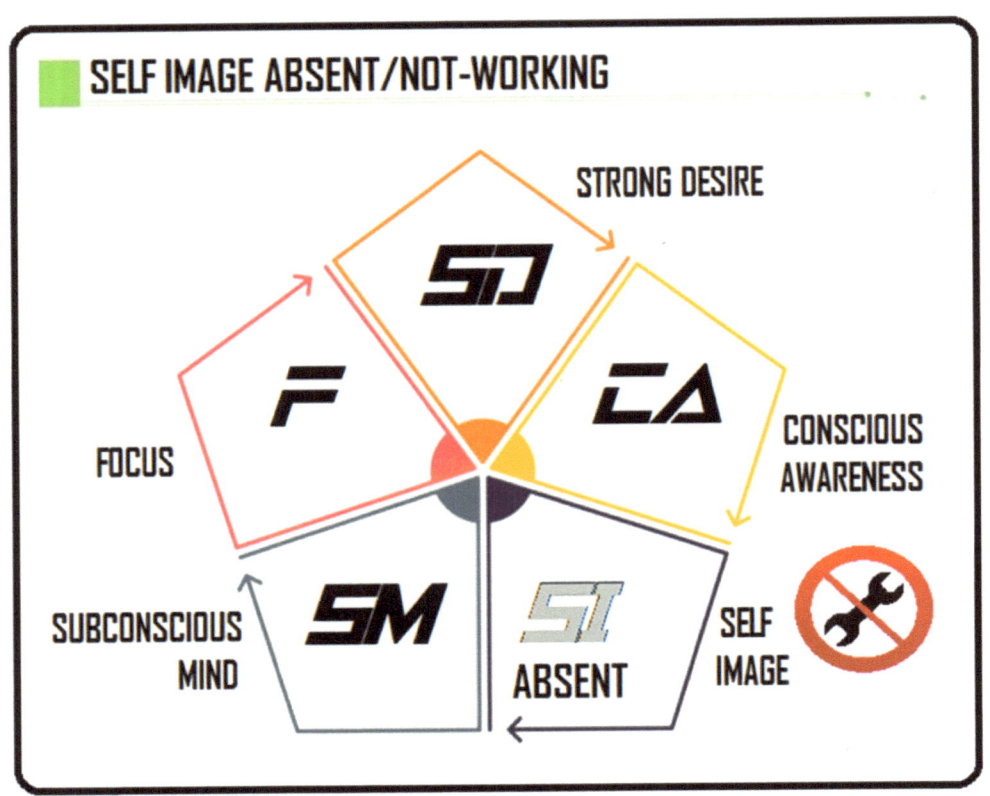

84 – The Silent Killer

The Silent Killer is provided with high or excellent potential but is not focused at all. The Silent Killer works very hard and always strives hard to be better, but he/she cannot manage to complete the ultimate goal: there is always a missing piece that is not completed. Cannot achieve the final purpose, cannot succeed, despite excellent potential.

Characteristics: The Silent Killer Profile Performer:

- Works harder than anybody else.
- Is not enough focused to complete the final purpose.
- Huge commitment and great devotion to training.
- Not provided with a proper direction.
- Focus is off.
- Lots of leadership potential.
- Applies the shotgun approach.
- Tends not to complete his/her *"Ultimate Goal"*.

Temperament: Balanced, determined, self-confident, ambitious.

Strengths: Motivation, determination, sacrifice, devotion, huge/natural physical potential.

Weaknesses: Everything is overwhelmed by rules and protocols, lack of consciousness and critical thinking, *good-soldie*r attitude, highly predictable.

Missing Mindset Tool: *FOCUS*

Call To Action: Development of FOCUS (→ Adaptation + Tactical/Strategic mental features):

- Needs to develop a seasonal strategic plan and apply it precisely, without switching (in the end).
- Needs to create the training scenario for applying only *"the last shot"*, to become familiar with the ultimate part of the goal.
- Needs to stay closer to the plan and apply it until the end (under the coach's control and supervision).

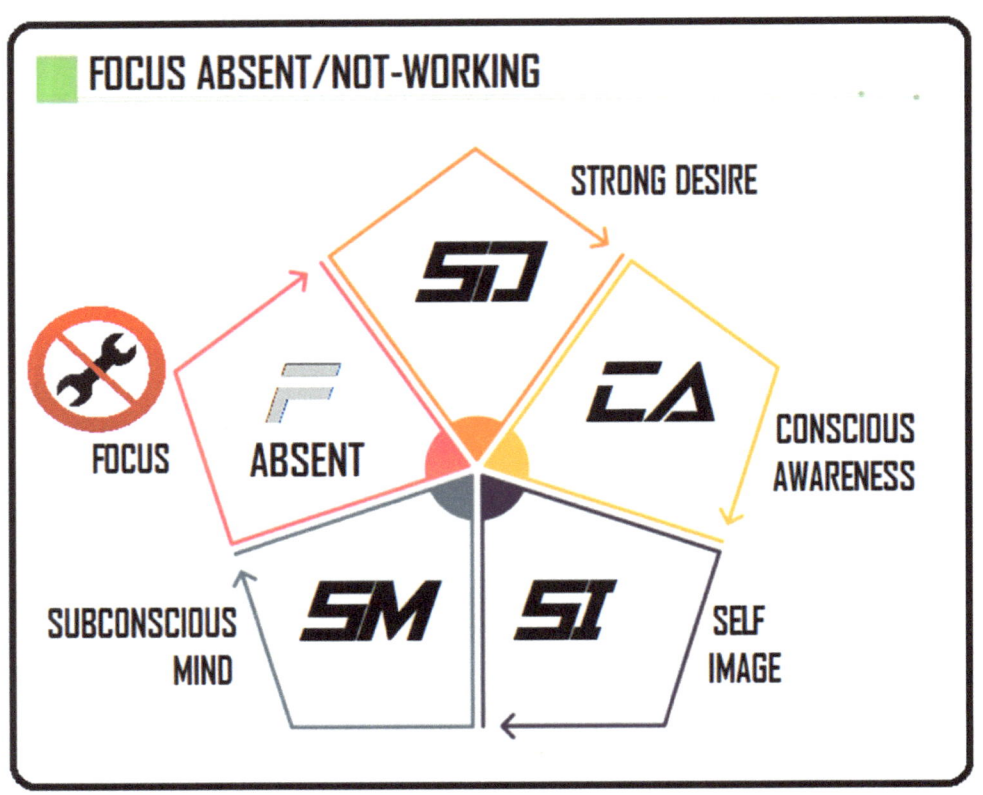

85 – The Subconscious Commando

The Subconscious Commando is that kind of uncommon athlete who only acts subconsciously: he/she is strongly forced to forget crucial details and is driven by a subconscious mind. Everything is executed in a state of physical and psychic hypnosis, in a sense. A kind of *automated machine* driven to complete a task.

Characteristics: The Subconscious Commando Profile Performer:

- The subconscious thoughts drive everything (Subconscious Mindset prevails all over the rest).
- He/she is driven by inner instincts and automated routines.
- Most of the residual mental tools work properly.
- Forgets crucial details which may affect the performance.
- Totally in auto-pilot.

Temperament: Calm (at the evidence), but in a state of constant and hidden anxiety, non-rational, emotional, reactive.

Strengths: High level of conditioning and technical automation, physically inexhaustible, getting fast in the flow.

Weaknesses: Emotional imprisonment, *Instinct-Trilemma* subdued, lack of awareness and rational thinking, oversized reactions.

Missing Mindset Tool: *CONSCIOUS AWARENESS*

Call To Action: Development of the Conscious Awareness (→ Self Consciousness):

- Start drafting and using a checklist (for any crucial activity/event).
- Empowering constructive and conscious self-talk.
- Evaluation of precision and details.
- Getting connected with the outside world (relationships, learning activities, social life).
- Exercises to empower focus, concentration, critical thinking, and analytical skills.

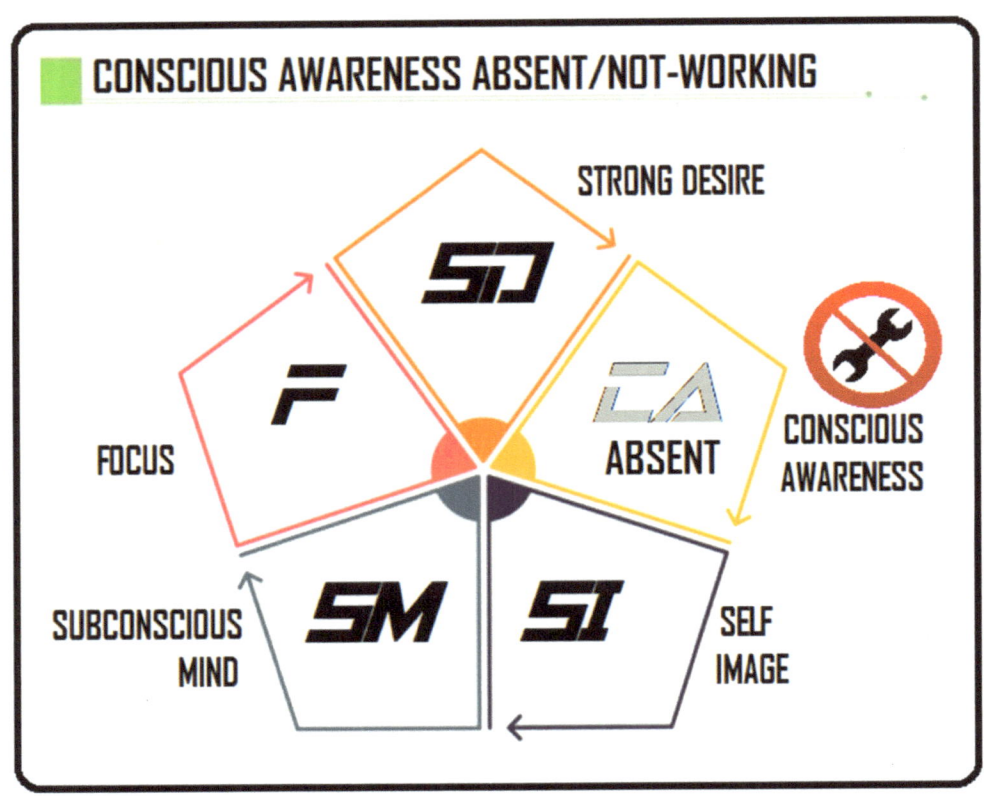

86 – The Contender

The Contender is the athlete who has developed all the *5 Mindset Tools* and knows how to manage, mix and make them work together in unison, consistently. Is the *ideal athlete*, who can apply to become the Champion. He/she can enter the winner circle of the Peak-Performers and become number one. It's up to him/her, it's only a matter of time before he/she succeeds.

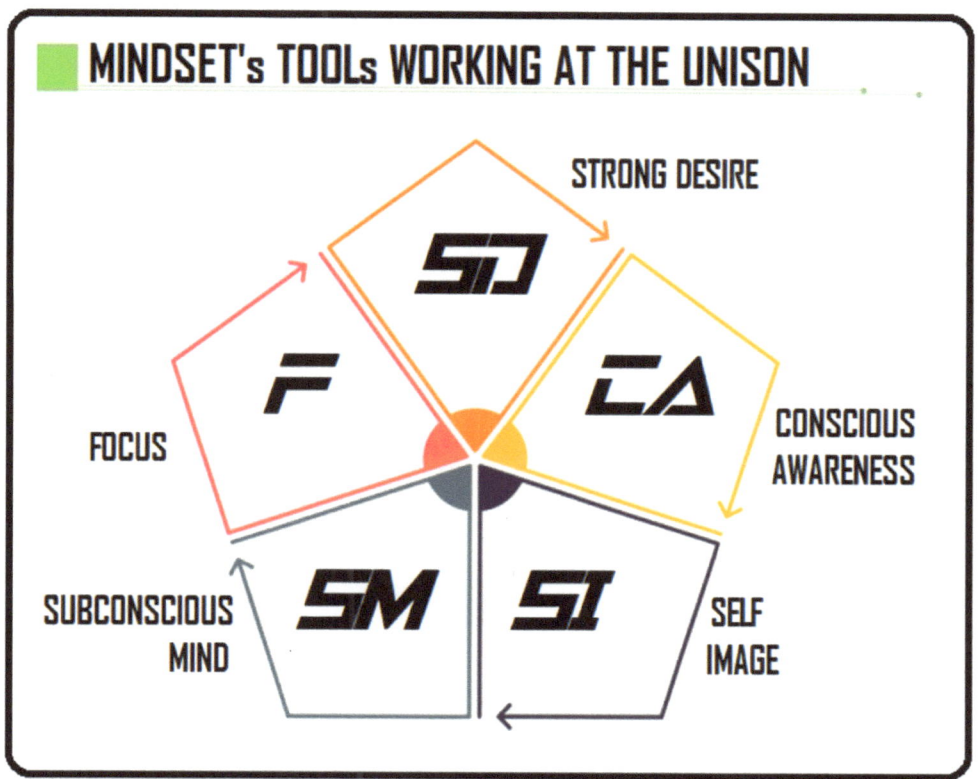

87 – The Champion and the Peak Performer

The Profile of the Champion starts with the *Contenders state*. You are provided with the whole of the tools needed and you have a conscious awareness of your *IPS*. You are provided with the awareness and you are also driven by a strong desire to succeed. You commit yourself all (*time + energy*) to succeed and continue investing in yourself. You take care of all the details. You're continuously in the *hearandnowness*, you entered the flow.

Stronger Desire:

- Your strong desire expresses itself through yourself and your motivation.
- You simulate competitions with your companions, for you love the challenges and you love winning.
- Your fears have become your best friend since you know how to put fears behind you until you embrace them all.
- You are not only *Goal-Oriented*, but even *Mission-Oriented*: you are a *Missionary of Success*
- You define and update and use your personal *performance logbook*: your bible to frequently check your state.

Greater Focus:

- You're always on the right track.
- You always know *Where, When, Why,* and *How.*
- You always plan it out.
- You are capable of huge visualization and imagery.
- You always pay attention to details.
- You are only focused on what you can 100% control and neglect the rest.
- You execute *one thing at a time*, striving for excellence.
- You have mental triggers which allow you to switch and react in the most appropriate way.

Subconscious Thought Improvement

- You got used dissecting everything you learn.
- You got used to recording everything you made in your *sports logbook* (subconscious flow, feelings, sensations, emotions).
- You know how to visualize the perfect outcome.
- You can visualize yourself performing perfectly.

Conscious Thought Improvement

- You empower your focus thanks to your Conscious Mindset.
- You always create checklists and use them effectively.
- You always take action and attack aggressively.
- You produce lots of quality, consciously: once you do great, you do lots and thousands of times.
- You are patient and concentrated.

Self-Image Improvement

- You investigate and try securing attitudes and habits of the Champions to your arsenal.
- You surround yourself with other champions and/or optimistic people.
- You know how to employ all the resources around you.
- You strive to force the world to answer you: you never settle for an unanswered question.

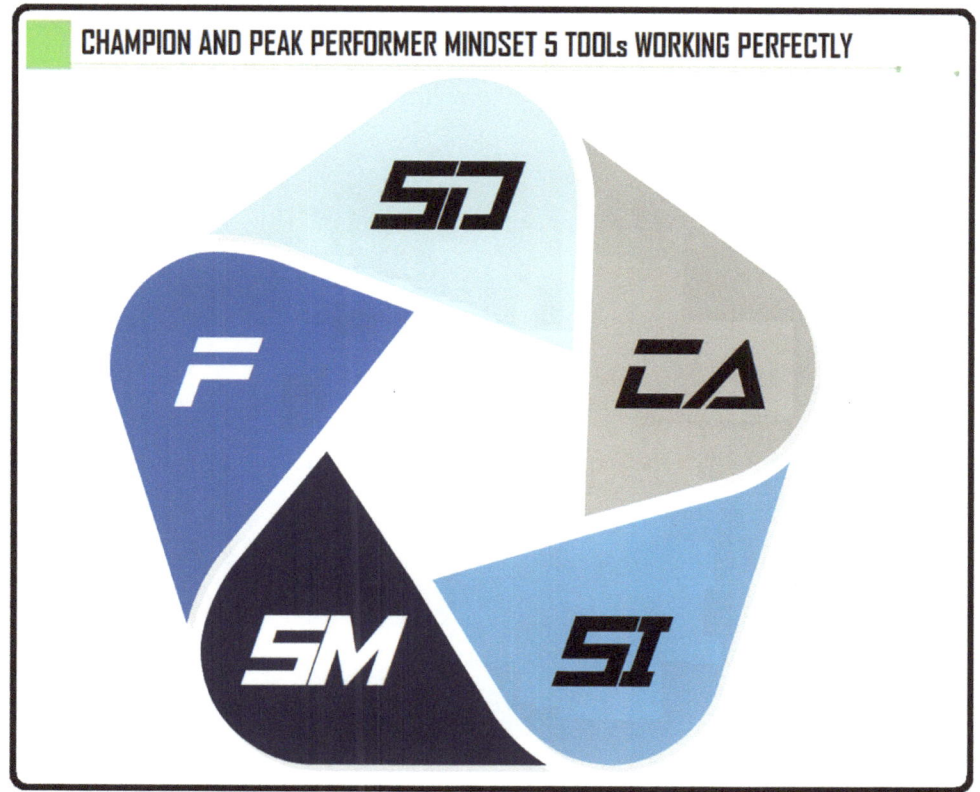

88 – The Habits of the Champion

The habit is any action (or *routine behavior*) you take, which is driven by a subconscious mind, even though has originally been developed through conscious repetition, over a period of time. Habits can be positive or negative, pushing you to do something or preventing you from doing the same thing, focus-oriented or barrier-oriented. What you have to know is that you can manage your habits, you can replace the ones which are barrier-oriented with new, productive ones. It's very difficult, and it takes time and energy, but it is possible and many athletes had did it effectively. As a starting point, you need to accept that you have a bad habit (if any) and that is your responsibility (ownership). Then you have to include the new action into your routine and follow the plan for at least 21 continuous repetitions (either 21 days or 21 sessions distributed in 2 months, at max). A conscious behavior (repetition) will activate a subconscious activity (habit). Then you ought to apply 4 main steps: (1) acceptance – (2) ownership – (3) repetition – (4) subconscious.

Champions have lots of habits, but there are few which occur more often than others The *winning Champion's Habits*:

- Do not postpone anything, which does not affect your plan. Take action and complete your task: no snoozing alarm is ever allowed.
- Get yourself organized both in sports, in business, and in your personal life: external order is the projection of your internal design.
- Pack your bags the same way every time.
- Dress for success: be always ready for great events and catch chances whenever they come.
- Show up on time, every time.
- Respect your rest, every time (physical/psychic relaxation and re-absorbent).
- Use your athlete's logbook daily.
- Be kind, be polite, and always use fair play.
- Be a leader, in any possible occasion: take control of the situation.

89 – The Attitudes of the Champion

Attitude refers to a set of emotions, beliefs, and behaviors towards a particular object, person, thing, or event. The attitudes are often the result of experiences or upbringing. They actually have a high impact on behaviors. Lots of sports and tactical actions are activated by attitudes. For this reason, attitudes are so much crucial for you if you really want to become a champion. Attitudes are resistant and enduring, but can change (and can be changed) as much as habits can do (better if you cope with both contemporarily, but similarly) if you take full ownership. Attitudes are formed as a result of a mix of 6 peculiar elements: experiences, social factors, learning, conditioning, observation, and inner beliefs: you should work on these aspects, as much as possible, to overturn bad attitudes and include new ones. Champions seem to have peculiar behavioral attitudes, which also influence the cognitive aspects of their mindset (thoughts and beliefs):

- Always take strong action to do your possible best on any occasion (attitude to precision and to excellence).
- Always do the right thing, because it's the right thing to do (the pragmatism of the PROs).
- Always enjoy the moment.
- Always courageously face fears head-on (*growth mindset*: they approach, rather than avoid).
- Always finish what you started.
- Always get up after getting knocked out (persistence).
- Always lead by example.

90 – Five Levels of Mental Toughness

There is a kind of evolutionary pattern that consists of 5 different levels of mental toughness: it includes any athlete's profile. Regardless of your intrinsic motivation, your original resources, or your hidden talents, any athlete starts from being an amateur, a simple practitioner of a specific sport discipline. Depending on the intensity and the frequency of the training sessions and learning programs, this athlete grows up and starts jumping to the relevant level: from amateur (as a starting point) to peak performer (as an ultimate target). During such a pathway the mental toughness level is enhanced. There is a strong connection between the enhancement of the mindset and the inner intention of the athlete when performing. Such a connection is described by the pyramid (see below). In short, the 5 levels present the following correlation (intention/profile):

- Level 5: *Playing not to lose* – The Amateur and the Low-Quality Athlete – The athlete applies the least quantity of energy needed to keep being considered an athlete, by him/herself and his/her sports community. At the same time, such an athlete knows that he/she has to start performing better, to improve his/her status and reputation.

- Level 4: *Playing to cruise* – The Semi-Professional Athlete – The Semi-PRO pushes something additional if compared to the amateur, but he/she is also convinced that he/she would continue to train and perform as long as he/she can cruise. This means mentally cruising through the job, without really engaging in any serious thought.

- Level 3: *Playing to improve* – The Professional Athlete – As a PRO, the athlete is systematically pushed both by internal and external solicitations and motivations. In such a state a first, significant mental snitch occurs: the PRO starts connecting emotions, feelings, and thoughts to engage his/her resources for improving the psycho/physical shape. The PRO continuously practices strong self-talk which sounds like this: *"Maybe I can accomplish more than I thought. Maybe I am better than I think I am"*. The PRO wants to win, but he/she also knows he/she has to improve his/her UPP to set to become something better. A new critical-thinking process is started.

- Level 2: *Playing to compete* – The Contender – The system of beliefs is definitely changed: The Internal Enemy has been won, an internal and strong desire has finally emerged, the willpower has overwhelmed the whole of hurdles, adversities, and problems have been overcome. The performer starts believing he/she is capable of achieving and becoming the best, the number one in his/her specialty. *"I think I can be the best"* is the mantra of the Contender, who may finally set to become the champion.

- Level 1: *Playing to win* – The Champion and the Peak-Performer – The Champion is a Contender who has finalized his/her sport pathway to victory. He/she has accomplished the tasks, has developed the whole of the skills, competencies, and mental capabilities to face all his/her opponents, and has achieved the hardest targets. Is driven by his/her inner spirit, rather than by material gratifications and rewards: has overcome his/her ego-needs and whims. He/she is fearless, by the time. The Champion is strongly convinced he/she cannot lose anymore. The mental jump consists of switching from competing to creating. The real challenge of the champion is with his/herself: expressing his/her best potential and proving him/her to be better than the previous season.

All of that said, you have to explore your inner motivations and investigate your real intentions, while you're training or performing, which are directly influenced by motivations. These intentions exactly describe your current level of mental toughness. Consider this a self-test to understand which is your current state and set yourself up for the next jump, accordingly.

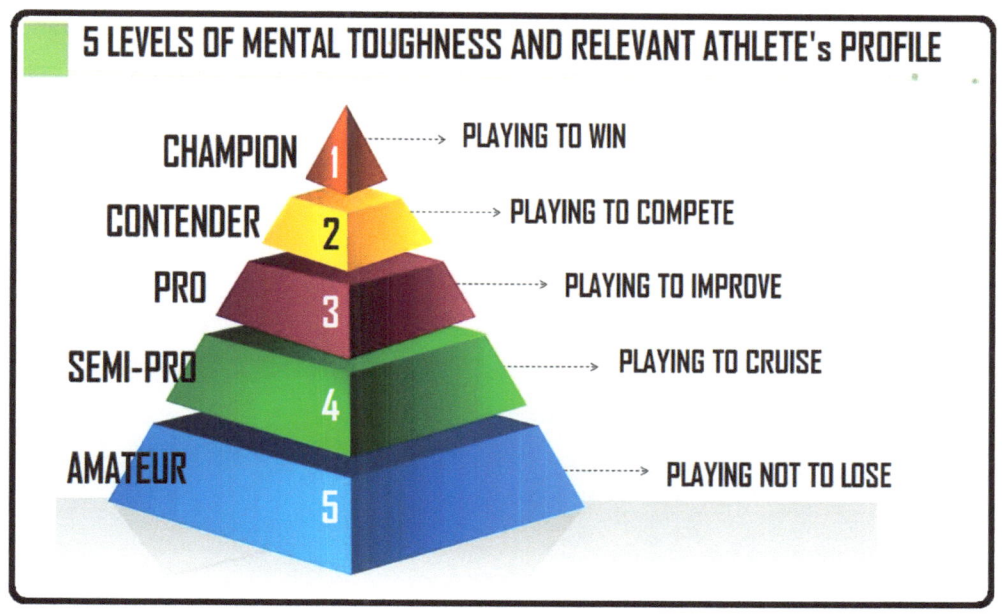

## CHAPTER ELEVEN

Action

91 – The MINDSET as a GOAL

If you are a semi-professional or a PRO, then you should have already developed a strong physical condition and a technical/tactical arsenal, which should not need any other significant improvement. A kind of motor and technical completeness, which does not mean you reached the perfection of the set of sports gestures of the entire available repertoire. You must keep on enriching the technical arsenal, of course, and training sessions ought to be focused on special tactics and hacks to enhance the athletics arsenal and to make the sessions more and more challenging. But we know, by that time, that this is not enough: we need to add something crucial.

The *Sport Mindset*, then, is the very best target to accomplish. A strong athlete who wants to apply him/herself for gold medals ought to have only one commitment: achieving mental toughness at any cost, the strongest possible mindset to overcome him/herself (the Ego), and overwhelm any other opponents, in the very crucial tournaments. As we already know, the only skill needed is a very strong will, focused, addressed in the right direction, straight driven towards the goal.

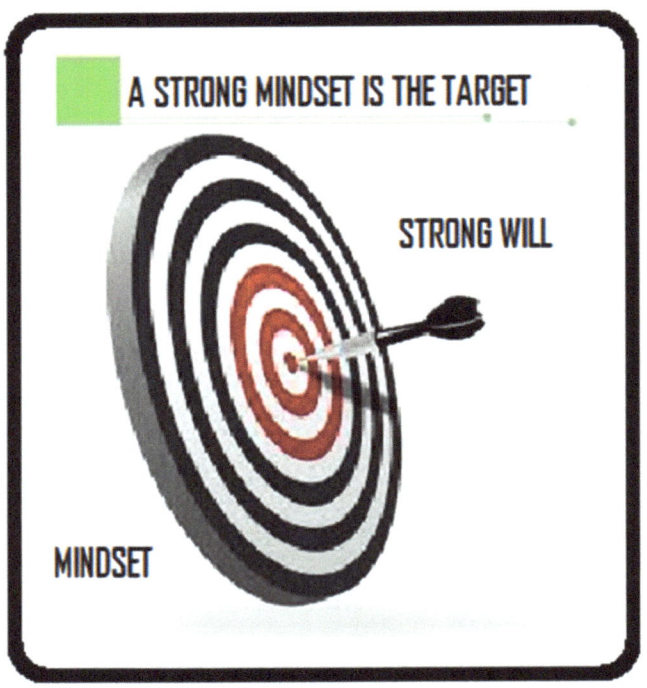

92 – Methodology

I have personally chosen and adopted a practical methodology to develop the end structure of my sport mindset, so far, and I also have applied such a way to several students of mine through the years and it revealed to be broadly effective and successful. We have to initiate the process, we have to develop something and we also have to finalize, e.g.: we have to structure our mindset. So a methodology is strongly needed and recommended.

ADDIE Methodology is a simple way to empower a single element of the Mindset-Mix. It actually consists of 5 steps:

1) *A – Analyze*: You have to isolate the element you want to develop/empower and you have to be clearly aware of it. No confusion, no doubts: you need to know in advance everything you need about this element, which might be considered *"your problem"* or *"what you actually need now"*.

2) *D – Design*: you have to brainstorm a few ways to hit the target, e.g.: you need to develop a short list of situations that lead to that specific *"state of mind"* which facilitates the workout. This stage needs your complete focus and specific creativity, e.g.: a kind of cognitive creativity related to your sport discipline (situation);

3) *D – Develop*: You finally made the right decision and selected the best exercises to hit the target. The Decision Making Process requires that you simulate the shortlist and select the right one based on effectiveness and difficulty (the more difficult, the better);

4) *I – Implement* the Introduction of the exercise into your routine. I is for Introduction and Implementation. The action consists of applying the exercise to a routine plan, every day (if possible). The secret of an effective implementation consists of introducing a kind of exercise in a systematic routine which is (1) technically feasible and (2) timely and sustainable;

5) E – *Evaluate*: You need to check and monitor the results. You have previously designed a few KPIs (at least two) related to this element and then you can check and compare the data, to better understand your progress on this specific feature.

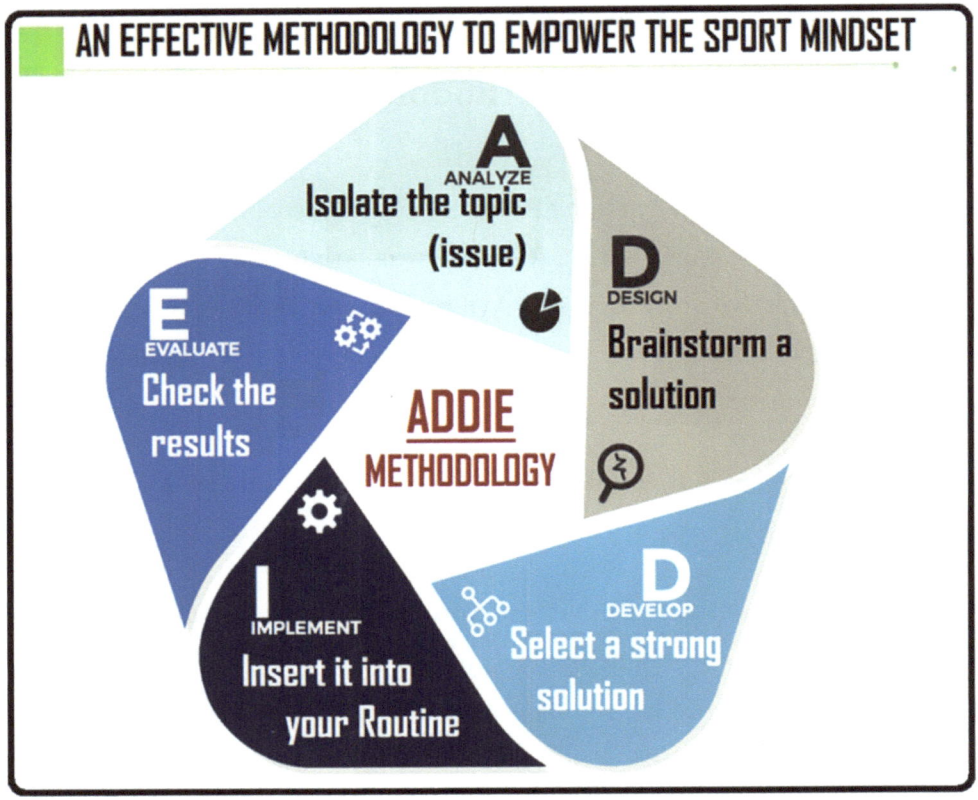

As intuitive *ADDIE-Methodology* is a kind of tool that ought to be developed personally, because: (1) only every single coach and athlete actually knows which are the missing pieces – (2) which are the best moments/exercises to apply – (3) for which, specific sports discipline. Nevertheless, I have developed some recommendation programs which may be applied to facilitate the acquisition of every feature.

Please find in the previous (and following) pages some patterns: each table refers to a specific Pillar and to the relevant factors:

TOPIC	GOAL	ACTION	EXERCISE	REPETITIONs

93 – The Main Principles and Methodologies to Achieve

As we already said, training is a long and complex process of adaptation: the physical body and the sports mental attitudes are systematically subjected to increasing loads and challenging stimuli; as a consequence, the body and mind adapt themselves and empower specific skills. From a motor and physical perspective, the conditional and coordinative skills are empowered, from a psychological and psychodynamic perspective the mental skills are empowered as well. The loads and exercises are the causes of such an adaptation, but the application of a such set of exercises must be executed in obedience to specific principles and methodologies. I want to present to you the main principles which ought to be applied for such a purpose. Some of them have been developed by Psychologists, Physiologists, and Pedagogues who have worked together and are mainly finalized to facilitate physiological attainments. Some others have been specifically developed to empower psychic attitudes and hacks. If you really want to become a Champion you cannot escape going through these methodologies, learning, and applying them to your training sessions and programs accordingly.

- Principle of Progressive Overload – It's a special combination of 2 principles: Overload & Progression. The overload principle is finalized to improve fitness and strength (conditional skills): the load/demand on the body must be greater than what the body is accustomed to. The load/stress must be outside your comfort zone. In other words, you have to put in some effort and push your body accordingly, during the exercise. The body will respond to the load by physiologically adapting to it. The progression principle is finalized to intensify the load: it basically consists of gradually increasing the load and the stress on the body. The progressive overload principle can be achieved by changing the F.I.T.T. parameters: *Frequency, Intensity, Time* of training, *Type* of training
- Principle of Regularity – Exercise must be done at regular intervals and be consistent. Consistency allows the body to adapt more efficiently and quickly. Ideally, exercises should be done 3-5 times per week. These figures are higher for the SEMI-PROs and the PROs (5-10 times per week).
- Principle of Specificity – Exercise should be designed based on your specific goals and needs. Specification depends on your peculiar sports disciplines: gestures, actions, tactics, strategies, ethical elements, and other specific features. Specific exercises elicit specific adaptations to create specific training effects. In other words, your body adapts to the specific demands on it.
- Principle of Reversibility – *Use it or lose it.* The effects of training and the body's adaptations are reversed if training sessions are too far apart or if there is a long break in exercise. Your training methodology ought to reduce or hopefully nullify the threat of such a principle being activated. The only way is continuity, persistence, and working hard.

- Principle of Variation & Adaptation – Over time, your body will completely adapt to a specific exercise routine to a point where your body will reach a training plateau. To limit reaching the training plateau, exercises must be varied and modified.

- Principle of Periodization – This principle is related to the long-term plan or goal of an individual. It refers to the changes or variations in the training program that are implemented over the course of a specific period of time, (the agonistic season = 1 year). It consists of the systematic planning of specific training goals or a specific sports discipline. The aim is to achieve optimal improvements in athlete performance at the right time while minimizing injury and burnout. As we already know periodization breaks training into days, weeks, and months.

- Principle of Repetitions – The only way to learn and master a technical gesture, a complex action, or a tactical/strategic solution is through repetition. *"Monkey sees, monkey does"* is not working, because the athlete must experience the technical requirements, and must execute one, 100, and one thousand times gestures before mastering it enough. For this reason, it's commonly recommended *"… once you do great, then do lots"*.

- Principle of Visualization and Imagery – Psychologists have proven that the human brain cannot differentiate between an actual experience and one imagined vividly and in detail. Mental rehearsal and visualization are one of the most important mental training skills to apply in order to increase performance. In fact, is very utilized by PROs and by Peak-Performers belonging to both sports disciplines, business, and politics. Visualization is most effective when the mind is relaxed.

- Mental Training for Mental Games – It consists of the creation of challenging situations and competitive scenarios. After that, you need to compete mentally, fix it all and succeed. It's a kind of visualization declination, in a sense, but more complex than expected, because it requires the construction of precise circumstances, compliance to specific rules (the rules of your sport discipline), and the mental application of an effective solution.

- Consciousness and Awareness – The principle according to which you need to know and understand the sense of any exercise, gesture, and action to better secure to your arsenal. Your knowledge and consciousness will enable you to apply the single exercise in the right way, thus you can learn the perfect gesture through lots of repetitions.

- Conscious activities feed the subconscious – This principle reminds you that the whole of the subconscious mind is influenced by conscious activities. The automated and conditional actions and reactions are fed by conscious training: exercises, applications, and efforts. If you want to improve your subconscious mind and make it support your purpose, in spite of resisting it, you must improve your conscious efforts.

- Conscious activities turn to the subconscious. The conscious gestures and actions turn to your subconscious and then can be activated by a mental trigger and keep going on, after a huge amount of repetitions, led by a conscious mind. Repetitions, after a specific amount that depends on the sports discipline and on the complexity of the gesture, enable you to turn to the subconscious and give you back additional energy to deal with strategy.

- Perfect Practice makes perfect – Such a principle is frequently adopted by Champions and Peak-Performers. They have a strong attitude to details and long for precise actions and gestures, at any time. You need to have a precise idea of the perfect gesture (*the nominal picture*) and you have to compare this picture to your performance (*the current picture*), then you can (must) fill the gap. Perfection is neither a dream nor a process, but a goal: if you practice perfection continuously, then you make it perfect.

- Resilience is developed through adversities – Learn to deal with setbacks or what you may perceive to be negative outcomes, both in the present moment and longer-term objectives. For instance, not finishing that final rep or last mile, or perhaps not reaching a weight loss goal within the exact time frame you have set yourself due to illness or injury. Focus on what is within your control; maintaining a positive and considered response to setbacks will ultimately lead to greater gains and performance success. You cannot empower your resilience without going through adversities.

- Principle of Resonance – As we already learned above, performance is always the precise projection of your state of being. There is a strong connection between your entire level of quality (being) and the event which you generate (performance and results). Such a connection is called "*resonance*".

- Principle of Cycle of Actions – According to this principle, any kind of action which is executed by an individual is the result of a specific process that unfolds in 4 main phases:

    o *Set of inner beliefs and convictions* (which depend on experiences, learning and culture, social state standards, internal bias, and barriers). This set activates a specific amount of resources and drives these resources to the confirmation of itself (e.g.: the beliefs activate only specific resources to confirm the original conviction).

    o *Resources activation* (the set of inner beliefs only activates special resources and which do autopilot towards a result, completely neglecting any other available tool or resource and any other kind of purpose, but the one which has been defined by the beliefs).

    o *Action and behaviors* (the action is driven towards the pre-specified goal).

    o *Results* (results follow. In the best case scenario these results actually confirm the original conjecture included in the set of beliefs).

Such a scenario, which oversees all kinds of human behavior, gives no chance to alternative options, but the ones which have been defined at the first stage: the beliefs. If you want to change the results, you ought to change the cause and the inner beliefs.

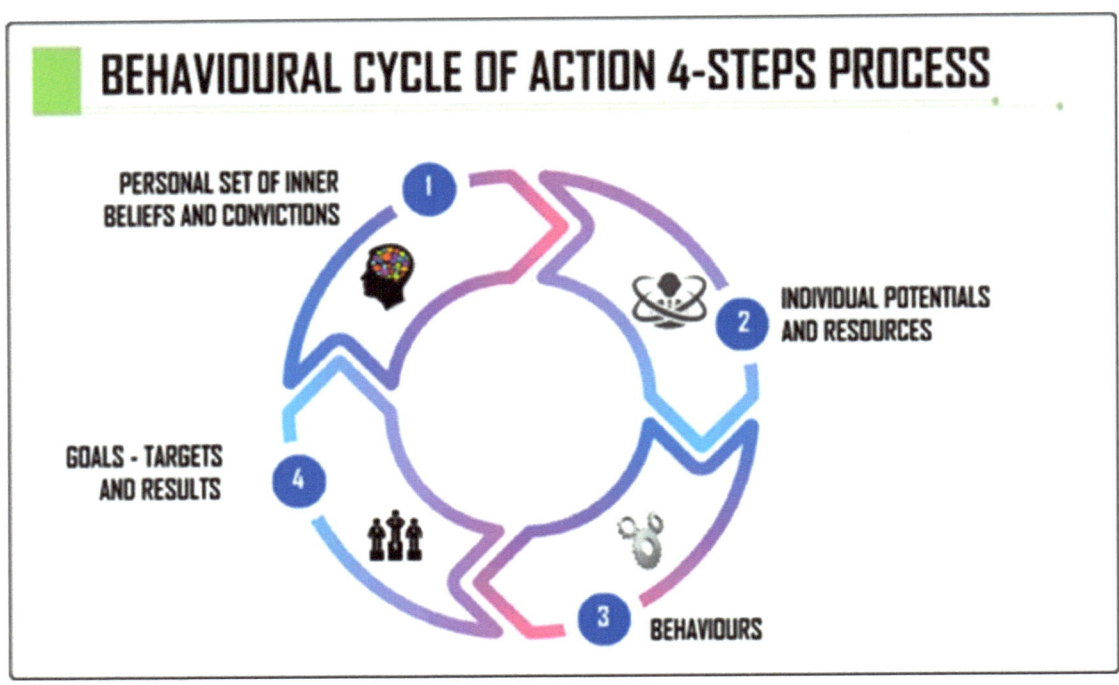

BEHAVIOURAL CYCLE OF ACTION 4-STEPS PROCESS

PERSONAL SET OF INNER BELIEFS AND CONVICTIONS

1

2 INDIVIDUAL POTENTIALS AND RESOURCES

GOALS - TARGETS AND RESULTS

4

3 BEHAVIOURS

THE MAIN PRINCIPLES AND METHODOLOGIES FOR A PHYSICAL AND A MENTAL TRAINING

Progressive Overload	Regularity	Specificity	Reversibility
Variation & Adaptation	Periodization	Repetitions	Visualization and Imagery
Mental Training for Mental Games	Consciousness and Awareness	Conscious activities feed subconscious	Conscious activities turns to subconscious
Perfect Practice makes perfect	Resilience is developed through adversities	Cycle of Actions	Law of Resonance

94 – SW-Analysis

SW-A is for *"Strengths and Weaknesses Analysis"* and comes from a more famous model belonging to the Marketing theory: *SWOT-Analysis* (Strengths, Weaknesses, Opportunities, and Threats). The Champion's mindset is naturally wired to catch these two crucial elements. We already know that weaknesses ought to be subdued to a process of empowerment which would firstly balance and then be finalized to cancel these weak points from the personality of the athlete. On the other hand, the strengths ought to be transformed into relevant *"Specials"*, e.g.: peculiar gestures which are so excellently mastered that we trust most and are used to overturn a bad or disadvantageous situation.

A strong mindset is based on the strategic utilization of these two elements. Any time the athlete knows which are these two and when the weak points may influence the performance or the strong points might be exploited to succeed.

As a final recommendation an unconventional model related to the generic Peak Performance must be explored.

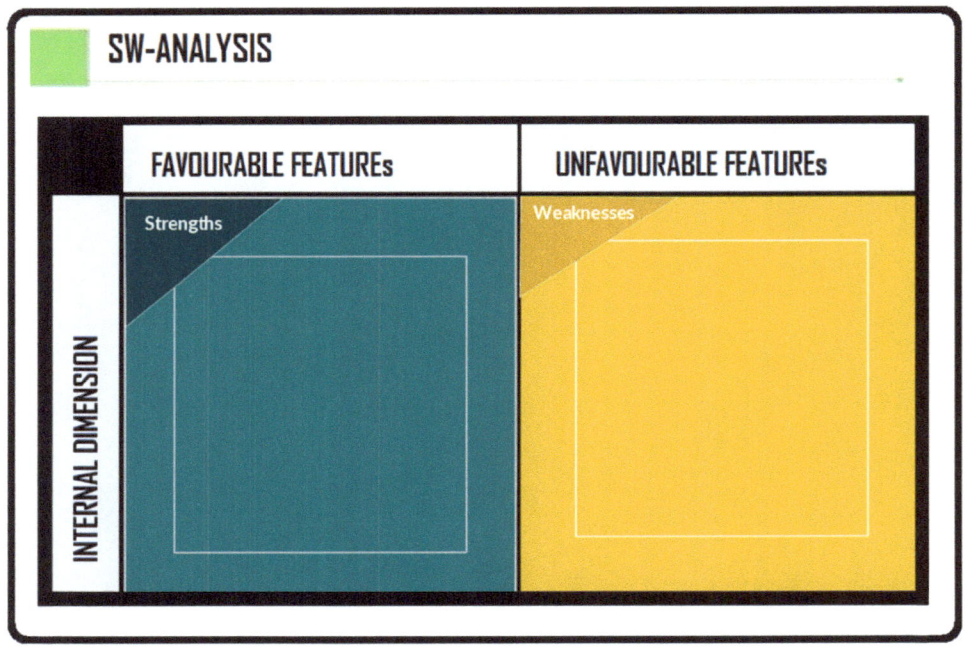

What you have to know is that when we seriously decide who we want to become we need to know who we really are. We need to catch the real gaps between our current state and condition (who we currently are) and the ideal one (the IPS: the *Ideal Performance State*). There are 4 segments of competencies we have to go through, depending on consciousness level:

1) Known Competences   (Results of the workouts)
2) Known Incompetencies   (1st level Gaps)
3) Unknown Competences   (Talents and Abilities)
4) Unknown Incompetencies   (2nd level Gaps)

The process of SW-Analysis should be pushed so deep to catch also the unknown/unconscious dimension (*Unknown competencies/incompetencies*). Very often they represent the gaps that do not allow the athlete to achieve: he/she neither knows what is missing nor the reason why is missing. There are a few ways to catch the unknown/unconscious and switch to the known/conscious: (1) Self-observation – (2) Mirroring – (3) Benchmarking with High-Level Athletes – (4) Applying to a Coach – (5) Peculiar treatment.

We know you are in lack some elements and the 8 Pillars surely include these factors you are in lack, but you do not know yet which are the crucial factors that you do not have (*Unknown incompetencies*).

The peak- performance requires you to catch these hidden factors, and manipulate and transform them as appropriate.

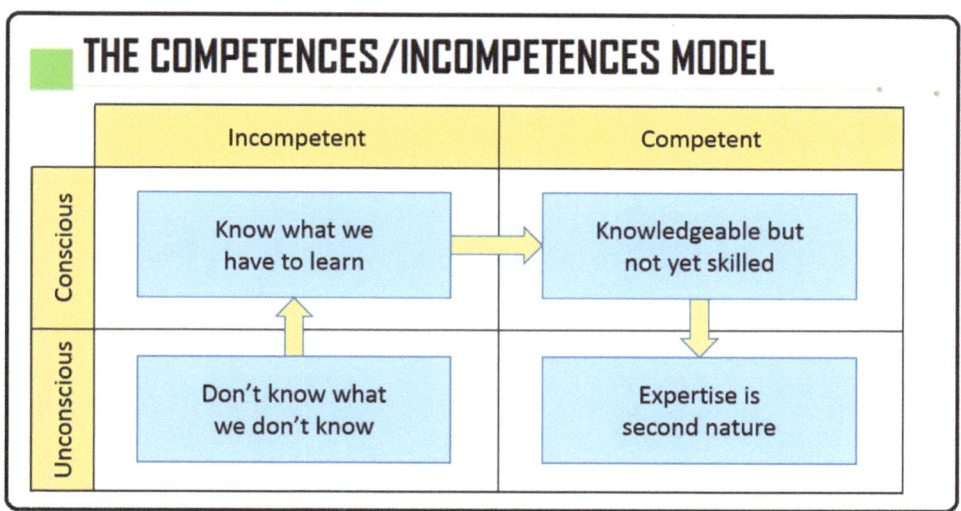

95 – MWR: Mental Workout Routine

The best way to ensure you are straight working in the right direction is that you practice the relevant exercises systematically, which means that you have introduced what is required to your workout routine. Mental toughness is nothing you can achieve once and for all, it is a daily work based on a daily commitment. After your first significant successes you going to get an additional switch. You will catch clearly in your mind which are the real elements that have helped you overcome specific hurdles and supported you to overturn, till the final victory. So you will be given additional motivation coming from such elements. You will have to strengthen a specific element of your mindset and this will be consolidated into your personality. So you will be able to switch to another purpose and will work for attaining another one you believe you're still missing (*known incompetenci*es or *unknown incompetencies* which are slowly becoming conscious and evident).

In a conclusion: the real task of an ambitious athlete who is provided with the aim of achieving the greatest possible goals is a full-time job: training your mindset, and applying your ultimate *Mental Workout Routine*, until victory will come.

This devotion is a common task for any athlete belonging to any kind of sports discipline: individual, collective, precision, combat, racket, speed, or contact. Any athlete practicing any kind of sport needs to be provided with mental toughness.

You have to develop a precise and solid Training Plan compliant with all the models and methodologies we have talked about so far and you have to mix your ordinary training held in the gym, with such solitary training specifically tailored to your special achievements. This is the real meaning of *the Mental Workout Routine.*

THE EXTENSIVE APPLICATION OF MINDSET RULES TO BOTH SITUATIONAL AND ROUTINARY SPORT DISCIPLINES

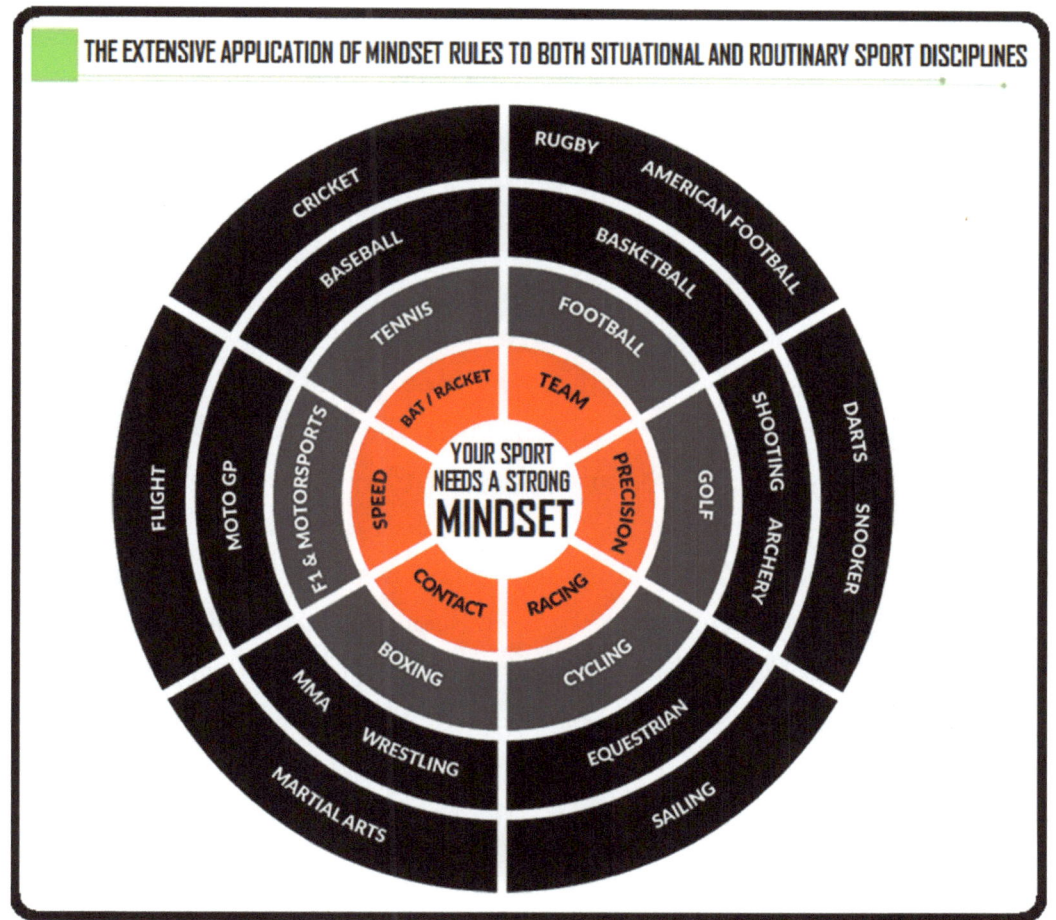

96 – Hurdles and Difficulties

I already knew from the start there will be problems in your future days.

I know there will be plenty of issues, doubts, and confusion in the upcoming training sessions. I already know that perfectly because I have been you, I have lived in your same house and I have walked in your shoes for years, in the past. I know everything and what I do not know, I can guess. The first risk you will be running consists of motivation and depends on the real power of your inner motivation. It's very easy to forget everything because most of all what has been said is *invisible, intangible, and doubtful.* You can only catch the real meaning of what we have talked about, inside. If you get closer to your heart and try to carefully listen to the noises, you would hear a lock that is rattling. Your inner talent wants to be unlocked and requires your consciousness. After you become aware, you will switch to action: *we need to work on the talked.* If your motivation is high, then you will start working, otherwise, you will forget anything we explored together and will condemn yourself to settle for the second, as long as your sports career will last. A second threat is related to your impatience: mindset enhancement requires time, effort, and repetition. You must accept the truth that you have to start the pathway and enter this self-improvement process without any quick expectation, otherwise, you will be going to be deluded, will lose your trust, and will finally reject this extra effort. The third and last threat consists of becoming so passionate about working on your mental toughness and relevant hacks that you will be neglecting the whole of your primary commitments which consist of training, training, and additional training sessions without being arrogant, keeping strong the focus on here and now, with a spirit of sacrifice and sense of responsibility. You must firmly keep in your mind that you cannot build anything great if you are in lack strong foundations. So keep in mind the step-by-step performance model and the relevant 6 stages and go back to basics when you think you are a great champion. Working on basics – first – means that you are building foundations to last. It means that you are building your arsenal on the rock.

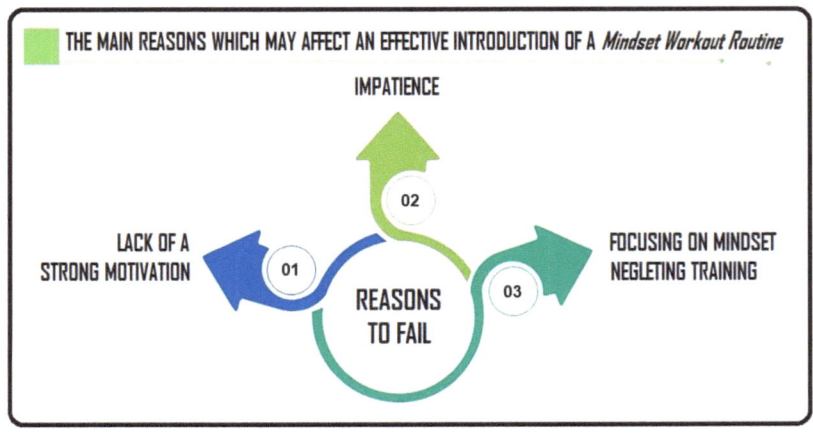

THE MAIN REASONS WHICH MAY AFFECT AN EFFECTIVE INTRODUCTION OF A *Mindset Workout Routine*

IMPATIENCE

02

LACK OF A STRONG MOTIVATION

01

REASONS TO FAIL

03

FOCUSING ON MINDSET NEGLETING TRAINING

97 – The Champion as a Super Hero

We have gone through the mindset of the Champion and we have realized that such a tough mindset is a mix of *a Conscious Mindset* and *a Subconscious Mindset*. We have learned that the generic Peak-Performer belonging to any kind of competitive contest is provided with special talents, skills, abilities, capabilities, and attitudes and that there are a few strong and positive habits that complete his/her profile. Ultimately we have also realized that the whole of the factors which compose such an incredible mix are learnable, developable, and achievable, as long as you have the strong will to transform yourself, step by step, and that you take full ownership of such a transformation.

Despite this, we remain suspicious of disbelief.

Whenever we recall the astonishing gestures and the incredible actions of one of our idols, we first appreciate them, but then we fall into a psychic trap: *Is that possible? Can a human being really strive so hard to achieve such a result? Couldn't this champion be supernatural (in a sense)?*

Very often it seems to be that our idol is not a human being, but a kind of *Sports Hero*. It seems that he/she is provided with peculiar supernatural skills. Let's go through this and explore these supernatural skills.

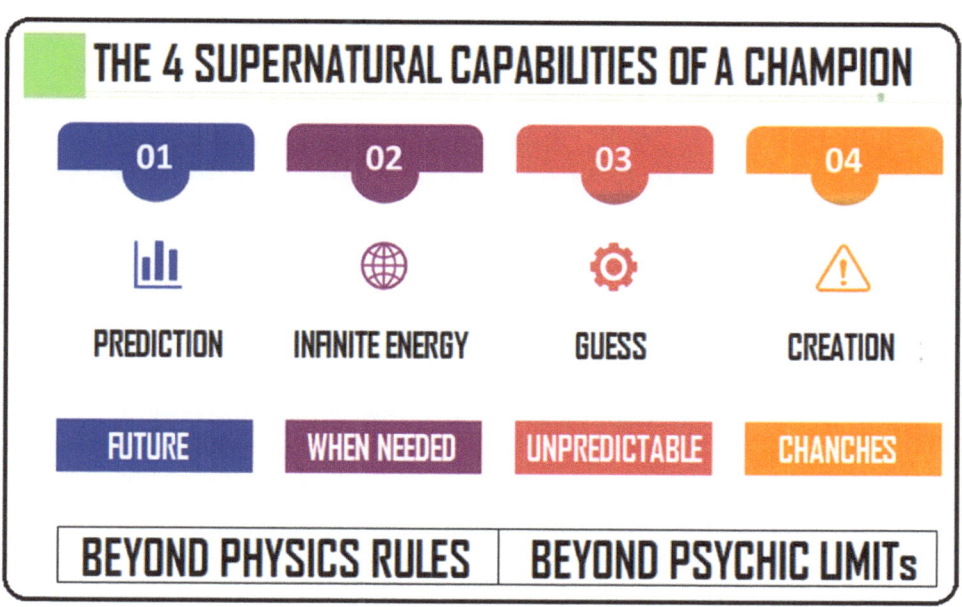

1) *The Champion is a prescient individual.* He/she can predict the future. There is no other way to interpret the Champion's ability to be always present whenever great things happen: such a capability enables the Champion always doing the right thing at the right time using the

right amount of energy, dramatically on time. The truth is that more often than expected and more often than we can realize in advance, the Champion has actually *"created"* that event, and has generated all the circumstances which have enabled him/her to perform that special and acrobatic action to succeed. The Champion *doesn't actually predict anything*, but secretly *creates the circumstances* to win and easily succeeds.

2) *The Champion is provided with an infinite amount of energy.* No matter how high is my commitment: I will never be able to train as much as needed to attain endurance, resistance to fatigue, power, strength, and speed to exploit whenever needed. I cannot reach the Champion's standards, because he/she is incredibly provided with infinite energy. That's what we may misunderstand and start to believe. The truth is that the Champion is a missionary, then he/she commits his/her full self to train, from one side. On the other side, we need to know that the Champion is naturally *"essential"*, this means that he/she knows how to distribute energy during the competition and that his/her subconscious mind precisely knows the right size of energy which any useful gesture requires, that knows when, where and how to engage extra-amount of energy whenever needed. Finally, we need to know that the Champion is strongly able to dissimulate his pulsions, emotions, and inner feelings: he/she is a master in dissimulating and feinting. You cannot catch if the Champion is tired unless the Champion decides to show up that feeling.

3) *The Champion is a soothsayer.* The Champion has the superhuman ability to guess what may be happening in very advance. Such competence is not superhuman, but can effectively be developed through mental training, visualization, imagery, and lots of repetitions. The Champions doesn't actually guess anything, but rather creates the circumstances, drives his/her opponents towards a specific direction (compliant to his/her strategy), takes the risk, bets on something, and then succeeds. No real superhuman skill, only strong will, training, and experience.

4) *The Champion is a Creator.* How can I compete with the Champion? He/she is a kind of God. He/she creates circumstances, chances, and opportunities as long as he/she expresses a desire. This is not human: the Champion can achieve whatever he/she wants in the preferred forms. As we already know this is true: the Champions *"create"* something according to a plan. To become a creator there's only needed very hard work, nothing else.

So in the very end we are encouraged in realizing that the Champion is not a Hero, is not a superhuman individual, but only an ambitious professional who has chosen the pathway for excellence. This means that he/she has worked like hell. Bus this also means that becoming the Champion is not an impossible mission: it is something within everyone's reach.

98 – Sport Mental Coaching for Peak Performers

No matter if you're an Athlete (who is applying to the next level), a Professional Trainer (who leads a team or drives a class of Athletes, in a specific individual/situational discipline), or a Professional Coach (who is used to support athletes in enhancing their performances and to unlock their potentials). Once you have understood the Mindset breakdown (8 Pillars, 55 Mindset Factors, 5 Model Factors), the forces which actually govern the whole of the mental drives, attitudes, and pulsations, the inner dynamics which regulate and determine the sports performances, you need to clear up your mind that all this awareness is yet not enough to enable significant progress. You need to take action: passionately, aggressively, and systematically. Do not forget that knowledge is still nothing, if not added to the action, while knowledge, added to the action, is real power. Whether you are an Athlete or you are a Coach, you need to take action in order to take real advantage of what we have dealt with until now. You need a Coaching Model (or Coaching Protocol) to implement the set of information to your workout routines.

Sports Mental Coaching is regulated by the same principles, models, and approach as any other coaching industry (ex: Business Coaching, Life Coaching, Performance Coaching). You need to develop your specific and personal Coaching Model, which is compliant with the Coaching protocols developed by ICF: International Coaching Federation). In the following paragraph, I will show you a simple and quick methodology that easily enables you to understand the basis of the Sports Mental Coaching process. Once you understand and secure such patterns to your arsenal, you can make your decisions and develop a methodology that better suits your attitudes, your code of ethics, your skills, and competencies as an Athlete or a Coach.

The SMC Protocol/Model is based on three steps:

- (*ZERO-SESSION*) – Preliminary Interview.
- (*STRATEGY*) – Development of a Masterplan + Reciprocal Trust Deal.
- (*ACTION*) – Provision of Coaching Sessions.

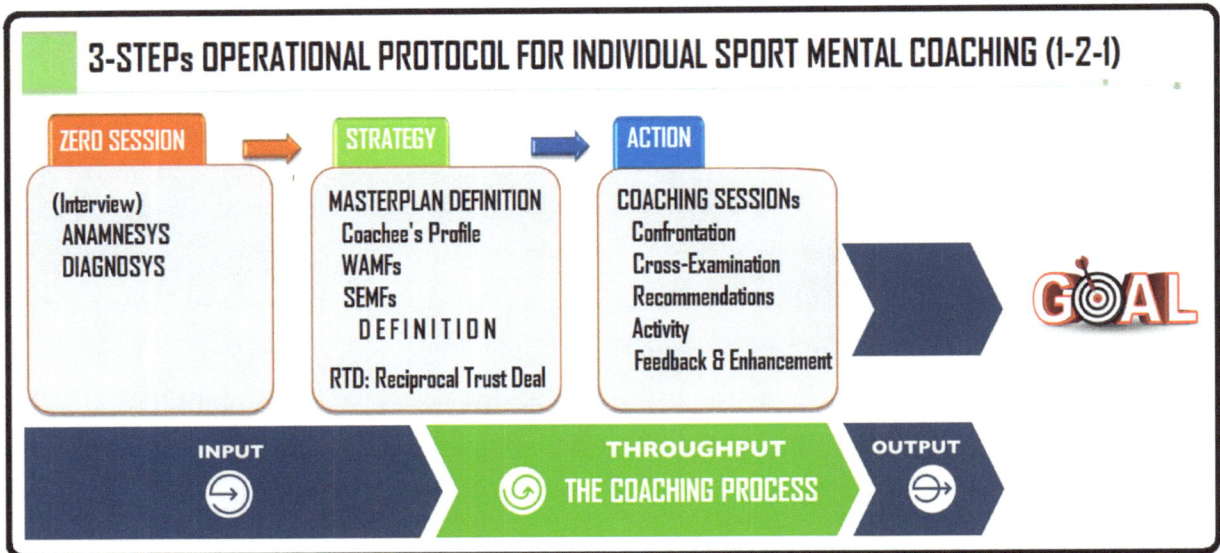

1st *STEP*. According to my personal view and approach, the first step is *free of charge*, which means that must be considered as an investment of the Mental Coach and is not charged to his/her possible/future Coachee. It basically consists of a 2 hours session (at max), which is finalized to explore specific elements pertaining to the Coachee, to get a lot of information through a special interview. The step consists of a multipurpose session. The Coach needs to go through the following items:

- Coachee's nature, disposition, and temperament.
- Absent or Weak factors related to the Sport Mindset.
- A global overview of the specific sport discipline practiced by the Coachee.
- Code of Ethics of the Coachee.

Apart from the technical and motivational exploration, the *ZERO-Session* is finalized to create the appropriate relationship between the two communication centers. From one side the Coach is required to facilitate the birth of a trusty and true relationship with the Coachee; on the other side, the Coach also needs to understand if he/she can actually support the Coachee in enhancing the final sports performance and in quickening the achievement of his/her final goal. If the Coach realizes that there are some biases, barriers, or hurdles related to the Coachee situation, which he/she is not capable to overcome, then the Coaching process cannot start. Same if the Coach realizes that the Coachee is driven by ambitions and expectations which do not really match his/her current situation/arsenal. If these two risks are clearly overcome, then the embryo of a *Reciprocal Trust Deal* can be born.

2nd *STEP*. The Second Step is focused on *Strategy*: based on the results and further exploration of the Coachee's past sports experiences, the Coach is required to develop a Masterplan (a *Grand Strategic Plan*) which includes the Coaching Goals, the protocol (frequency/methodology), the first 10 Factors on which the Coaching Process must be focused and started over. In addition to that, the Coach also needs to clearly define which is the profile of the Coachee, according to the 5-Factors Model.

When ready, the Coach submits the Masterplan to the Coachee. If the Coachee is willing to start the Coaching Process, then the whole of the elements of the Masterplan can be partially reviewed and finally agreed upon. The Coach and the Coachee together submit documents which include a Masterplan and the terms and conditions of payment for the Coaching Sessions. Such a document is called a *"Reciprocal Trust Deal"*. It necessarily must include a *Non-Disclosure Clause*, which sounds like an intrinsic guarantee for the Coachee (privacy).

3rd STEP. The third step is *Action*: The Sports Mental Coaching process is started and both the Coach and the Coachee are fully committed to following the rules and the standard protocols. Especially: the Coachee is required to apply and follow the recommendation of the Coach, as they naturally emerge during the coaching sessions.

99 – Preliminary Check and Strategy Definition

The first step is crucial because, in a limited slot of time, the Coach needs to catch the actual talents of the Coachee, his/her intrinsic motivations and drives, the possible intrinsic vulnerabilities, the mental barriers, and many other elements, without being tough and too much invasive. In fact, this first session is also finalized to create a trusty and honest relationship between the both, so it takes lots of energy, patience, and a kind of generosity from the Coach's side.

The whole of this information can be gotten through a special interview, led by the Coach, which is structured into three main parts:

1) Questions/Answers
2) Specific Test
3) Evidence

1) Questions/Answers

The *Questions/Answers box* is finalized to understand the main features of the Coachee's nature, without neglecting his/her mental barriers, bias, fears, talents, and any other skill/capability, which is related to the 55 Sport Mindset Factors. Such an interview ought to include the following items (*open questions*):

- the definition and the role of fate and fortune and the Coachee's opinion about that;
- the Coachee's LOC (*Locus of Control*: internal/external): the Coach needs to understand the size of the sense of control of the outside world;
- the code of ethics of the Coachee (the Top-5/Top-10 ranking);
- the Coachee's character and temperament;
- Coachee's reaction to adversities;
- Coachee's propensity to risk;
- Coachee's willingness to tolerate uncertainties;
- Coachee's strengths and weaknesses;
- Coachee's decision-making process (drivers, critical items).

2) Specific Test

The *Specific Test box* consists of providing the Coachee with peculiar tests, which enable the Coach better profiling the Coachee as an Athlete (his/her current status). One of the *Must-Be* tests is related to the 5-Factors Model. It consists in forcing the Coachee to sort the 5 factors, from the one he feels weakest to the strongest, and assign the relative score (1-10). The Coachee needs to complete the pyramid by entering the names of the relevant factors.

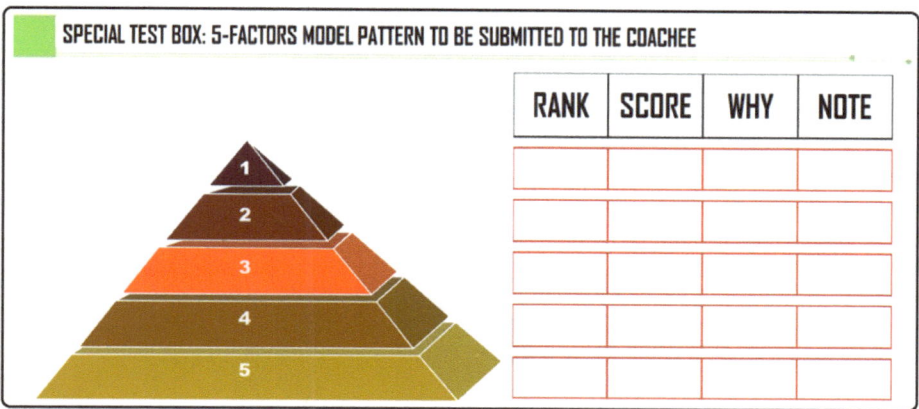

3) Evidence

The *Evidence box* is finalized to catch a few information related to the Coachee (from one side) and to corroborate or disprove specific opinions/beliefs got through the first two boxes. The Coach can test the Coachee through his/her experience as a coach, a trainer, and a sportsman. This crucial set of information is gotten through deep and careful observation of the following items:

- behaviour;
- punctuality;
- way of dressing;
- voice tone;
- way of confronting;
- language and choice of verbs/adjectives;
- emotional reactions to specific topics/questions;
- body language;
- response time.

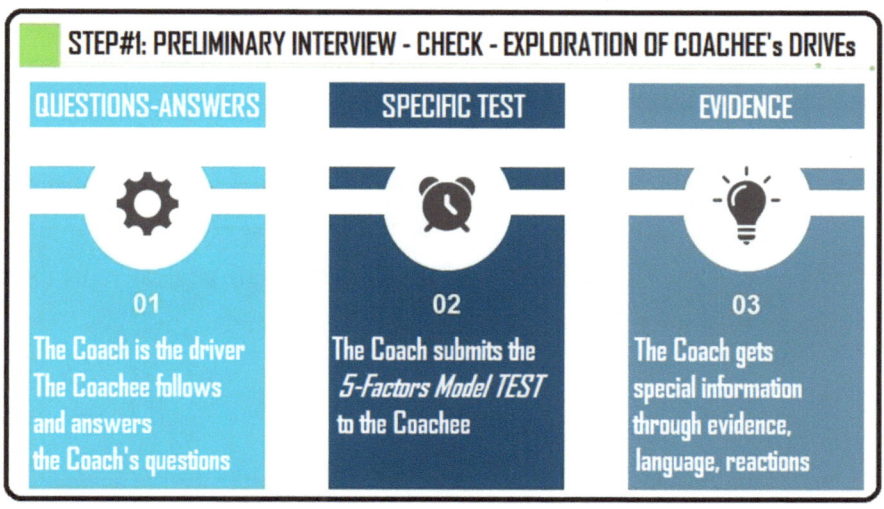

100 – Athletes' Profile, WAMFs & SEMFs Definition

Based on the results of the First Step (*ZERO-Session*), the Coach should be provided with enough information to decide if the case is a BID/NO-BID (or *GO/NO-GO*). In short, the Coach can decide to accept the Coachee or refuse to start a training process, for special reasons.

If the Coach has decided to accept the case, then he/she has to develop a Masterplan of the (Sports Mental) Coaching Program which consists of an articulated document that would include the following items:

1) Attendance frequency (Coaching Sessions);
2) Intensity (session's duration);
3) Periodization (targets/timing);
4) Targets to start with;
5) Methodology.

The results coming from the first step (*Interview*) must be used and exploited to define the following:

- The Coachee's most crucial elements which are weak or even absent (WAMFs: *Weak or Absent Mindset Factors*) – 5 at max;
- The Coachee's most crucial strengths or elite skills (SEMFs: *Strong and Elite Mindset Factors*) – 5 at max;
- The Coachee's "*Current State*", according to the 5-Factors Model taxonomy: *The Rookie – The Spectator – The Participant – The Prima Donna – The Silent Killer – The Subconscious Commando – The Contender.*

These three crucial elements represent the founding basis of the Coachee's growth strategy and of the entire Mental Coaching process which he/she will have to undergo.

In facts:

- The work related to both the WAMFs and the SEMFs can be easily performed according to the technical recommendations which have been presented above;
- The work related to the "*Current State*" of the Coachee can be easily performed according to what has already been described and explained in the above pages.

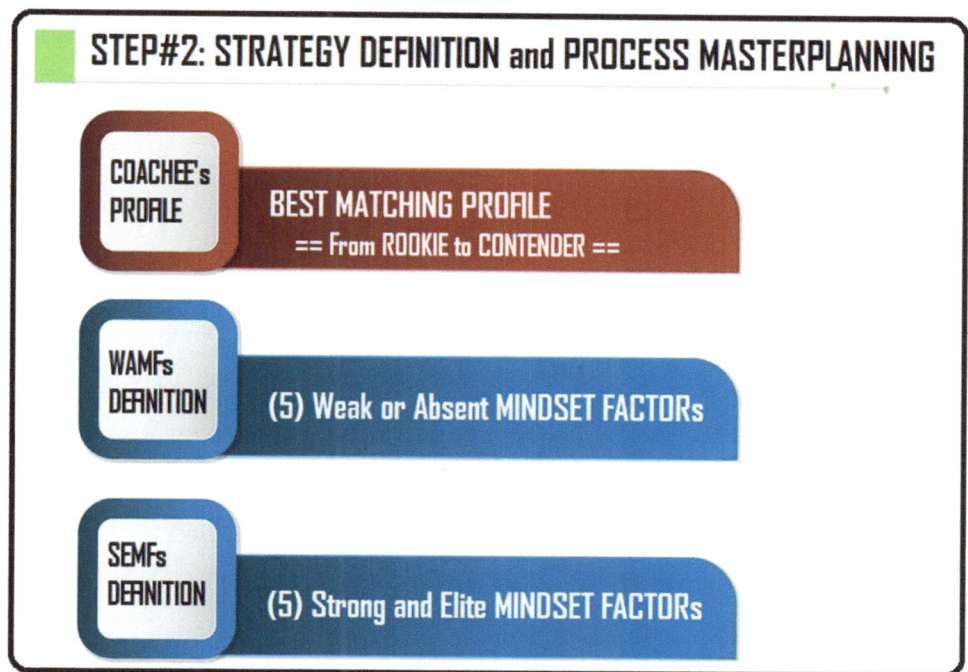

101 – Coaching in Action

The third and final step of a generic Sports Mental Coaching Program consists of the Coaching Sessions which are provided to the Coachee.

As you already know this Manual has been conceived and written to describe, explain and highlight the whole of the mental factors which actually affect Sports Performance in any competitive discipline. In fact, the final purpose of this book consists of exploring the Sport Mindset and trying to facilitate the pathway of any athlete who wants to achieve his/her best goals of glory and to recommend specific topics and operational recommendations to the Coaches and to the Sports Trainers while performing their role. I have no intention to recommend any Coach how to coach their Coachees and their Athletes for two main reasons.

The first one is that any Coach has developed his/her own model, approach, and methodology and I guess if they really coach their Clients, this approach must be effective enough. The second reason pertains to experience: any Coach should be drawing on his/her own experiences to define the coaching approach and methodology.

These are the reason why I will not recommend anything to them: ICF protocols and standards are already enough to ensure the work is carried out in a workmanlike manner. Must be plainly understood that the Coach needs to be certified and provided with the legitimacy to operate. Do not forget that each of the chapters related to the Sport Mindset Pillars (Chapters 2 to 9) includes the paragraph *"Powerful Questions"*: each of those questions – which are segmented by topic – has been developed according to the Coaching Methodology standards, and can be considered tools *ready-to-use*, for any Coach.

 Same process, same steps, same commitment for an Athlete: if you are an athlete and you want to become a world champion or you only want to enhance your performance, you have to apply the same procedures and take the same commitments and follow the pathway that I have described above. *Acceptance (of your gaps)* → *Knowledge* → *Exploration* → *Strategic Masterplan* → *Action*: these are the main steps to transform an Athlete into a World Class Peak Performer in any sport Discipline.

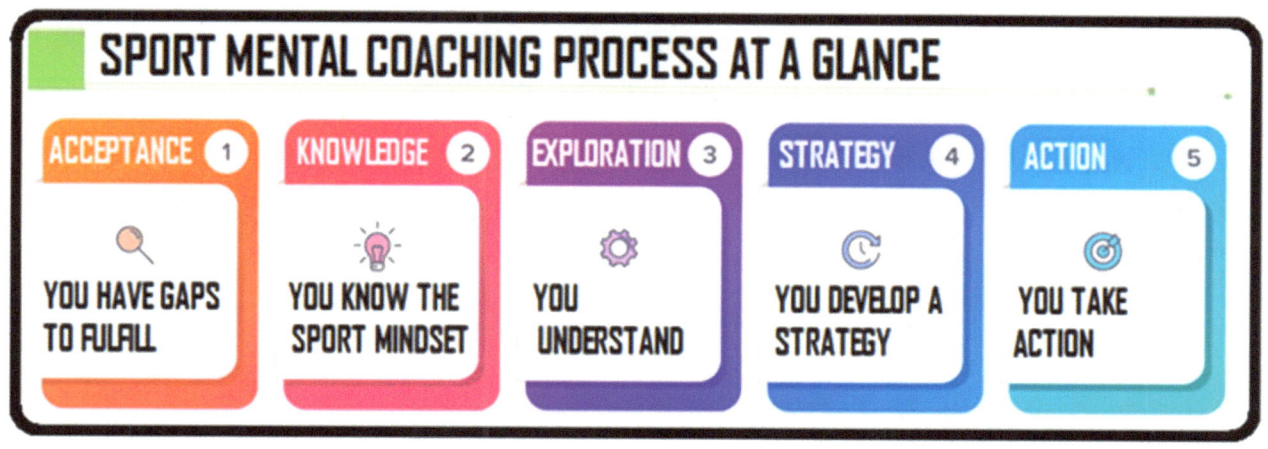

SPORT MENTAL COACHING PROCESS AT A GLANCE

ACCEPTANCE 1	KNOWLEDGE 2	EXPLORATION 3	STRATEGY 4	ACTION 5
YOU HAVE GAPS TO FULFILL	YOU KNOW THE SPORT MINDSET	YOU UNDERSTAND	YOU DEVELOP A STRATEGY	YOU TAKE ACTION

COACHING BEHAVIOURS (from U.K.-COACHING CLUB)

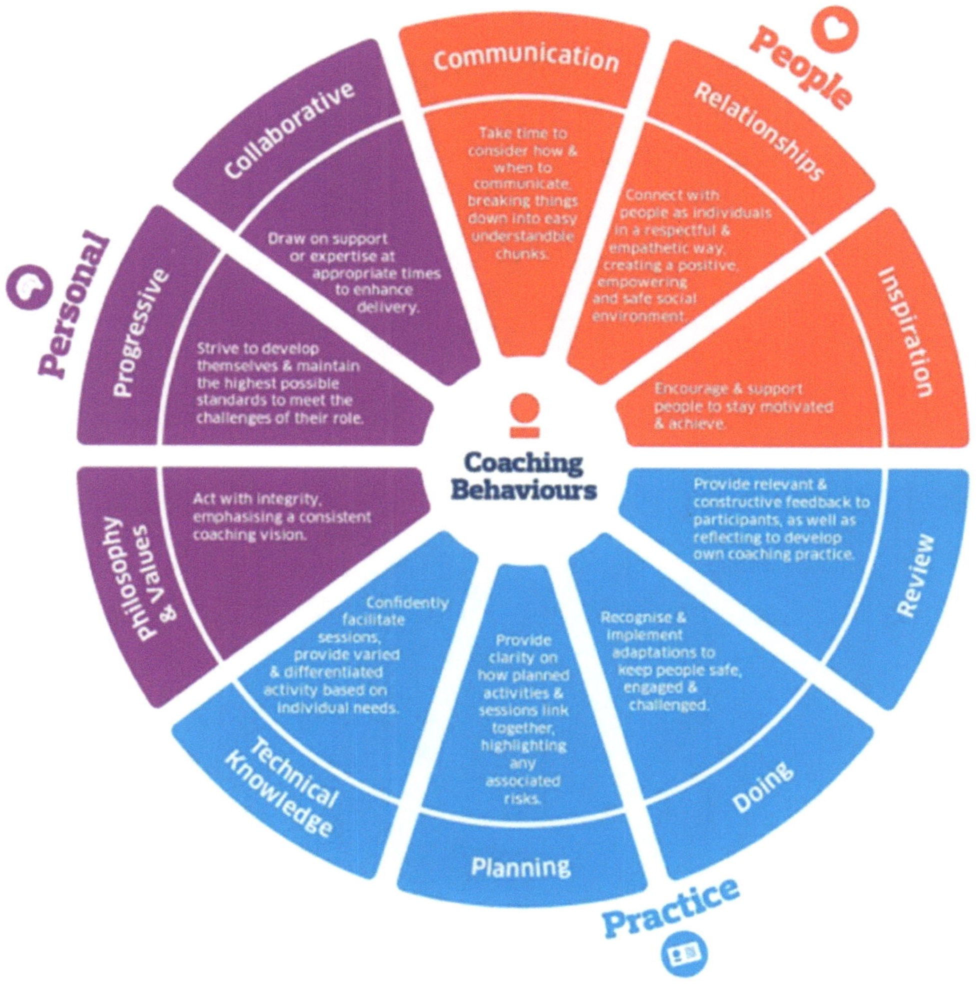

Communication
Take time to consider how & when to communicate, breaking things down into easy understandble chunks.

Collaborative
Draw on support or expertise at appropriate times to enhance delivery.

People

Relationships
Connect with people as individuals in a respectful & empathetic way, creating a positive, empowering and safe social environment.

Inspiration
Encourage & support people to stay motivated & achieve.

Personal

Progressive
Strive to develop themselves & maintain the highest possible standards to meet the challenges of their role.

Philosophy & Values
Act with integrity, emphasising a consistent coaching vision.

Coaching Behaviours

Review
Provide relevant & constructive feedback to participants, as well as reflecting to develop own coaching practice.

Technical Knowledge
Confidently facilitate sessions, provide varied & differentiated activity based on individual needs.

Planning
Provide clarity on how planned activities & sessions link together, highlighting any associated risks.

Doing
Recognise & implement adaptations to keep people safe, engaged & challenged.

Practice

Conclusion

Afterward one may believe that the whole of the skills needed for becoming a champion is a set of psychic attitudes, coordinative and conditional capabilities, and something additional, whom we use to name *"talent"* and nothing else. Many high-level athletes, champions, and coaches, use to say that all of that might be summarized in a simple sentence: *"The will to win"*. I personally do not agree with that. There is something that is missing, something enormous which we have already dealt with in the book, about which we need to be clearer because it actually includes the real secret, the magic of becoming a world-class athlete and a champion. It contains the enchantment of the *Peak Performance.*

You need to have the will and the willingness to suffer.

This internal quality is crucial for both physical, psychic, and strategic training and enhancement of your arsenal as an athlete and as a man. You can have the will to win – everybody has this – but if you really want to succeed you must have the will to suffer, which is related to the will and instinct of survival.

If you want to switch to a higher level, if compared to your current average level of performance, you need to feel threatened and then you need to rely on your inner instinct of survival and on your adaptation skills: these two elements can provide you with a real will to suffer, to tolerate anything, to move faster, to achieve.

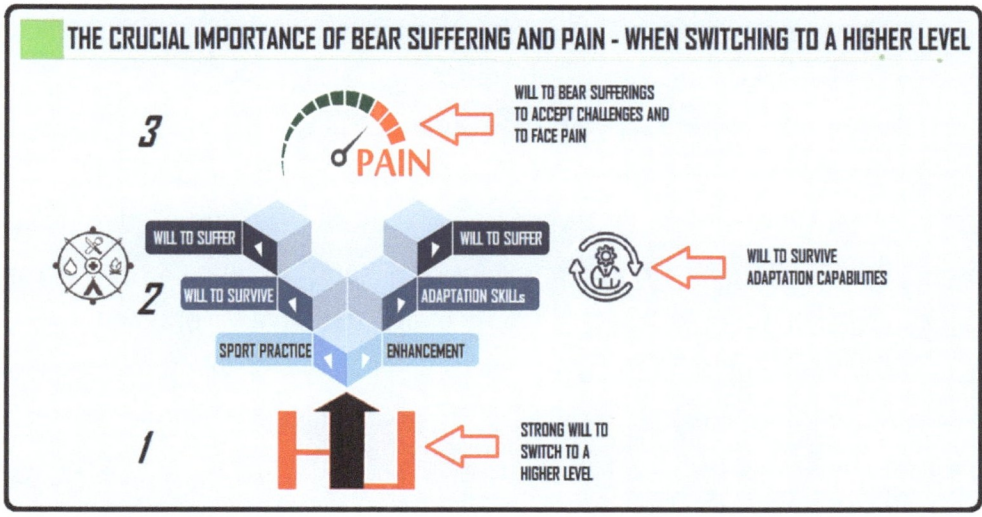

If you really feel threatened, then a psychic process is started inside: your strong belief looks for internal resources and it addresses the most ancestral part of our being. The instinct of self-preservation, will for survival, and adaptation skills are quickly awakened and give you back all the energy and resources to deal with pain and to find a solution, in the meantime. The problem is that *we ought to feel threatened*, somehow, and is very infrequent that an athlete feels such kind of perception if he is only practicing a sport discipline or if he is involved in an official performance. This may only happen if you believe your discipline is *"your life"* when you are completely and entirely committed to that.

What we have to accept is that pain and suffering are factors which we undeniably need to be prepared to handle, because there is a huge truth in Sport, which is true for any other area of human activity: *No/Pain—No/Gain*. There is no real possibility to achieve huge goals without going through the pain. Based on my personal experience I can assure you have to face your inner fears and overcome them completely, understand the real causes which determine your fears, and go through pain and suffering if you want to switch to a higher level and become a world-class athlete. If you explore the biographies of the biggest Champions of any sports discipline you would realize that no one has had an easy life, none of them has managed to become the best version of themselves without facing the pain. No one ever said it would have been easy: if someone did, he/she simply lied because he/she had never been a champion, or because he/she had some interest in communicating this lie, in making things easier for you. Words cannot transform reality.

Pain is something tangible. Pain presents a few forms through which reveals itself to you. It only comes when you decide on a strong, robust switch in your career: if you settle yourself for a mediocre level or you are satisfied with an average yield, you would not know the pain, because it will not be necessary: comfort zone avoids pain. The pain is caused by special friction: this friction depends on the desire to achieve a higher result even though you have resources not yet aligned for that level. When pain arrives you have to be prepared to live with it: if you fail to prepare to handle pain, you'd better prepare to fail and you can be sure you will never achieve those peak performances which you are longing for, to become a Top Player in your sport discipline. The real problem is that such kind of skill cannot be taught, cannot be learned, cannot be transferred: either you are already endowed with it, or you will never be endowed at all. The willingness to suffer and accept pain is something that you cannot learn, is a kind of prequalification skill to become a champion. If you're already provided with such a psychic attitude, then you will find many ways to meet it, to test and to enhance it: this will enable you to face any kind of adversity. This will give you back the toughest mindset you never thought you may attain in your life. During your training sessions, tournaments, and sports career you will have to get acquainted with multiple sources of pain: humiliation, frustration, fatigue, lack of money, abandonment, inability to accept defeat, shame, serious injuries, completely wrong self-image, rush to arrive, impatience, difficulty in committing yourself to goals, inability to concentrate, acceptance of your weaknesses, bad looks and bad performances in important competitions, loss of self-confidence.

Any of these elements will cause you pain and if you are not willing to go through this, you will never learn the lesson.

The pain is nothing but a test: it is not coming to hurt you, but only to verify the strength of your will and ambition to be stronger and stronger, until you become the number one.

There is a *conscious pain* and an *unconscious pain*. Conscious pain is more useful because the awareness of the pain you are suffering constantly reminds you what you are fighting for, your final purpose. Do not forget that the word *"champion"* comes from the ancient Latin word *"campus"*: the battlefield, then champion means *"fighter"*, in a sense. Conscious pain may also be generated voluntarily. Unconscious pain must be interpreted and managed appropriately, otherwise is only a lack of energy and may cause a lack of motivation. In both cases, you have to go through your pain, learn the lesson and get back up.

So my personal recommendation is not to avoid pain, but to go through that, any time it is coming, because a big training period is coming to you, both physical and psychic. When pain is coming, it means that time is ripe for an enrichment of your sports arsenal, so do not go away, but approach it and live it completely: abandon yourself to it and make it your Master. Just consider that your opponents are not doing the same, but remember that any champion, before becoming a champion, did the same, he faced his nightmares, he knew the pain and he got over it. Just remember that pain is weaknesses leaving your body.

Post Factum

As a matter of fact, to become a Champion a special mix of events should join together, on that special day. First of all, you have to be alive. In the second instance you have to be present that day, that place, that time, lucid, motivated, and clearly oriented towards your goal. On the third and last you have to perform at your best and YPB (*Your Personal Best*) should be stronger or quicker or better than one of all your opponents, at least that particular day. Does an athlete know that will be the day? Does he really know that will become the World Champion of his sports specialty? Sometimes he knows, sometimes he does not, but he always "*feels*" something, he clearly feels inside that will be the right day. Does he feel scared? Sometimes he does, sometimes he does not, but the one who will become Champion knows how to manage his/her emotions and he/she takes control of internal vibrations, quickly regains calmness, and goes straight to the point, the competition, the reason why he/she is there that day, that time: *the victory*. What does he/she need to prove and whom is he/she going to convince? Nobody exists but him/herself. He/she has to prove that the lesson was learned and that is now ready to be the Champion. He/she only has to prove his/her status of being the champion to him/herself. Before the competition, he/she is still no one, but when the competition is off he/she is the Champion. How can the same person be no one and the world champion on the same day, in the same minute? This might seem so strange, but in fact, it is not, is very simple. That athlete "*is already*" the world champion, but nobody knows this, yet. He/she has worked hard, he/she is prepared, he/she learned the lessons well, and he/she is ready. That athlete *is already the champion*, but an official competition is needed to confirm this in the world of humans: *pure bureaucracy*. Being a Champion is a matter of "*being*", and is a spiritual condition, not a qualification. Nobody can give you such a title: is a matter of internal qualities, of the level of being. So you are already the Champion, but you need to be recognized as a champion, then an official tournament is necessary to convince the audience. Let's quickly get to the point. So what? Can anyone become successful in Sports? Can anyone become "*the World Champion*" of his/her sport discipline? We spoke about the 4 areas which affect and determine Sports Performance: if a good athlete works hard and empowers each of those areas, may he/she apply to become a World Champion? On one side there is a technicality, which also includes psychic and mental attitudes and capabilities. On the other side, there is magic, something which cannot be explained and which is directly connected to radical motivation, aspiration, and will. As a result, we can conclude that is really difficult to become a World Champion or a World Class Athlete in any sports discipline, but there are individuals who can handle the whole of these difficulties and achieve. Each tournament always returns a winner, each world championship always returns a World Champion. Getting on the highest podium is a human event, a chance that is offered to any athlete, theoretically. Is a goal within our reach? Both average and top performers have exactly the same chances and resources: it's up to them.

Who is that person who actually knows if you're going to become a Champion or not? Who is the person who may judge your potential? Who is this special person? A World Class Coach? Your Personal Coach and Master? Your Fan or Followers? Who is this person?

The only truth you have to know is very simple.

It's up to you. That person is you.

Nobody can say anything about your future, because your destiny is in your hands. So take care: decide the man/woman you want to become and become that person. Decide the goals you want to reach and act accordingly: prepare yourself and go take your World Title, because is just there, in a still undetermined future, waiting for you.

I leave you here, after this long and interesting journey that we have done together. I hope that all my experiences and recommendations can be useful to enable you to attain your goals, one day. Please find below my 12 golden rules. I have developed this short list during the last 30 years, one sentence after the other, very slowly. Each new sentence was generated by a long experience of years and I granted it to become a rule only after evaluating its effectiveness on my skin. I know the sense of each of those 12 sentences because each of them clearly resonates with a specific event, failure, victory, or difficulty. Hope you find my personal list useful and effective. I owe these rules to all my sports and personal achievements. Thanks for your kind interest and attention.

1) Have a clear goal and keep moving in the right direction $=$
2) Work like hell $=$
3) Give a single-minded devotion to your goal $=$
4) Keep trying until you succeed $=$
5) When competing, *"Be Here and Now"* $=$
6) Never Complain $=$
7) Believe in yourself and in what you do $=$
8) Don't listen to Naysayers, learn how to manage other's criticism $=$
9) Don't be afraid to fail $=$
10) Go through your pain and overcome fears $=$ •
11) Be humble, but don't ever settle to be the silver medalist $=$
12) Don't ever quit ▬

BEING A WORLD CLASS ATHLETE IS ONLY UP TO YOU - DON'T LISTEN TO THE NAYSAYERS

YOU ARE THE

CHAMPION

(1) SET YOUR GOAL
(2) MAKE YOUR COMMITMENT

(3) TRAIN LIKE HELL
(4) PUT YOUR NAME ON THE GOLD CUP

Good Luck – Joe Santangelo

July 14th – 2021

www.ingramcontent.com/pod-product-compliance
Lightning Source LLC
Chambersburg PA
CBHW040439150626
46551CB00025B/136